Clinical Concepts and Practical Management Techniques in Dentistry

Edited by Aneesa Moolla

Published in London, United Kingdom

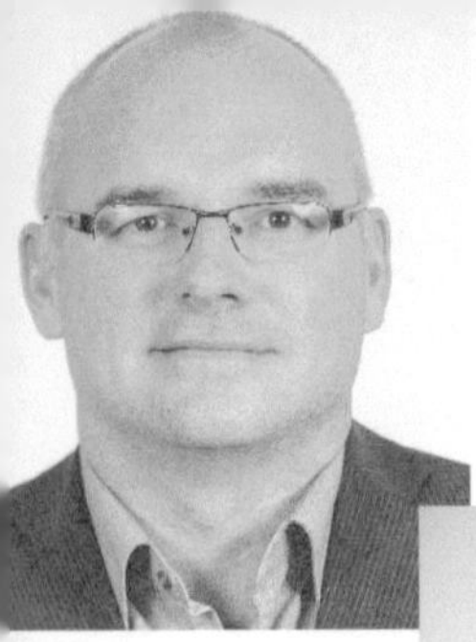
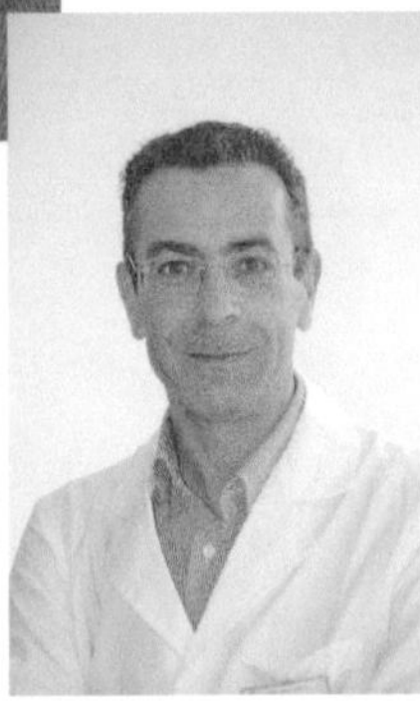
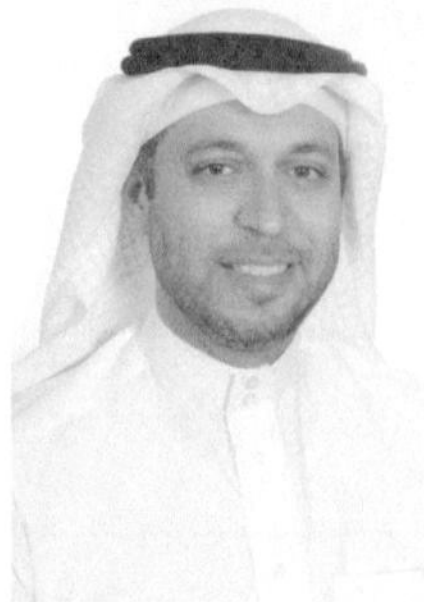
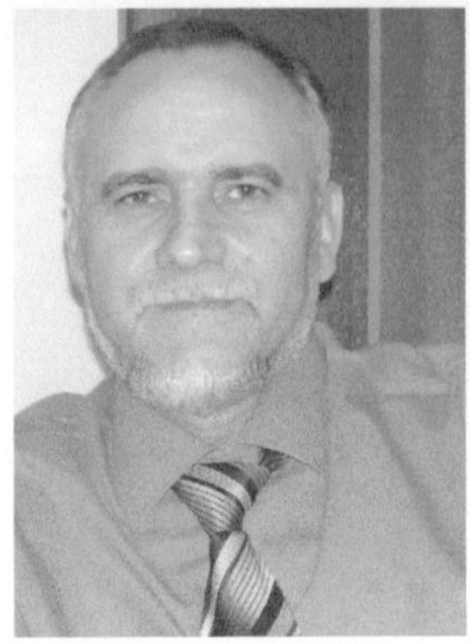
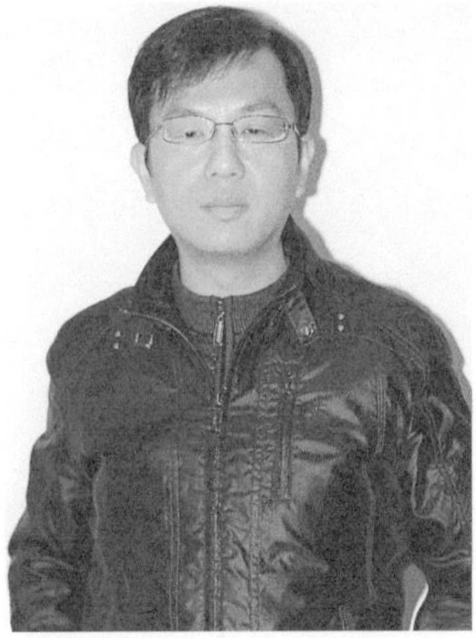
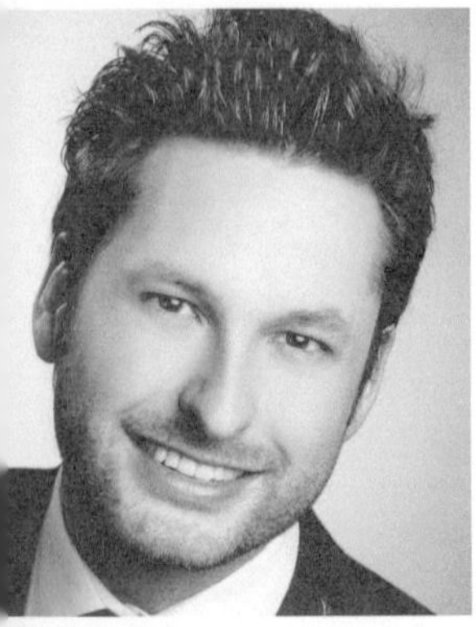
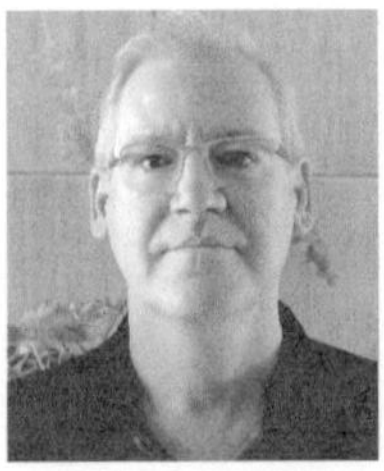

IntechOpen

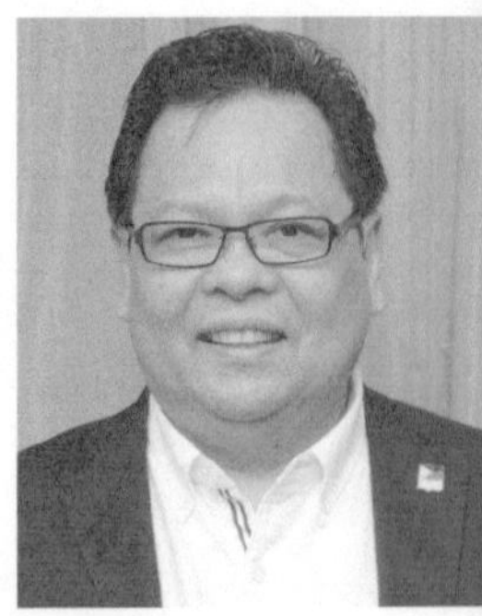
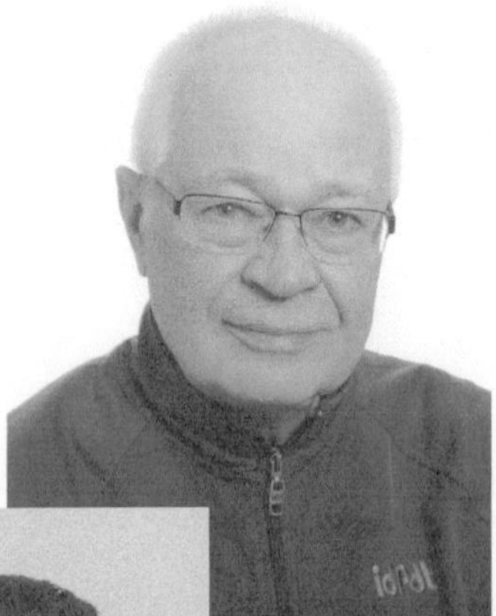
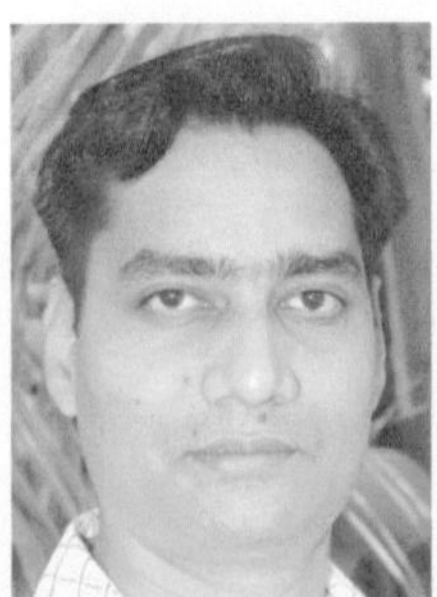
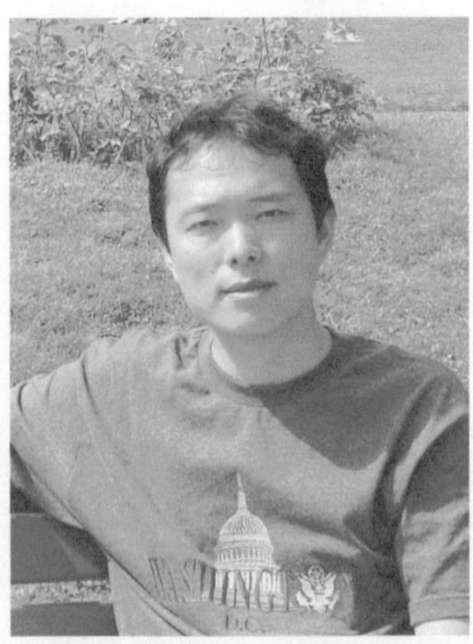
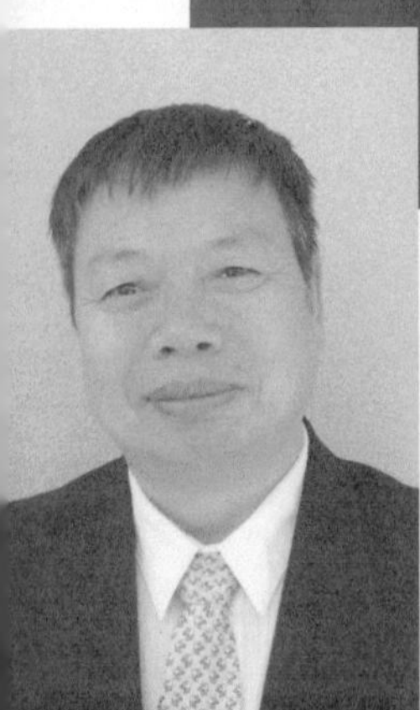
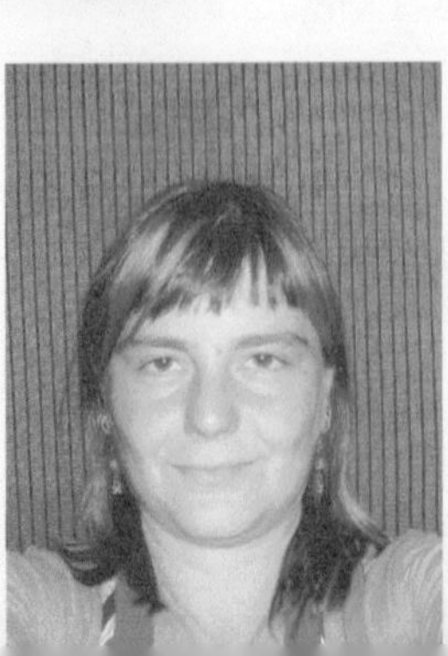

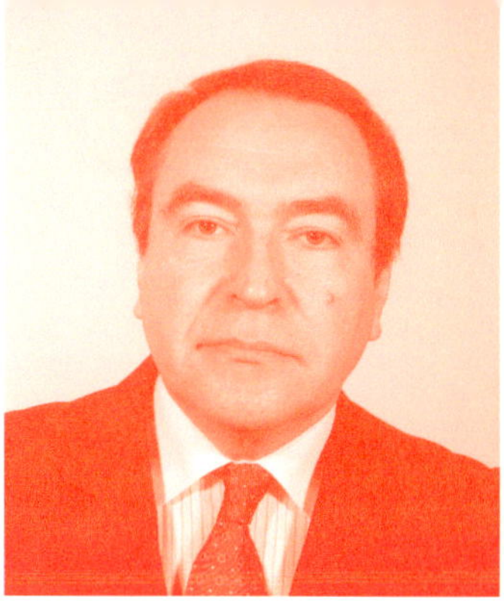
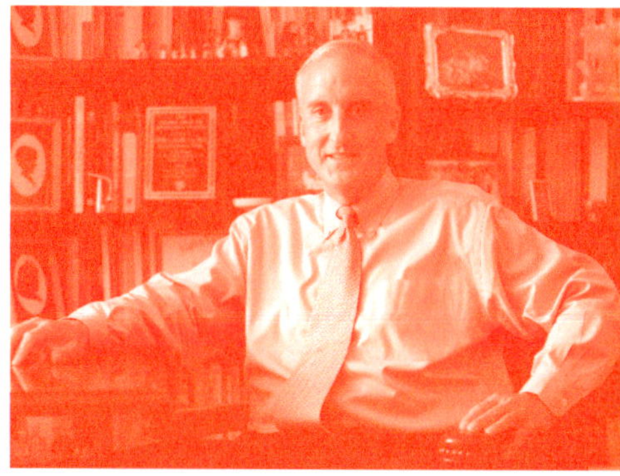
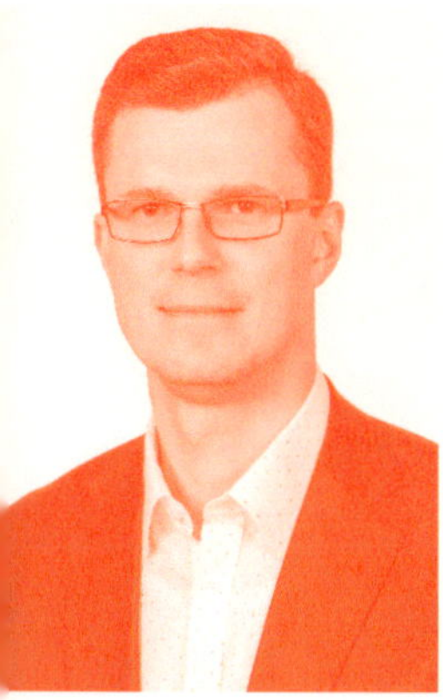
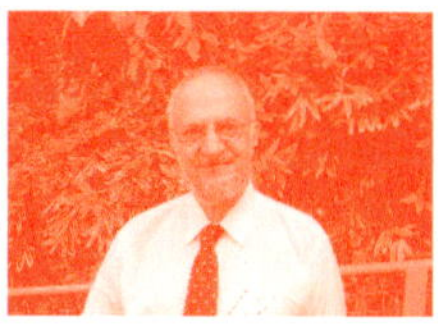
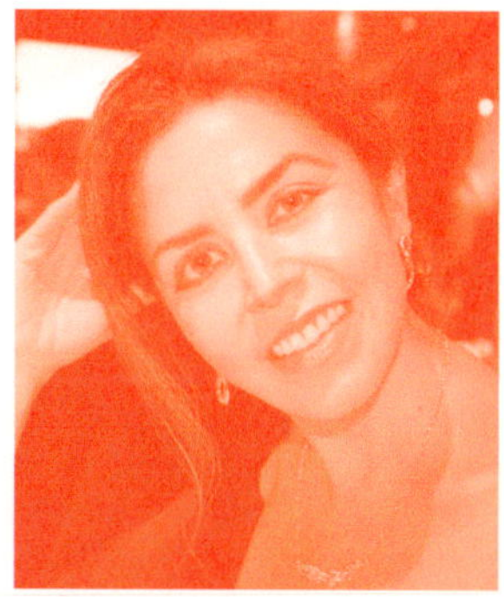

Supporting open minds since 2005

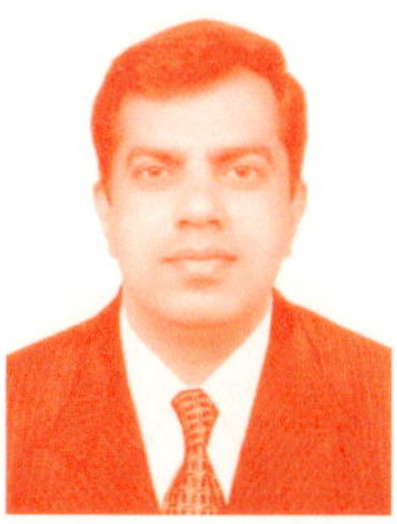
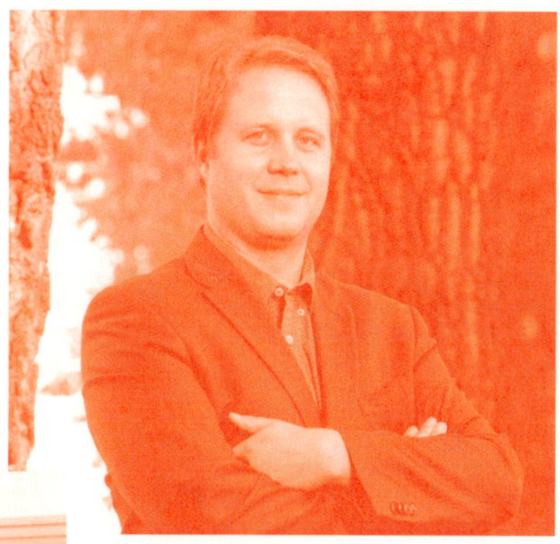
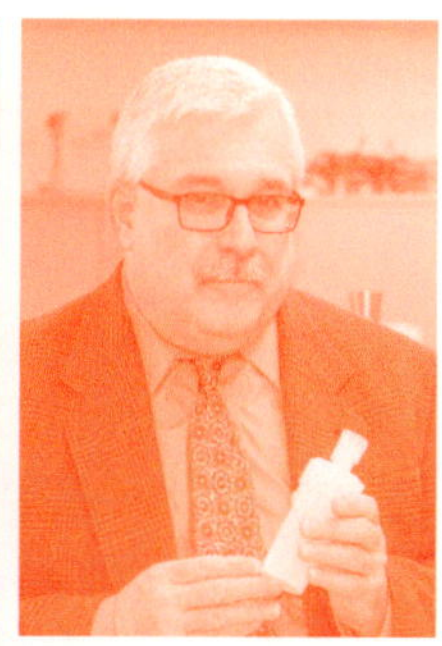
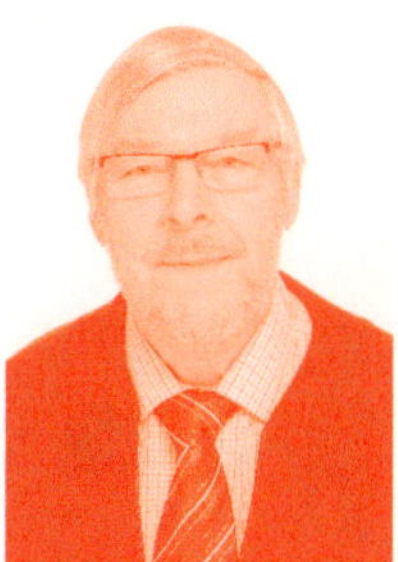
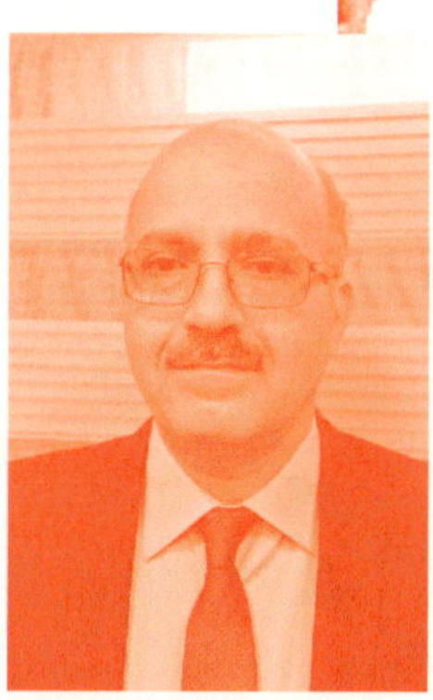
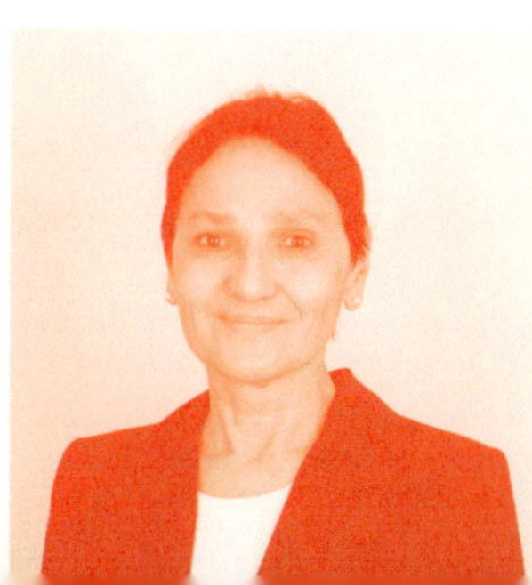
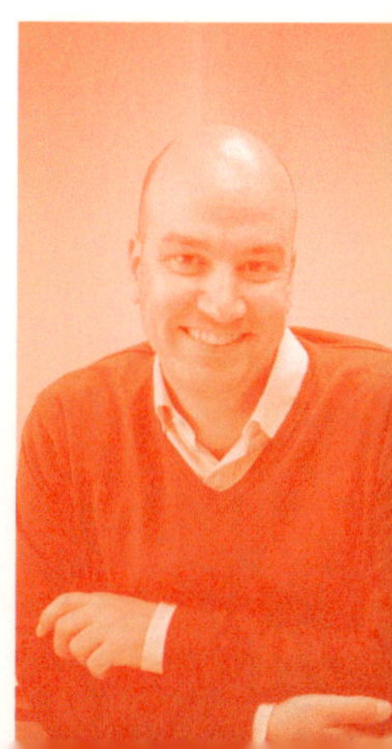

Clinical Concepts and Practical Management Techniques in Dentistry
http://dx.doi.org/10.5772/intechopen.87384
Edited by Aneesa Moolla

Part of IntechOpen Book Series: Dentistry, Volume 7
Book Series Editor: Zühre Akarslan

Contributors
Vishakha Grover, Amrit Baweja, Aman Bhagat, Ashish Jain, Anchal Ohri, Neeta V. Bhavsar, Deepak M. Macchindra Vikhe, Girish Suragimath, Ashwinirani SR, Aneesa Moolla, Sankeshan Padayachee, Tshakane R.M.D. Ralephenya, Sizakele Ngwenya, Keisuke Nakano, Toshiyuki Kawakami, Kiyofumi Takabatake, Hotaka Kawai, Hidetsugu Tsujigiwa, Hitoshi Nagatuka, Ali Khan, Shakeela Yousaf, Muhammad Saad Shaikh, Meshal G. G. Al-shammari, Feng Luo, Hongyan Luo, Ruyi Li, Changxing Qu, Guang Hong, Qianbing Wan, Kelebogile A. Mothupi, Christopher Olubode Ogunsalu, Natthamet Wongsirichat, Ann Chianchitlert, Diane Selvido, Irin Sirisoontorn, Bishwa Prakash Bhattarai, Dinesh Rokaya

First published in London, United Kingdom, 2022 by IntechOpen
IntechOpen is the global imprint of INTECHOPEN LIMITED, registered in England and Wales, registration number: 11086078, 5 Princes Gate Court, London, SW7 2QJ, United Kingdom
Printed in Croatia

British Library Cataloguing-in-Publication Data
A catalogue record for this book is available from the British Library

Additional hard and PDF copies can be obtained from orders@intechopen.com

Clinical Concepts and Practical Management Techniques in Dentistry
Edited by Aneesa Moolla
p. cm.
Print ISBN 978-1-83962-842-9
Online ISBN 978-1-83962-846-7
eBook (PDF) ISBN 978-1-83962-847-4
ISSN 2631-6218

For EU product safety concerns:
IN TECH d.o.o., Prolaz Marije Krucifikse Kozulić 3, 51000 Rijeka, Croatia, info@intechopen.com or visit our website at intechopen.com.

IntechOpen Book Series
Dentistry
Volume 7

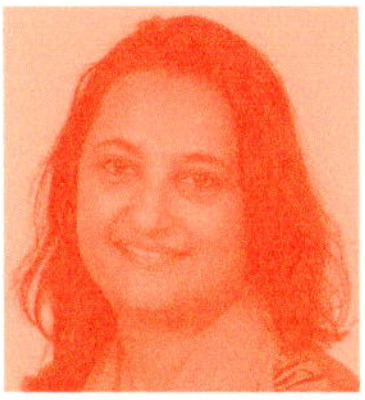

Dr. Aneesa Moolla has extensive experience in the diverse fields of health care having previously worked in dental private practice, at the Red Cross Flying Doctors association, and in healthcare corporate settings. She is now a lecturer at the University of Witwatersrand, South Africa, and a principal researcher at the Health Economics and Epidemiology Research Office (HE2RO), South Africa. Dr. Moolla holds a Ph.D. in Psychology with her research being focused on mental health and resilience. In her professional work capacity, her research has further expanded into the fields of early childhood development, mental health, the HIV and TB care cascades, as well as COVID. She is also a UNESCO-trained International Bioethics Facilitator.

Editor of Volume 7: Aneesa Moolla
University of Witwatersrand,
Health Economics and Epidemiology Research Office
Johannesburg, South Africa

Series Editor: Zühre Akarslan
Gazi University Faculty of Dentistry, Turkey

Scope of the Series

The major pathologies which dentists encounter in clinical practice include dental caries and periodontal diseases. Diagnosis and treatment of these pathologies is essential because when untreated, abscess could occur and it can even lead to the extraction of the tooth. Extracted teeth can be replaced with implants. Dentists and patients are nowadays more familiar with dental implant treatments. As a result, advanced diagnostic tools which aid in pre-operative treatment planning (cone-beam computed tomography, computer aided implant planning etc..), new implant designs improving the success of osteointegration, new materials, and techniques are introduced in the dental market.
Conditions which dentists frequently encounter in their clinical practice are temporomandibular joint (TMJ) disorders. These disorders include degenerative musculoskeletal conditions associated with morphological and functional deformities. Accurate diagnosis is important for proper management of TMJ pathologies. With the advance in technology, new materials, techniques and equipment are introduced

in the dental practice. New diagnostic aids in dental caries detection, cone-beam computed tomographic imaging, soft and hard tissue lasers, advances in oral and maxillofacial surgery procedures, uses of ultrasound, CAD/CAM, nanotechnology, plasma rich protein (PRP) and dental implantology are some of them. There will be even more new applications in dentistry in the future.

This book series includes topics related to dental caries, dentomaxillofacial imaging, new trends in oral implantology, new approaches in oral and maxillofacial surgery, temporomandibular joint disorders in dentistry etc.

Contents

Preface

This book includes important information for comprehensive treatment planning for a wide variety of dental procedures. Written by internationally recognized oral health specialists, this book offers information on revised concepts of oral diseases and disorders, including insights and diagnostics for each category. Readers will learn about radiology for diagnosis, retrospective studies, and planning considerations for periodontics, endodontics, oral surgery, and restorative dentistry. Additionally, the book includes practical guidelines for detecting child abuse within the dental practice, as well as the basics of statistical methodologies in dentistry.

The first section discusses treatment modalities for impacted molars as well as the radiology of developmental defects. Chapters in this section include a wealth of updated clinical information. The interesting use of radiographs to explore variations in periodontal status among different gender groups is also a focus of this section. The subsequent section provides in-depth coverage of pertinent endodontic and restorative clinical concepts and dental management techniques. Chapters address regenerative endodontic procedures as well as restorations of endodontically treated teeth. Another interesting concept discussed within this section is the use of zirconia as a restorative material.

Zirconia has been overlooked as a restorative dental material for many decades. It consists of zirconium dioxide, which has maximum mechanical strength and fracture resistance when compared to all other non-metallic materials. Besides its high strength, zirconia is widely favored for its superior surface smoothness. Despite these beneficial characteristics, zirconia is not as widely used as it could be. This is likely due to cost and knowledge. Most local dental laboratories cannot afford to invest in high-tech, computerized, advanced CAD/CAM systems needed for clinical procedures using zirconia. Additionally, these laboratories do not have enough skilled or knowledgeable personnel to utilize this new technology. However, this has slowly started to change as clinicians learn about this material and begin investing in the technology linked to the usage of zirconia.

Another salient point in dentistry is dental trauma. The role of a dental hygienist becomes key in scenarios of dental trauma, as they often are the first points of care in such scenarios. As such, they are key players in emergency treatment modalities that could ensure success of subsequent endodontic or restorative procedures in cases of dental trauma. Dental trauma is not always accidental, however, and this brings us to the role of all oral healthcare professionals in detecting cases of abuse. Cases of abuse usually pertain to young children who have no means of self-defense and almost always have nowhere to turn for help.

It is only recently that society has become increasingly aware of the problem of child abuse across all socioeconomic groups. Abuse often results in immeasurable tragedies involving the emotional, physical, or cognitive impairment of a child that often has far-reaching consequences and impacts on healthy adulthood. The wellbeing and safety of some children across the world are threatened daily by neglect and child abuse. All oral healthcare professionals thus have a key role to play in recognizing and reporting abuse cases. Creating awareness of how to properly recognize abuse, especially child abuse, is critically and legally important to all oral healthcare professionals globally.

Finally, since epidemiology and public health in oral healthcare are about monitoring general oral health at the population level, the final chapter focuses on probability and sampling in dentistry. It highlights how clinicians can understand the bigger picture of oral health within their respective communities and populations.

I sincerely hope that this book provides readers with the helpful knowledge it intends to bring forth.

Aneesa Moolla
University of Witwatersrand,
Health Economics and Epidemiology Research Office,
Johannesburg, South Africa

Section 1

Oral Medicine, Periodontology and Radiology

Chapter 1

Review in the Treatment Decision of Modalities for Impacted Second Molar

Ann Chianchitlert, Diane Selvido, Irin Sirisoontorn, Bishwa Prakash Bhattarai, Dinesh Rokaya and Natthamet Wongsirichat

Abstract

Impacted permanent tooth can occur on any tooth in the dental arch. The incidence of retention and impaction of the second molar lies between 0 and 2.3%. It is infrequently found in normal dental patients because most of the second molar impactions are asymptomatic. However, it is a common occurrence in orthodontic practice. The impacted second molar may provoke many pathologic disorders to the adjacent and opposite teeth, eventually malocclusions. There are many treatment modalities in facilitating the eruption of the second molar impaction. Early diagnosis and early treatment are crucial for the successful treatment of mandibular second molar impaction. This article presents an overview of various treatment modalities for an impacted second molar.

Keywords: Second molar, Treatment modality, Unerupted tooth, Impacted tooth, Diagnosis, Surgery

1. Introduction

Unerupted or impacted permanent tooth can involve any tooth in the dental arch. According to many authors, the teeth that are usually involved are the maxillary and mandibular third molars, the maxillary canines, and the mandibular second premolars, respectively. The delayed eruption of second permanent molars is an infrequent occurrence; however, it has clinical impacts when it occurs.

The frequency of occurrence in the impacted second molars is rare and can vary within 0% to 2.3% [1–3]. Permanent molars are exceptionally crucial for the dentition to develop normally and for the facial growth synchronization, along with providing occlusal support for masticatory functions. Any disturbance in the eruption path of permanent molars can lead in a short lower facial height [4].

Most of the time, the pathology from the impacted second molar may provoke many pathologic disorders to the adjacent and opposite teeth. Caries, periodontitis, roots resorption, or pericoronitis may occurred to those neighboring teeth. Other results may form the follicular cyst, tilting of neighboring teeth, and eventually malocclusions [5, 6].

The treatment modalities for unerupted second molars depend on the impaction's severity and the stage of development of the patient [5], which often requires a multidisciplinary approach. The treatment options include surgical procedures [7, 8], orthodontic methods [9, 10], and combined surgical and orthodontic [11]. Some authors suggested extracting the unerupted molar and following orthodontic approaches [10, 12, 13]. Each method has its advantages and disadvantages.

Timely early diagnosis and treatment of permanent second molars' impaction contribute to the most satisfactory consequences with promising and lasting prognosis [14]. Later treatment will be more problematic because not only will the clinical divergence increases with time, but also, the ability to adjust the existing dentition is less.

There are various treatment modalities of the second molar impactions. However, there are no clear guidelines for the clinician to follow when dealt with such cases. Therefore, this review will explain the etiology and incidence of impacted second permanent molars, emphasize the need for earlier diagnosis, and focus on treatment options that can guide the decision-making process.

2. The eruption of permanent molar

The eruption of permanent molars diverges on or after the eruption of other permanent teeth because the former primary teeth are absent. The formation of permanent molars is consecutively originated in the maxillary tuberosity and at the connection of the mandibular ramus and body of the mandible. The jaws' development results in the respective position of the first permanent molar to shift forward at the time of the development of the second molar. The occlusal surface of the mandibular molars is mesially inclined while the occlusal surface of maxillary molars is distally inclined during the beginning of the formation. The crowns then slowly shift to a more vertical position. Notably, there is an inherent close association between the eruption of a tooth and the stage of root development. Moreover, three-quarters of the roots of the tooth will be formed right after emergence. Remarkably, half of the roots of central incisors and lower first permanent molars have been developed by this time [5].

The concept of eruption failure is different from the delayed eruption. It is reflected as the incapacity of the tooth to erupt in the oral cavity [15]. This may occur in one or more teeth, with primary or the permanent dentition, and could possibly be incomplete and complete eruption failure. Bone or soft tissue may cover the teeth. In more ways, the failure is reliant on the pre-existing etiology [16].

3. Eruption disturbances and ectopic eruption

A disruption in the eruption path means the second molar erupts into contact apical to the eminence on the first permanent molar's distal surface, and from this occurrence, the second molar can be locked [17] (**Figure 1**). Impaction, by definition, is tooth retention owing to an obstruction in the tooth germ's eruption path or ectopic position in the dentition [11]. Impaction is deemed to be the termination of the eruption of a tooth. The obstruction can be detected clinically or radiographically in the route of eruption or due to the tooth's malposition. Primary retention stops the eruption of a customarily situated and developed tooth before the emergence, without a visible obstruction in the eruption path. Secondary retention is the ending of the tooth eruption after the emergence devoid of a physical barrier [2, 5, 18]. There are distinct treatment approaches for the eruption disturbances [5].

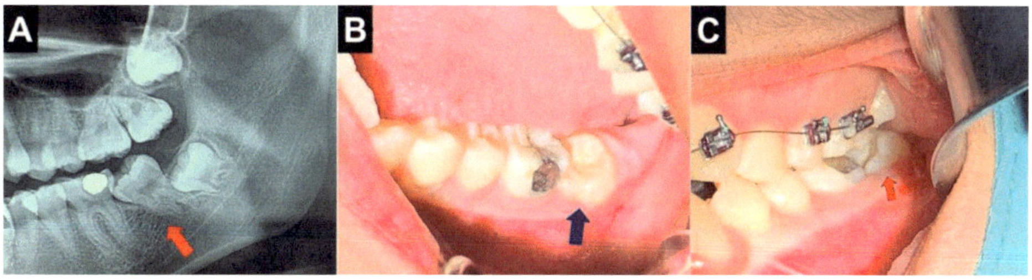

Figure 1.
The impacted second molar that occur (arrow) A: a part of panoramic radiograph on the left side B: in the oral cavity C: the occlusion of the lower impacted second molar and upper second molar.

4. Discussion

4.1 Incidence

The diagnosis of impacted second molars has been made typically between 10 and 14 years of age. Helm and Seidler defined ordinary emergence for the second molar at 12.4 and 11.9 years in the maxilla and 11.9 and 11.4 years in the mandible for boys and girls, respectively [19]. The late emergence of the second molars is seldom the primary reason for an orthodontic recommendation [20].

4.2 Prevalence of impacted second molars

The frequency of impacted second molars is only minimal and it varies from 0% to 2.3% [2]. Brondemark and Tsiopa found 2.3% of the wide-ranging prevalence of eruption disturbances of the permanent second molar. Cho et al. reported that the impaction mandibular second molars in Chinese children was only 1% [21]. The impacted second molars are usually overlooked whenever there is clinical examination, and radiographs might not be routinely taken for all cases. Furthermore, these impacted the second molar teeth are ignored by asymptomatic patients [22].

However, a greater incidence of second molar impaction is more common in orthodontic patients [23]. The prevalence of impacted second mandibular molar from orthodontic records of young caucasian was relatively high (1.36%) as the study was conducted on the orthodontic population [24]. The age of the individuals with impacted second molar varies from 9 to 26 years [1, 2]. Second molar impaction often ensues much more in the mandible than in the maxilla, which may arise for the reason that there is a later development of the upper third molar [25]. These impactions tend to be more unilateral than bilateral [2, 25]. Second molar impaction and retention are habitually detected during orthodontic treatment as a supplemental finding and are infrequently the main reason for referral to an orthodontic clinic [26].

4.3 Etiology

Many factors are elaborated with the failure of eruption, affecting prognosis and treatment [20]. The impacted second molar is an asymptomatic pathology. Failure of eruption is also more likely to be a secondary finding during orthodontic treatment [27]. Andreasen et al. [4] concluded that three leading factors are drawn in the eruption interference. These causes incorporate position of the ectopic tooth, barriers in the eruption path, and failures in mechanism of the eruption [17, 28]. Posterior crowding is thought to be the most common cause of mesially angulated lower-second-molar impactions [11].

Heredity is also brought up as a secondary etiological factor [29]. Patients with specific syndromes may involve some systemic factors [16]. In the patients with a disturbance of local eruption, only one or a few teeth may be affected. The early diagnosis of eruption disturbances is crucial. It is essential to provide treatment at a suitable time and minimize complications [5, 25, 30].

An ectopic eruption of the maxillary first molars impaction is often related to a mesial angle path to the expected direction of eruption. It may also affect the second molar's failure to upright from its mesial inclination during the emergence. Supernumerary teeth and odontogenic tumors or cysts can be the major physical barriers of the eruption path [5].

The eruption of mandibular second premolar and second molar usually in competition for space of the dental arch. When this posterior space in the arch is inadequate, the earlier emergence second premolar may cause the failure of eruption of the second molar [31].

4.4 Diagnostic approach and treatment time

The impacted second molars are diagnosed between 10 and 14 years of age [32]. Rapid diagnosis is crucial in improving prognosis and alleviating the effect of the failure of eruption. It requires a full clinical and radiographic examinations including previous medical record, which are enough to differentiate between impaction, primary, and secondary retention [5, 15].

As the time of eruption may differ among each child, follow-up at six-month intervals of children with mixed dentition is recommended to guide the pattern of eruption and the development of the teeth. The posterior crowding cases and the uncertain of the molar retention should be more concerned [21]. The orthodontist should be alerted if one erupted lower second molar without the contralateral molar is observed in the clinic. The number of teeth with delayed eruption compared to the contralateral teeth should be one of the cautions.

In a preadolescent patient, a panoramic radiograph showing a lower-third-molar follicle positioned on top of the developing second molar crown may give early warning of future impaction [32].

If the eruption of a permanent mandibular second molar is six-month delayed compared with its contralateral molar or both molars show a year delay in eruption, the dubitation of molar retention must necessitate further radiographic investigation [21]. The cone-beam computed tomography is a tool that can be employed to identify ankylosis [28].

Unerupted molar may be found in a panoramic radiograph thru a regular dental check-up or orthodontic assessment and treatment planning [20]. The radiological examination must focus on the follicles of unerupted molars, dental abnormalities, root abnormalities, dilacerations, taurodontism, invagination, resorption, or dental caries in both neighboring primary molar and first permanent molar [30].

The treatment option depends on the mandibular second molar impaction dictated by the degree of mesial angulation and its vertical depth, which could be seen in a panoramic radiograph. The inclination of impacted teeth is calculated from the angle between the first and second lower molars' long axis. The impacted second molar is in mesial inclination if the angle between their long axis is more than 40°. If the angle of the long axis of both molars is between 40° and – 20°, the impacted second molar is in a vertical position, and if the angle is less than –20° means the impacted second molar is in distal inclination [20]. The vertical depth of impacted teeth will determine by the distance between the distal marginal ridge of the first molar to the mesial marginal ridge of the impacted second molar [22].

4.5 Treatment modalities

The treatment modalities for the second molar impaction depend on the variety of abnormalities of the eruption and the patient's age. Treatment options may incorporate observation, repositioning or surgical exposure, orthodontic uprighting, and the extraction of unerupted molar. Each modality has its indications, contraindications, advantages, and disadvantages [20].

The orthodontic or surgical approach is indicated only when the etiologies are from impacted ectopic erupting teeth and primary retention [17]. However, a prior observation time is essential to confirm the diagnosis through a radiographic follow-up before any intervention. The natural eruption may occur in normal occlusion in a few cases [11].

The intervention should be deliberated after an observation period of 12 months when the possibility of self-correction is ruled out [21]. Abnormally positioned tooth germ of the third molar may create a physical barrier that causes the second molar impaction. The suggested treatment is removing the third molar at the 11–14 years age old together with a in-depth follow-up for the second molar [5].

Once there is no chance for self-correction, the parents and patients should be informed about the treatment option for the impacted molars. The treatment options may include orthodontic uprighting, surgical repositioning, the impacted second molar extraction and letting the third molar drift into the second molar position, and transplanting the third molar into the extraction site of the impacted second molar [21].

4.6 Orthodontic treatment

Diagnosis made early on and prompt treatment are vital to an effective treatment of mandibular second molar impaction. The orthodontic treatment is recommended for impacted or ectopically erupted teeth and in cases of primary retention [17]. Although orthodontic treatment is usually given in the mandibular arch the success rate is the same for both the arches [11].

The individuals between 11 and 14 years in which the roots of second molars are still incomplete are suggested to treat the impaction. The poor prognosis is the impacted molars with fully formed roots [5]. The success of orthodontic treatment relates to numerous local considerations such as the impacted tooth 's angulation, the third molar position, and the severity of crowding or follicle collision [11]. There are several methods to treat the second molar impaction. However, there are some limitations, specifically in the treatment of severely deep impacted teeth.

4.6.1 Conventional appliance

At the first stage of conventional orthodontic treatment, during the alignment and leveling, a tube is bonded to the molar's buccal surface. It will be engaged with a continuous archwire. Super-elastic archwire and a push coil spring will ensure the alignment and distalization. The super-elastic archwire used for alignment and leveling of the teeth is curved distally of the impacted second molar. It is inserted in the tube to help uprighting the impacted second molar [31].

4.6.2 Orthodontic uprighting cantilever spring

The techniques of uprighting the impacted mandibular second molar with a cantilever spring are optional treatments besides extraction or surgical repositioning of the tooth. The treatment can be directed with or without the removal of the adjacent third molar. It needs surgical exposure of the crown of the impacted second molar, followed by bonding an orthodontic attachment for uprighting the impacted tooth [33].

It is a straight forward way to upright the angulated and impacted second molar using an uprighting cantilever spring attached to a bonded tube on the distobuccal cusps of the affected tooth [31].

The cantilever mechanics designed was useful for the correction of an extremely tipped and deeply impacted molar. When the cantilever mechanics is used, the tipped molar will have an uprighting moment and an extrusive force.

Thus, an occlusal interference with the opposing tooth may occur. Morita et al. suggested utilizing a compression force with a two-step bend incorporated into a NiTi archwire for cases in which the molar was slightly tipped and extruded [34].

4.6.3 Orthodontic uprighting and distalized segmented wire

Several orthodontic techniques utilize the distalized segmented archwire to upright the impacted molar. Before the bonding of fixed orthodontic appliances, a segmented wire is engaged between the impacted second molar and the adjacent first molar. The segmented archwire for the technique must have super elasticity characteristics. The wire will be bent and bonded to the occlusal surface of the first permanent molar [35].

Bach technique is one of the non-surgical technique for uprighting mesially impacted mandibular molars. The technique used an .014" x .025" Copper NiTi wire.36 Whereas other developed a technique using .016" x .016" NiTi wire [36]. Fu et al. developed a polearm using 0.016"x 0.022″ titanium molybdenum alloy wire [22]. A major advantage of these techniques was that they could be utilized on both bonded and unbonded mandibular arch.

4.6.4 Temporary anchorage devices

Temporary skeletal anchorages devices have some superior advantages. They could provide vertical and distal traction forces at the same time with a good moment and line of action. They could also diminish the side effects related with dental anchorage. There are two methods of utilizing a temporary anchorage device for uprighting molar impaction, direct and indirect anchorage.

Direct anchorage is when the teeth moved directly towards or against the mini-screw. Chang et al., reported the use of a ramus screw to upright the complex impacted second molar [37]. An indirect anchorage refers to stabilizing certain teeth via a rigid connection with the mini-screw and subsequent use of these stabilized anchors to move other teeth in the dental arch [38].

4.7 Surgical approach

Because these impacted teeth have limited access, surgical approaches should be considered to help with their necessary uprighting. Techniques are as follows:

4.7.1 Surgical exposure without orthodontic traction

Surgical exposure of the buccal surface bonded with a bracket has been done by Going and Reyes- Louise in 1999 for an impacted second molar. The exposure resulted in the successful positioning of the second molar of 40 patients. They applied this technique for seven years with an acceptable prognosis [39].

Usually, the buccal surface will be exposed via soft tissue removal or drilling into the bone covering the tooth. Care must be given to drilling into the bone to not traverse through the second molar's cementoenamel junction and root areas [39]. This method was discussed as the most successful treatment by Magnusson and Kjellberg. These researchers conducted a clinical trial involving 87 patients ranging from 11 to 19 years old. The study gained 70% favorable results, making it a recommended modality [11].

4.7.2 Surgical exposure and luxation

As mentioned above, the procedure to expose the second molar is to remove the buccal bone to gain the tooth's surface visibility. In patients where, orthodontic treatment is not an option or contraindicated, luxation is the next step. Using a straight elevator, the second molar is gently and slightly manipulated to the tooth's position, luxating occlusally and distally, reaching the approximate level of the occlusal plane.

Kravitz et al. claimed that this technique is suitable for conserving the apical blood supply since the tooth will remain within the socket [32]. Hence, the tooth can have a favorable prognosis, especially when there is still incomplete root formation [32, 40]. Disadvantages would be fractures and pulp necrosis due to the manipulation employed in this method [20].

4.7.3 Surgical uprighting

To achieve the upright position of the impacted second molar, the extraction of the third molar might be necessary. The removal of the third molar can be done with a standard approach in these cases [41–43]. According to McAboy et al., a trough is made on the second molar's distal to compensate for the distal movement. Two hands are recommended in doing this procedure: one hand on the elevator to change the position of the tooth occlusal and distally, less than 75 degrees, five while the other hand will be for the cortical plate and alveolar ridge support [41].

The surgeon was said to feel a "snap" into the trough provided in the distal area, possibly indicating a stable position [44]. However, the tooth was advised to be placed off-occlusion slightly to avoid trauma on the site, and necessary stabilizing techniques can be performed if there is mobility [41]. This technique was widely evidenced to have a good prognosis and claimed to have no unfavorable sequelae in long-term follow-ups [43, 44]. Furthermore, other authors supported that removing the third molar might not be required in these cases [24, 40].

Autogenous bone grafting or any bone substitutes can be applied in this technique for stabilization in some cases where there are areas devoid of bone [41, 44]. On the other hand, Boynton and Lieblich suggested that bone grafts are not necessary for the stabilization process [45].

4.7.4 Extraction

Subsequently, suppose all other minimally to moderately invasive surgical modalities fail. In that case, the prognosis is poor, and pathology has commenced— then extraction can be an option [33]. This method was said to be the most unsuccessful among all the modalities tested by Magnusson and Kjellberg since it was reported that the third molars that replaced these teeth resulted in a mispositioned state. Once this treatment is indicated, proper patient education on untoward outcomes is suggested [11].

4.7.5 Autotransplantation

Immediate transplantation of the third molar into the intentionally extracted second molar site is also an indicated management. Still, it possesses immense risk as there will be periodontal and pulpal complications after the procedure [32, 41]. Successful outcomes depend on the generation of new periodontal ligament and cellular structures, suggesting that the tooth should be transplanted right away to make way for a better prognosis.

According to Tsukiboshi, this treatment's indications include the donor and recipient teeth should be morphologically analogous to each other; both teeth should be prepared with less invasive procedures; if endodontic treatment is deemed necessary, the therapy completion should be completed after two weeks [46]. In this procedure, failure happens when there is a pulpal infection, ankylosis, and resorption on the transplanted tooth [47]. The use of a piezosurgery machine in autotransplantation has been developed and resulted in an effective modality in harvesting the third molar to replace a second molar [48].

4.8 Timing of uprighting

Preferably, the literature suggests that surgical repositioning approaches should be made in a second molar with half or two-thirds of root formation. Dessner [49] described that there is minimal root fracture that can happen in this development stage. Intervention in the earlier stages of root formation rather than the recommended one results in a displaced, unstable, and less than the second molar's desired position.

5. Conclusion

Second molar impaction and retention are infrequently the initial reason for orthodontic treatment recommendation because they are rare and asymptomatic. It may be discovered in a regular panoramic radiograph during routine orthodontic evaluation. The diagnosis and treatment planning, which should consider the patient's age is crucial. The treatment options include observation, surgical extraction of unerupted permanent molars, and a number of orthodontic and surgical methodologies for purposely uprighting the impacted molars. Though there are no definite guidelines for managing the second molar impaction, this literature can assist in the decision-making process and treatment planning of such clinical cases.

Acknowledgements

The authors would like to thank the staff, colleagues, and dental assistants including co-workers in Walailak University International College of Dentistry.

Finally, the authors would like to thank Christian Estacio from Walailak University International College of Dentistry for editing and revising the language of this manuscript.

Author contributions

Conceptualization: Irin Sirisoontorn, methodology: Irin Sirisoontorn, validation: Irin Sirisoontorn, formal analysis: Irin Sirisoontorn, investigation: Irin Sirisoontorn, resources: Dinesh Rokaya, Bishwa Prakash Bhattarai, data curation: Irin Sirisoontorn, writing—original draft preparation: Ann Chianchitlert, Diane Selvido, writing—review, and editing: Irin Sirisoontorn, visualization: Irin Sirisoontorn, supervision: Natthamet Wongsirichat, final approval: Irin Sirisoontorn.

Funding and sponsorship

This study did not receive funding by a research grant or any sponsorship.

Conflict of interest

The authors declared the conflict of interest.

Ethics approval

This study did not require ethical approval because it is a review literature.

Declaration of patient consent

There is no need for patient consent.

Author details

Ann Chianchitlert, Diane Selvido, Irin Sirisoontorn*, Bishwa Prakash Bhattarai, Dinesh Rokaya and Natthamet Wongsirichat
Walailak University International College of Dentistry, Bangkok, Thailand

*Address all correspondence to: irin.sirisoontorn@gmail.com

References

[1] Farman AG, Eloff J, Nortje CJ, Joubert JJ. Clinical absence of the first and second permanent molars. Br J Orthod. 1978;5(2):93-97.

[2] Bondemark L, Tsiopa J. Prevalence of ectopic eruption, impaction, retention and agenesis of the permanent second molar. Angle Orthod. 2007;77(5):773-778.

[3] Grover PS, Lorton L. The incidence of unerupted permanent teeth and related clinical cases. Oral Surg Oral Med Oral Pathol. 1985;59(4):420-425.

[4] Proffit WR. Equilibrium theory revisited: factors influencing position of the teeth. Angle Orthod. 1978;48(3):175-186.

[5] Raghoebar GM, Boering G, Vissink A, Stegenga B. Eruption disturbances of permanent molars: a review. J Oral Pathol Med. 1991;20(4):159-166.

[6] Albert H B Schuurs AHB. Pathology of the dental hard tissues. 2012:225-55.

[7] Haralabakis NB, Tsianou A, Nicolopoulos C. Surgical correction of mesially impacted mandibular second molars. J Clin Orthod. 2003;37(4):209-212; quiz 4.

[8] Johnson JV, Quirk GP. Surgical repositioning of impacted mandibular second molar teeth. Am J Orthod Dentofacial Orthop. 1987;91(3):242-251.

[9] Miao YQ, Zhong H. An uprighting appliance for impacted mandibular second and third molars. J Clin Orthod. 2006;40(2):110-116.

[10] Johnson E. Managing second molars. Am J Orthod Dentofacial Orthop. 2011;140(2):269-273.

[11] Magnusson C, Kjellberg H. Impaction and retention of second molars: diagnosis, treatment and outcome. A retrospective follow-up study. Angle Orthod. 2009;79(3):422-427.

[12] Bach RM. Non-surgical uprighting of exposed, mesially impacted lower molars. J Clin Orthod. 2012;46(8):480-485; quiz 91-2.

[13] Alessandri Bonetti G, Pelliccioni GA, Checchi L. Management of bilaterally impacted mandibular second and third molars. J Am Dent Assoc. 1999;130(8):1190-1194.

[14] Salentijn EG, Ras F, G Mensink G, van Merkesteyn JPR. The unerupted maxillary second molar, due to an overlying and malformed upper third molar: Treatment and follow-up. J Orthod. 2008 Mar;35(1):20-24

[15] Palma C, Coelho A, Gonzalez Y, Cahuana A. Failure of eruption of first and second permanent molars. J Clin Pediatr Dent. 2003;27(3):239-245.

[16] Ahmad S, Bister D, Cobourne MT. The clinical features and aetiological basis of primary eruption failure. Eur J Orthod. 2006;28(6):535-540.

[17] Andreasen JO PJ, Laskin DM. Textbook and colour atlas of tooth impactions. 1997.

[18] Raghoebar GM, Boering G, Jansen HW, Vissink A. Secondary retention of permanent molars: a histologic study. J Oral Pathol Med. 1989;18(8):427-431.

[19] Helm S, Seidler B. Timing of permanent tooth emergence in Danish children. Community Dent Oral Epidemiol. 1974;2(3):122-129.

[20] Sanaa Alami HA, Bellamine M, Quars FE. Impacted First and Second Permanent Molars: Overview. IntechOpen. 2019:1-25.

[21] Cho SY, Ki Y, Chu V, Chan J. Impaction of permanent mandibular second molars in ethnic Chinese schoolchildren. J Can Dent Assoc. 2008;74(6):521.

[22] Fu PS, Wang JC, Wu YM, Huang TK, Chen WC, Tseng YC, et al. Impacted mandibular second molars. Angle Orthod. 2012;82(4):670-675.

[23] Owen AHI, Early surgical management of impacted mandibular second molars. J Clin Orthod. 1998;32::446-50.

[24] Cassetta M, Altieri F, Di Mambro A, Galluccio G, Barbato E. Impaction of permanent mandibular second molar: a retrospective study. Med Oral Patol Oral Cir Bucal. 2013;18(4):e564-e568.

[25] Varpio M, Wellfelt B. Disturbed eruption of the lower second molar: clinical appearance, prevalence, and etiology. ASDC J Dent Child. 1988;55(2):114-118.

[26] Evans R. Incidence of lower second permanent molar impaction. Br J Orthod. 1988;15(3):199-203.

[27] Srinivasan MR, Poorni S, Venkatesh A, Vasanthi B. Prevalence of impacted permanent mandibular second molars in South Indian population: A cross-sectional study. Indian J Dent Res. 2016;27(5):540-543.

[28] Proffit WR, Fields HW, Larson B, Sarver DM Contemporary Orthodontics. 6 ed., St. Louis, Mosby, 2018.

[29] Fu PS, Wang JC, Chen CH, Huang TK, Tseng CH, Hung CC. Management of unilaterally deep impacted first, second, and third mandibular molars. Angle Orthod. 2012;82(3):565-571.

[30] Suri L, Gagari E, Vastardis H. Delayed tooth eruption: pathogenesis, diagnosis, and treatment. A literature review. Am J Orthod Dentofacial Orthop. 2004;126(4):432-445.

[31] Vedtofte H, Andreasen JO, Kjaer I. Arrested eruption of the permanent lower second molar. Eur J Orthod. 1999;21(1):31-40.

[32] Kravitz ND, Yanosky M, Cope JB, Silloway K, Favagehi M. Surgical Uprighting of Lower Second Molars. J Clin Orthod. 2016;50(1):33-40.

[33] Shpack N FT, Lai YH, Kuftinec MM VA, Shapira Y. Mandibular permanent second molar impaction treatment options and outcome Open J Dent Oral Med. 2013;1:9-14.

[34] Morita Y, Koga Y, Nguyen TA, Yoshida N. Biomechanical considerations for uprighting impacted mandibular molars. Korean J Orthod. 2020;50(4):268-277.

[35] DiBagno D BL, Rinchuse DJ. Uprighting impacted mandibular second molars using NiTi wire. Orthod Practice. 2015; 6:40-44.

[36] Bach RM. Non-surgical uprighting of mesially impacted lower molars. J Clin Orthod. 2011;45(12): 679-681.

[37] Chang CH, Lin JS, Roberts WE. Ramus screws: the ultimate solution for lower impacted molars. Semin Orthod. 2018;24:135-154.

[38] Magkavali-Trikka P, Emmanouilidis G, Papadopoulos MA. Mandibular molar uprighting using orthodontic miniscrew implants: a systematic review. Prog Orthod. 2018;19(1):1.

[39] Going RE, Jr., Reyes-Lois DB. Surgical exposure and bracketing technique for uprighting impacted mandibular second molars. J Oral Maxillofac Surg. 1999;57(2):209-212.

[40] Padwa BL, Dang RR, Resnick CM. Surgical Uprighting Is a Successful Procedure for Management of Impacted Mandibular Second Molars. J Oral Maxillofac Surg. 2017;75(8):1581-1590.

[41] McAboy CP, Grumet JT, Siegel EB, Iacopino AM. Surgical uprighting and repositioning of severely impacted mandibular second molars. J Am Dent Assoc. 2003;134(11):1459-1462.

[42] la Monaca G, Cristalli MP, Pranno N, Galluccio G, Annibali S, Pippi R. First and second permanent molars with failed or delayed eruption: Clinical and statistical analyses. Am J Orthod Dentofac Orthop. 2019;156(3): 355-364.

[43] Pogrel MA. The surgical uprighting of mandibular second molars. Am J Orthod Dentofacial Orthop. 1995; 108(2):180-183.

[44] Shipper G, Thomadakis G. Bone regeneration after surgical repositioning of impacted mandibular second molars: a case report. Dent Traumatol. 2003;19(2):109-114.

[45] Boynton T, Lieblich SE. Surgical uprighting of second molars. Atlas Oral Maxillofac Surg Clin North Am. 2013;21(2):235-237.

[46] Tsukiboshi M. Autotransplantation of teeth: requirements for predictable success. Dent Traumatol. 2002;18(4): 157-180.

[47] Rohof ECM, Kerdijk W, Jansma J, Livas C, Ren Y. Autotransplantation of teeth with incomplete root formation: a systematic review and meta-analysis. Clin Oral Investig. 2018; 22(4): 1613-1624.

[48] Zufia J, Abella F, Trebol I, Gomez-Meda R. Autotransplantation of Mandibular Third Molar with Buccal Cortical Plate to Replace Vertically Fractured Mandibular Second Molar: A Novel Technique. J Endod. 2017;43(9): 1574-1578.

[49] Dessner S. Surgical uprighting of second molars: rationale and technique. Oral Maxillofac Surg Clin North Am. 2002;14(2):201-212.

Chapter 2

The Radiology of Developmental Dental Defects Demystified: An e-Based Learning System

Christopher Olubode Ogunsalu

Abstract

The purpose of this perspective-type chapter is to provide the readership with in-depth knowledge in the area of developmental abnormalities with special emphasis on radiology together with its clinical implications. The intention of this chapter is not only to be descriptive of the radiology of the developmental dental defects, but to provide the readership with the various possible differential diagnoses and how to arrive at a definitive diagnosis and being mindful of the fact that some of these radiological presentations can be pathognomonic while others are variable in presentation. The ultimate goal of this chapter is to provide the prerequisite knowledge to the clinicians to enable them to arrive at a definitive diagnosis based on radiology and radiographic presentation without the need of any other investigation if possible. It is as such important that in this chapter the readership will be elevated to a level of realistic, yet clinician with the reasoning and interpretation of a radiologists in the area of developmental dental defects (DDD) since by understanding the basis of utilizing radiography to arrive at the definitive diagnosis of these developmental defects amidst of the various differential diagnoses, they would have gained full knowledge and control of the pertinent use of terminologies in this specific and unique area of dentistry. Conventional radiography such as periapical radiographs, bitewings and dental panoramic tomography will be utilized largely in this chapter, without the need for computerized tomography or CBCT. Certain conditions such as concrescence (not fusion and germination) and enamel pearl may be very difficult to identify or distinguish using conventional radiography and the role of advanced imaging technique will be mentioned. It is as such the intention of this unique book chapter to display in an *Atlas work note* format, the radiology of the developmental dental defects, with the intention to bring in the knowledge required to the undergraduate students of dentistry and postgraduate dentists and inclusive of the practicing clinicians in the field of dentistry.

Keywords: pathognomonic, variable, features, dental, defect, differential, diagnosis, radiographic, atlas, work note

1. Introduction

In this chapter, the radiographs of important developmental dental defects (DDD) will be displayed and important radiologically related questions will follow together with the answers. This is to assist the reader in understanding not only the radiology of the DDD and also the clinical significance, but also the various possible differential diagnoses. It is my intention to clinically (clinical significance) and radiographically demonstrate to the readers that correlation matters between the later and the former since some clinically obvious DDD can in fact not have any specific or pathognomonic radiological presentation. The case of multiple bilateral parapremolars that was recently managed by me is replete of this statement, "*the more you look at the X-ray, the less you see of the clinically significant presentation of the developmental dental defects*."

In this chapter, the questions posed which follows the presented radiograph will be in black and brown and the answers are in red. This is to aid the sound understanding of the radiology of the developmental dental defects at a glance. Each radiograph is as such within a plate.

This chapter will end with the developmental dental defect called regional odontodysplasia. The regional odontodysplasia is very rare and I have decided to correlate the radiology with the clinical findings and histological findings by encouraging the readers to read the classical article of Jahanimoghadam et al. [1] on the subject and for them to utilize such knowledge obtained to present a power point lecture for presentation on regional odontoplasia with the expectation that they will be opportune, 1 day to make such presentation to an audience of dental practitioners and academics.

2. Methods

The author for the first time provides a self-directed dento-maxillofacial radiology atlas with focus on the developmental dental defects. The atlas that aims at demystifying the reporting and the differential diagnosis and diagnosis of the subject area utilizes a collection of radiographs to report radiographic images and arrive at both a differential diagnosis and a definitive diagnosis.

Each radiograph is depicted as a plate and as such consecutively numbered from 1 to 37.

Each plate is given a heading that concurs to the definitive diagnosis. This heading is depicted in RED.

The radiographic images are then followed by specific questions including instructions for the reader to point at specific areas of the images. These questions are depicted in BLACK.

The questions are then repeated in BOLD BROWN with the answers to the questions displayed adjacent to it and depicted in RED.

At the foot of each radiographic plate is a reference or list of reference that is aimed at providing obvious reference to each plate. These references are highlighted in Green.

All questions are strictly radiographically oriented and has strong clinical inclination and to include the use of both the radiographic and clinical information to arrive at a definitive diagnosis and clinical treatment or management. All questions and pointers are completely answered for the benefit of the student's e-based learning without the need of a lecturer.

All the wordings of the manuscript are those of the author and have not been copied from any previous text.

The students on repeated reading of the text and correlation of such information with each preceding radiographic image will completely understand the topic without the need of a tutor.

1. Point at the anomaly.

2. What is it called?

3. List two clinical considerations of this condition.

4. Point at the anomaly.

   See arrow A.

5. What is it called?

   Dens invarginatus (dens in dente).

6. List two clinical considerations of this condition.

   a. Dental infection without any carious lesions.

   b. Inaccessible root canal, hence treatment of teeth usually infected is by extraction and replacement of extracted teeth by removable or fixed prosthesis (**Figure 1**) [2].

1. Describe the lesion.

2. What is it called?

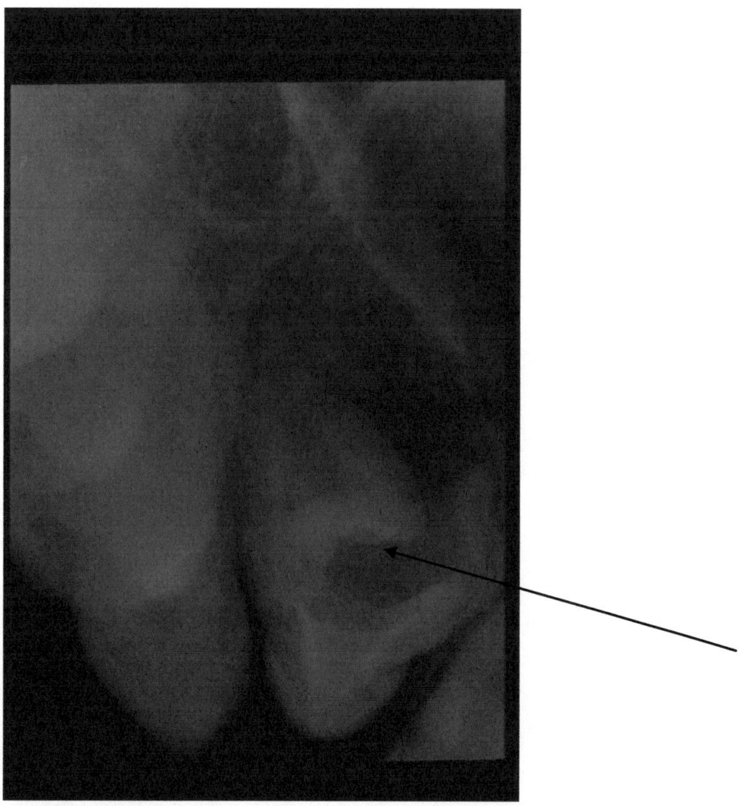

Figure 1.
Periapical radiograph showing dens inverginatus.

3. How is it usually discovered?

4. Is it a developmental dental defect?

5. Describe the lesion.

   The occlusal radiograph shows a well-defined and well-corticated, heart-shaped unilocular radiolucent lesion with septations within it in the anterior region of the palate. The lesion is about 35 × 25 mm and intimately related to the apical region of the anterior teeth.

6. What is it called?

   Nasopalatine duct cyst or the incisive canal cyst.

7. How is it usually discovered?

   a. Routine radiography (occlusal radiograph)

   b. Swelling under a denture

   c. Painful or infected swelling in the anterior maxilla

8. Is this a developmental dental defect?

   No, it is actually a developmental non-odontogenic cyst? (**Figure 2**) [2].

1. Use an arrow to point at the developmental dental defect.

2. What is it called?

3. What are the clinical implications for this condition?

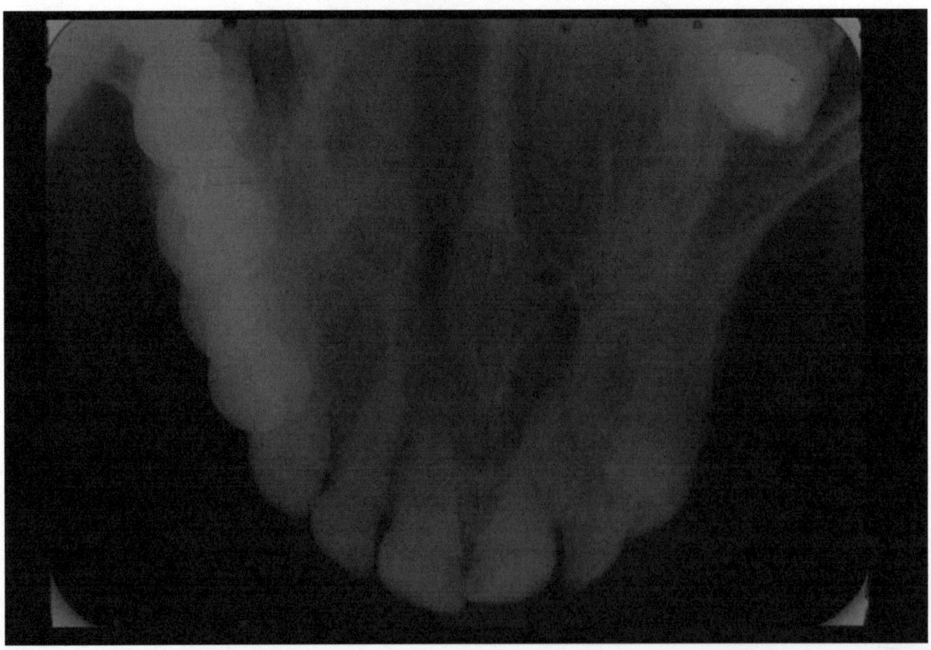

Figure 2.
Occlusal radiograph showing nasopalatine duct cyst (see arrows).

4. Use an arrow to point at the anomaly.

   See white arrow B.

5. What is it called?

   Anodontia.

6. What are the clinical implications for this condition?

   Since the permanent successor is missing the bone in the area is usually deficient and extraction and implant placement may not be effected easily unless bone grafting is done. Fortunately, this tooth may remain in occlusion throughout life despite it being prone to caries formation and periodontal disease (**Figure 3**) [2].

This patient has had no extractions

1. Point at all the anomalies with arrows.

2. What is this condition called?

3. Explain your findings.

4. Point at all the anomalies with arrows.

   See the arrows.

5. What is this condition called?

   Hypodontia.

6. Explain your findings.

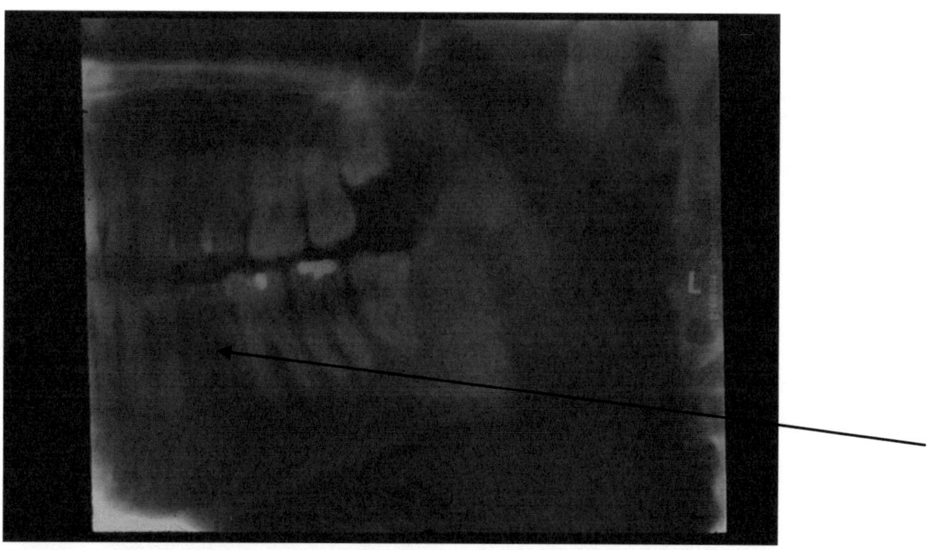

Figure 3.
Part of a dental panoramic tomogram (DPT) showing over-retained deciduous second molar and missing second premolar in the lower jaw (see arrows).

In all the four quadrants, some deciduous teeth are over retained with the permanent successors absent in the bone. These over-retained deciduous teeth are the canine teeth in the upper jaw and the first molars in the mandible. It is not unlikely that the edentulous space in the maxilla is as a result of permanent teeth that never formed (**Figure 4**) [2].

1. Point at the main anomaly.

2. What is it called?

3. What do you see clinically?

4. Do a report on this radiograph?

5. Point at the main anomaly.

   See the arrow.

6. What is it called?

   Mesiodens.

7. What do you see clinically?

   A diastema caused possibly by a rotated miniature/defective supernumerary incisor.

8. Do a report on this radiograph.

   This is a dental panoramic tomogram (DPT) of a child in mixed dentition stage—the upper jaw in the anterior region presents with a microdont supernumerary tooth with an upwardly directed crown, which is impinging on the root of the central incisor on the right side to cause the incisor to rotate.

   Diagnosis: Mesiodens that is causing a pressure effect on the central incisor **(Figure 5)** [2].

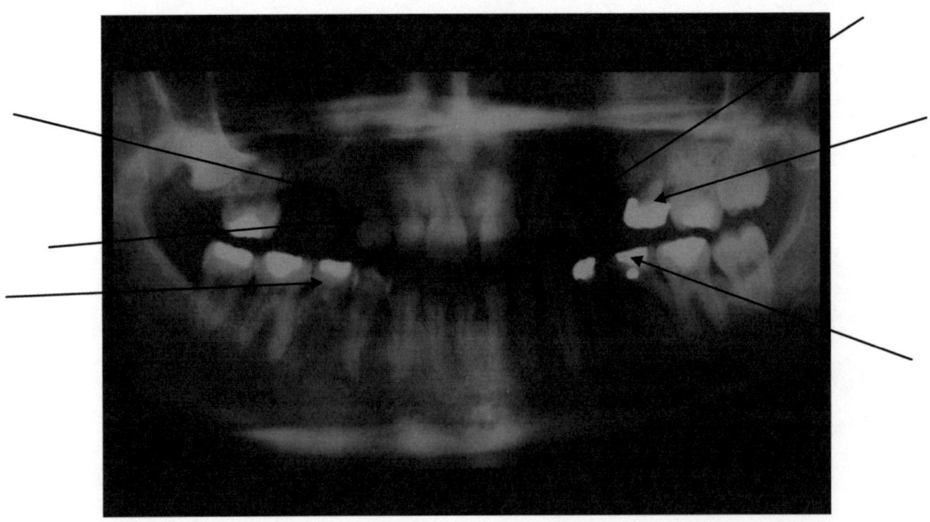

Figure 4.
DPT showing numerous missing permanent teeth and over-retained deciduous teeth. (See arrows).

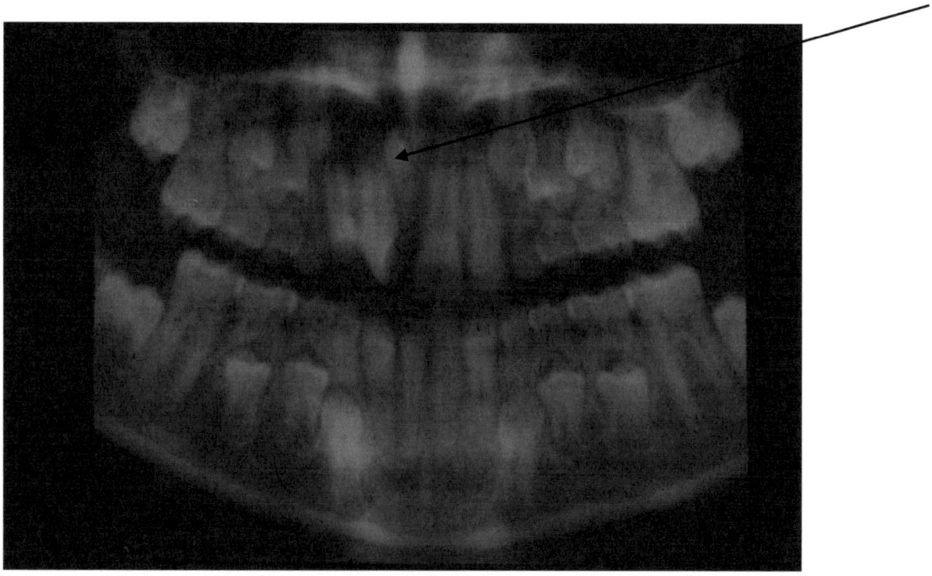

Figure 5.
DPT of a patient in mixed dentition stage showing a maxillary mesiodens tooth (see arrows).

1. With an arrow, point at the anomaly.
2. What is this called?
3. Explain the clinical considerations of this particular situation.
4. With an arrow, point at the anomaly.

   See arrow.
5. What is this called?

   Macrodont.
6. Explain the clinical considerations of this particular situation:
   1. Inability to erupt into the arch.
   2. Possibility of forming a dentigerous cyst or ameloblastoma.
   3. Difficulty in the surgical extraction of the tooth if needed.
   4. Creation of an oro-antral communication following extraction (**Figure 6**) [2].

1. With an arrow, point at the anomaly.
2. What is this called?
3. What are the clinical considerations for this particular case?
4. With an arrow, point at the anomaly.

   See the arrow.

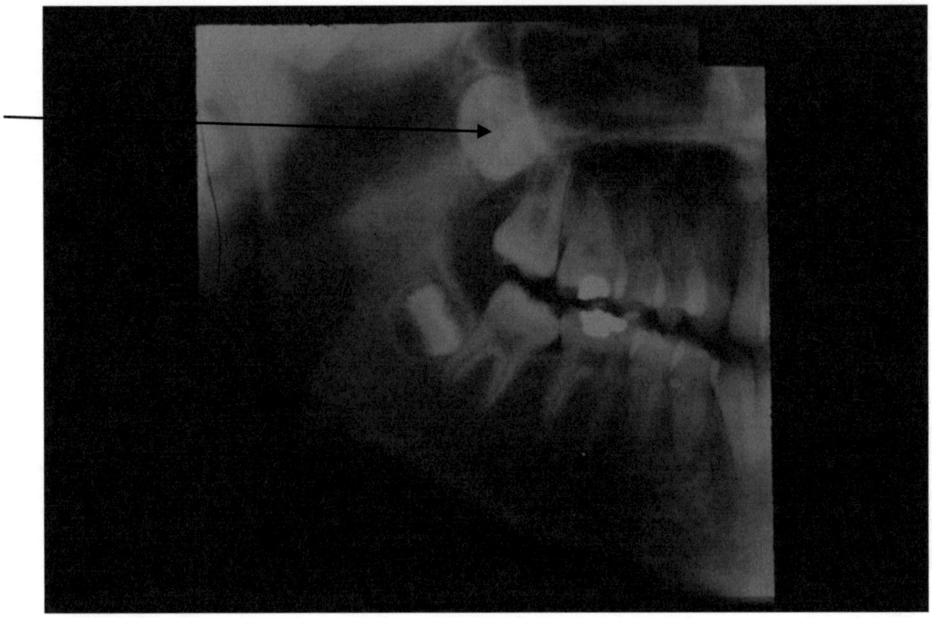

Figure 6.
Part of a DPT showing a Macrodont (see arrows).

5. What is this called?

   Microdont.

6. What are the clinical considerations for this particular case?

   1. High possibility of development of periodontal disease.

   2. High possibility of forming a carious lesion.

   3. Technical extraction, should it be a part of the surgical extraction of four wisdom teeth **(Figure** 7) [2].

1. Use an arrow to pin point at the anomaly.

2. Give two differential diagnosis.

3. What is the common name for the conditions you have named?

4. How do you confirm a diagnosis?

5. Use an arrow to pin point at the anomaly.

   See arrow.

6. Give two differential diagnoses:

   1. Germination

   2. Fusion

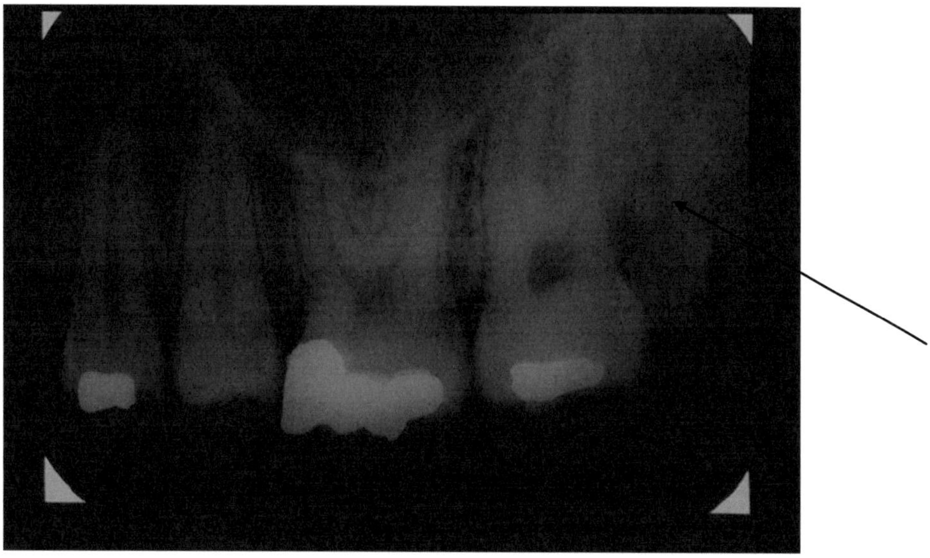

Figure 7.
Periapical radiograph showing a microdont tooth (see arrows).

7. What is the common name for the conditions you have named?

   Both differential diagnosis above are called double teeth or twinning.

8. How do you confirm a diagnosis?

   The confirmation is purely clinical—this is by counting the number of teeth in the arch. If the numbers of teeth is normal, then it is fusion; however, it is germination if the number of teeth is more (**Figure 8**) [2].

1. Apart from the buried canine tooth, point at the anomaly on the periapical radiograph.

2. What is it called?

3. What are the clinical implications of this condition?

4. Apart from the buried canine tooth point at the anomaly on the periapical radiograph

   See the arrow.

5. What is it called?

   Dens inverginatus.

6. What are the clinical implications of this condition?

    1. Infection of the periapical tissues without any carious lesion.

    2. This infection may spread fast leading into cellulites.

    3. Inability to access the root canal during a proposed endodontic treatment, hence the need for extraction and immediate implant or crown and

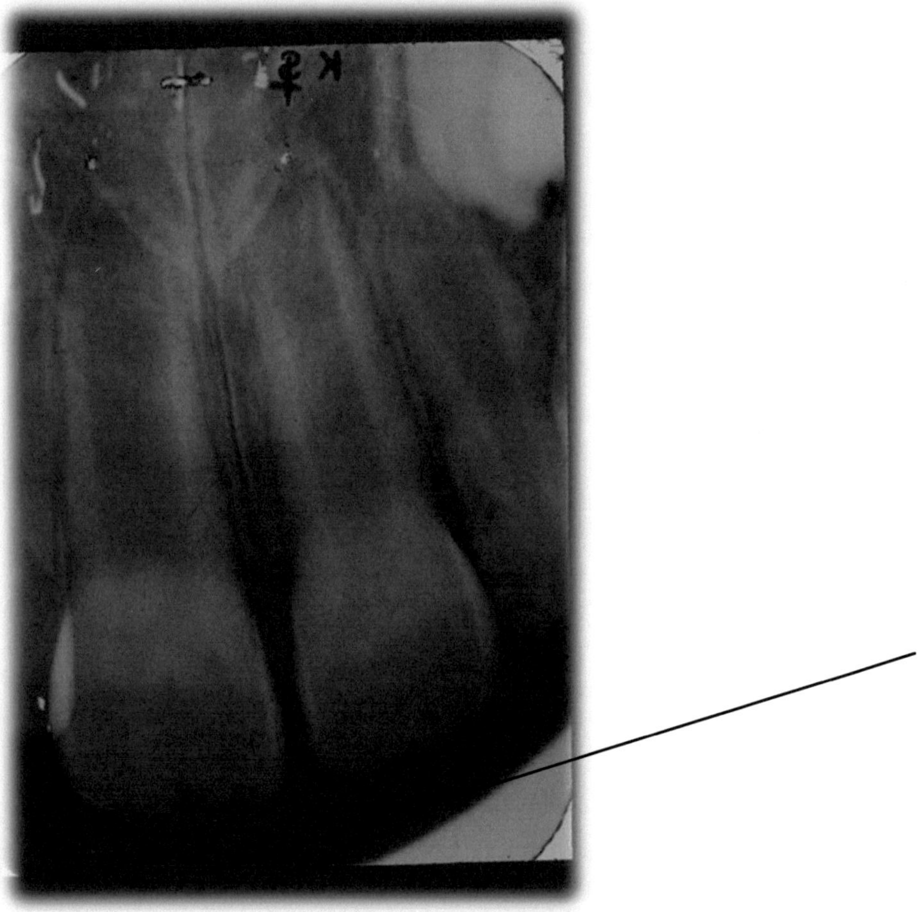

Figure 8.
Periapical radiograph double teeth in relation to the upper central incisor tooth (see arrows).

bridge. Usually, root canal treatment is commenced, only to fail because of the structural defect (DDD), which existed and was undetected before the commencement of root canal (**Figure 9**) [2].

1. Explain the anomaly and point at it.

2. What is it called?

3. What are the clinical implications of this condition?

4. What other implication is this condition ascribed to?

5. What is it termed?

6. Explain the anomaly and point at it.

    1. Large root canal of the tooth (pointed to).

    2. Large pulp chamber and canal.

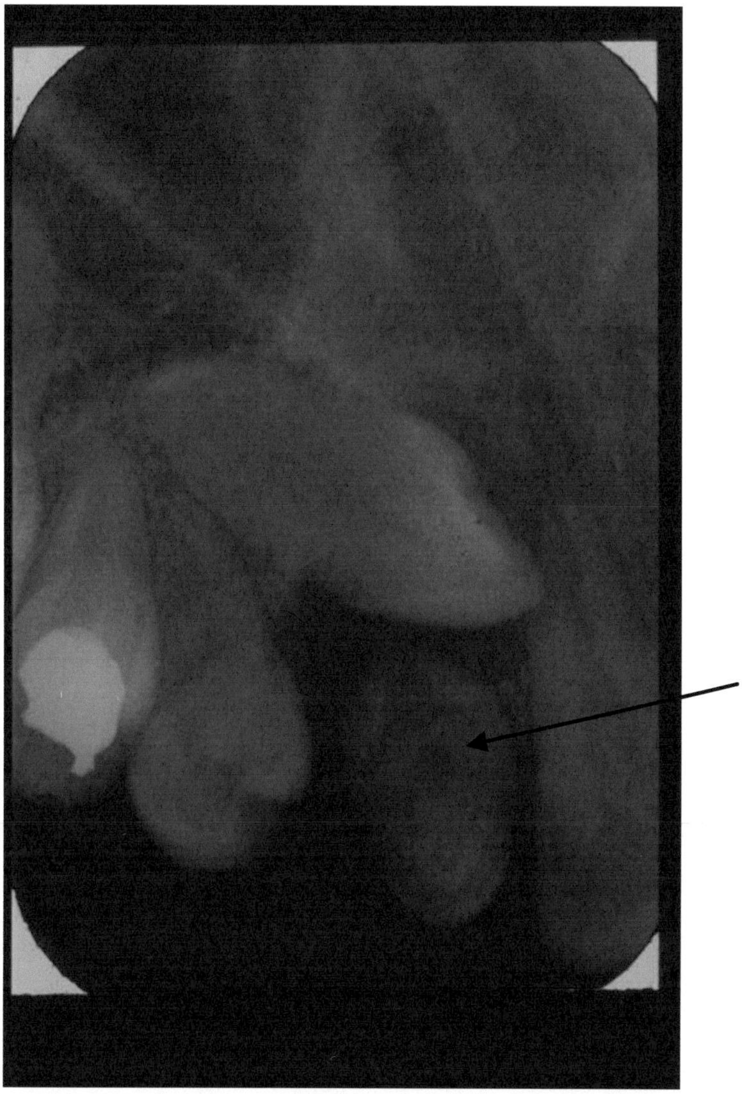

Figure 9.
Periapical radiograph showing s dens inverginatus (see arrows).

3. Rectangular pulp cavity.

4. The inter-radicular bone/furcation area is low in location.

5. Triangular inter-radicular bone.

7. What is it called?

Taurudontism.

8. What are the clinical implications of this condition?

1. Difficulty in extraction.

2. Difficulty in endodontic treatment (obvious).

9. What other implication is this condition ascribed to?

   Forensic implication.

10. What is it termed?

    Unique non-coincidental forensic finding at postmortem (**Figure 10**) [2].

1. List five differential diagnosis of the above condition.

2. What are they collectively called?

3. Use an arrow to point to a tooth tissue that will require radiological monitoring for the progression of this disease.

4. Which of these list in #1 above are developmental dental defects?

5. What do you expect to see in this tissue?

6. Do you now understand that tooth tissue loss is both a clinical and radiological diagnosis and that amelogenesis and dentinogenesis inperfecta are tooth tissue loss?

7. List five differentials diagnosis of the above condition:

   1. Attrition,

   2. Abrasion,

   3. Dentinogenesis imperfect,

   4. Amelogenesis imperfect,

   5. Erosion.

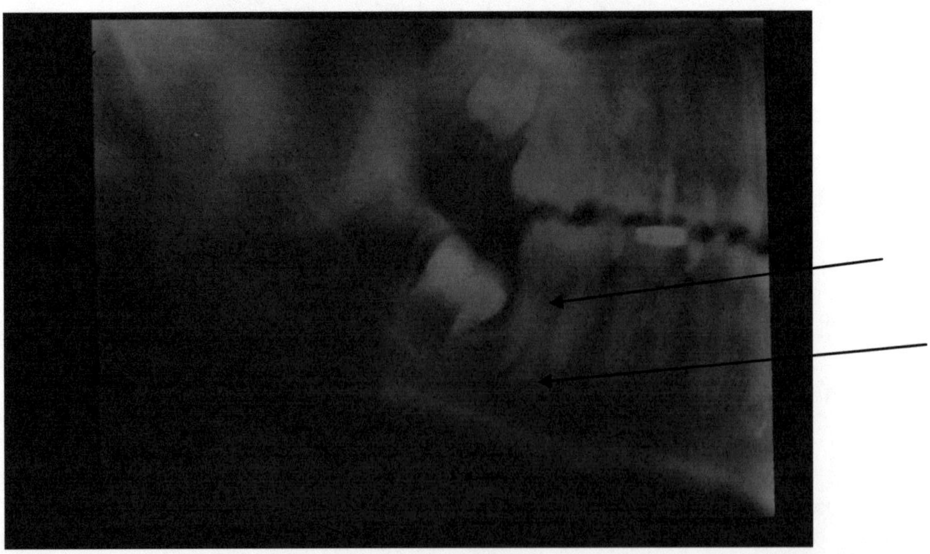

Figure 10.
Part of a DPT showing the lower second molar affected with taurodontism (see the arrow showing the enlarged and rectangular pulp chamber and low furcation involvement).

8. What are they collectively called?

   Tooth tissue loss.

9. Use an arrow to point to a tooth tissue that will require radiological monitoring for the progression of this disease

   See the three arrows pointing to the pulp.

10. Which of this list in #1 above are the developmental dental defects?

    Amelogenesis imperfecta and dentinogenesis imperfecta.

11. What do you expect to see in these teeth?

    Obliteration of pulp canal/cavity.

12. Do you now understand that tooth tissue loss is both a clinical and radiological diagnosis and that amelogenesis and dentinogenesis imperfecta are conditions with tooth tissue loss?

    Yes! (**Figure 11**) [2].

1. What is the arrow pointing at?
2. Is this tooth still developing?
3. Why do you think it is or not developing?

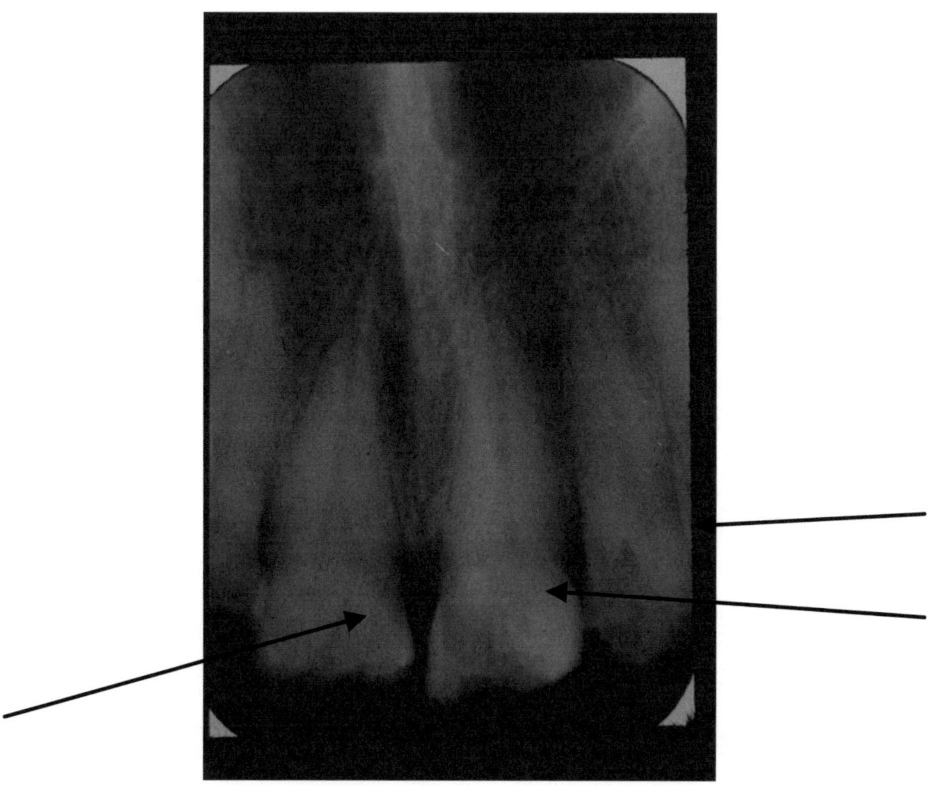

Figure 11.
Periapical radiograph showing tooth tissue loss (see arrows).

4. Point to other pathology relating to this tooth and explain it briefly.

5. What is the arrow pointing at?

   A microdont tooth (third molar).

6. Is this tooth still developing?

   Yes.

7. Why do you think it is not developing?

   The roots are not fully formed.

8. Point to other pathology relating to this tooth and explain it briefly?

   There is a pericoronal radiolucency (arrow #1), which may be the initial stage of a cystic degeneration—should a cyst form, it is likely to be a dentigerious cyst. Also, an ameloblastoma may develop around the tooth. However, because the roots are still developing, there may be some eruptive force, which may direct the tooth to occlusion (**Figure 12**) [2].

1. Point to the main anomaly in this radiograph.

2. What is it called?

3. Indicate three (3) clinical considerations of this anomaly.

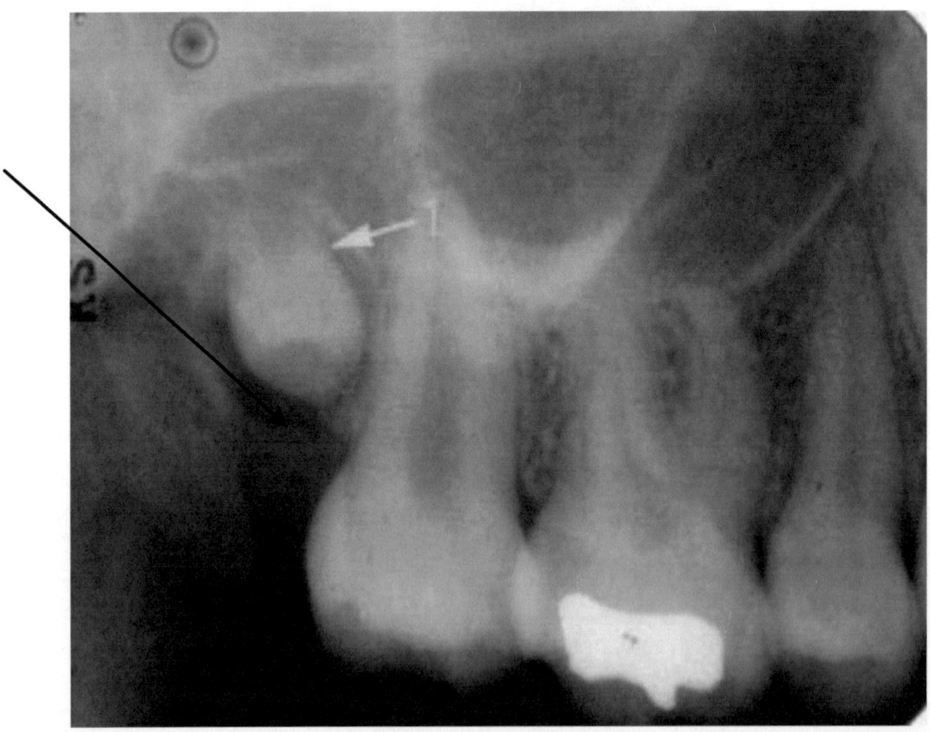

Figure 12.
Periapical radiograph showing a microdont third molar tooth. See the yellow and black arrow delineating the boundaries of the developing cyst. (see arrows).

4. Point to the main anomaly in this radiograph.

   See arrow pointing to the bent tooth.

5. What is it called?

   Dilaceration of an upper central incisor tooth.

6. Indicate three (3) clinical considerations of this anomaly:

   1. The need for a surgical extraction,

   2. Difficulty in the surgical extraction with the possibility of fracture of the apical 1/3rd of the roots,

   3. Inability to effect a root canal treatment (**Figure 13**) [2].

1. Point at the developmental dental defects.

2. What is it called?

3. Explain it.

4. What other name is this condition called?

5. Point at the developmental dental defects.

   See the two arrows.

6. What is it called?

   Regional odontodysplasia.

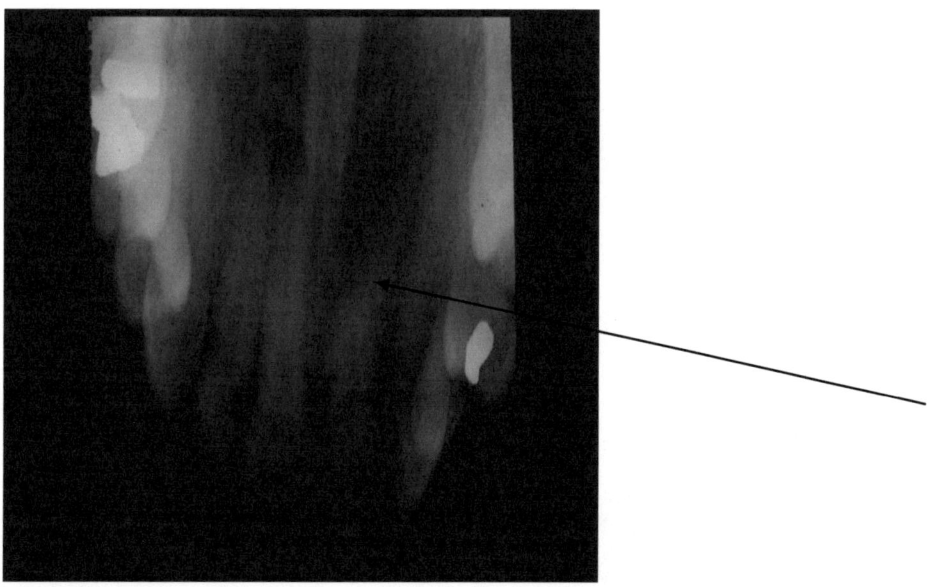

Figure 13.
Occlusal radiograph showing a dilacerated maxillary central incisor (see arrows).

7. Explain it.

   This is a very uncommon developmental dental defect that is usually localized to a quadrant of the mouth/jaw. It is a condition with no hereditary affiliations, with no race predilection, but affecting more females than males. The enamel, dentine, and pulp of the teeth are affected to the extent that the affected teeth do not develop properly. The teeth will as such appear more radiolucent than normal.

8. What other name is this condition called?

   Ghost teeth (**Figure 14**) [2].

1. Describe this radiograph.

2. What is your diagnosis?

3. What are the main reasons for making this diagnosis?

4. What are your differential diagnoses?

5. Describe this radiograph.

   A dental periapical radiograph of the anterior teeth showing malformed central and lateral incisors with enlarged pulp cavity and with severe teeth tissue loss of developmental origin. The coronal enamel is very inadequate; the dentine and pulp cavities are also poorly developed.

6. What is your diagnosis?

   Regional odontodysplasia or dentinogenesis imperfecta.

7. What are the main reasons for making this diagnosis?

   Poorly developed enamel, dentine, and pulp tissue with tooth tissue loss. The changes in the pulp cavity can be construed as obliteration of the pulp cavity.

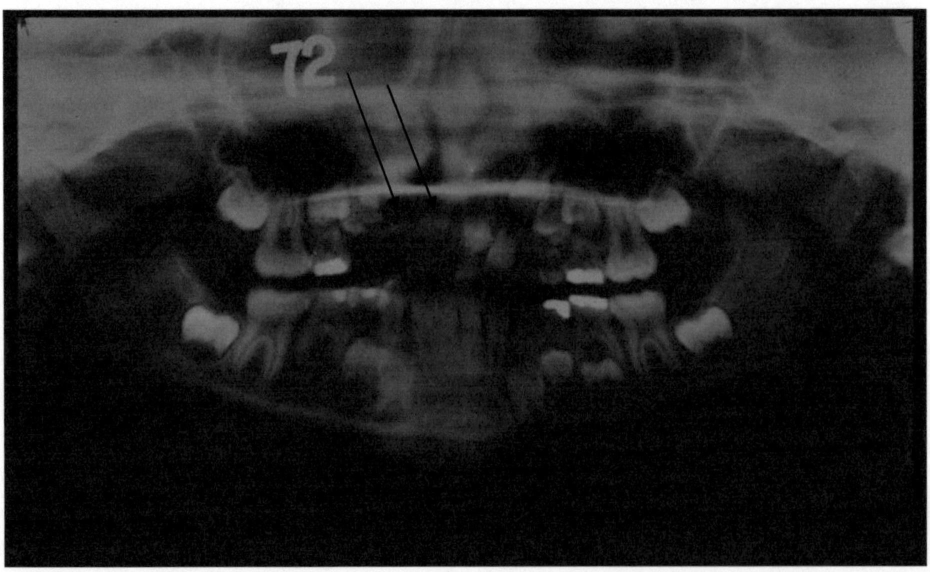

Figure 14.
DPT of a child showing ghost teeth in the anterior region of the maxilla. (See arrows).

8. What is your differential diagnosis?

    1. Non-syndrome dentine dysplasia.

    2. Osteogenesis imperfect.

    3. Dentinogenesis imperfect (**Figure 15**) [2].

1. Point at the buried tooth.

2. What is it called?

3. List the possible causes of this situation.

4. List the possible sequel of this condition.

5. Point at the buried tooth.

   See the pointing arrow.

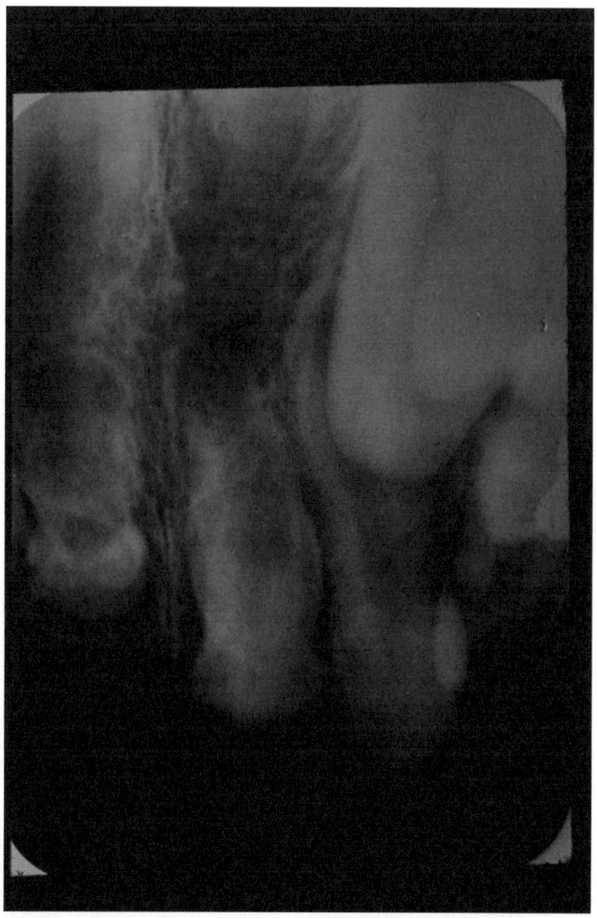

Figure 15.
Periapical radiograph showing upper central incisors with obliterated pulp cavity, tooth tissue loss as in dentinogenesis imperfecta.

6. What is it called?

   Wondering tooth.

7. List the possible causes of this situation:

   1. Infection,
   2. Loss of coronal eruptive force,
   3. Associated lesion/tumor,
   4. Congenital or hereditary.

8. List the possible sequel of this condition:

   1. Resorption of adjacent root,
   2. Bucco-lingual expansion/swelling of the mandible,
   3. Formation of dentigerous lesion,
   4. Ameloblastoma formation,
   5. Weak point in which fracture can easily occur following slight trauma (**Figure 16**) [2].

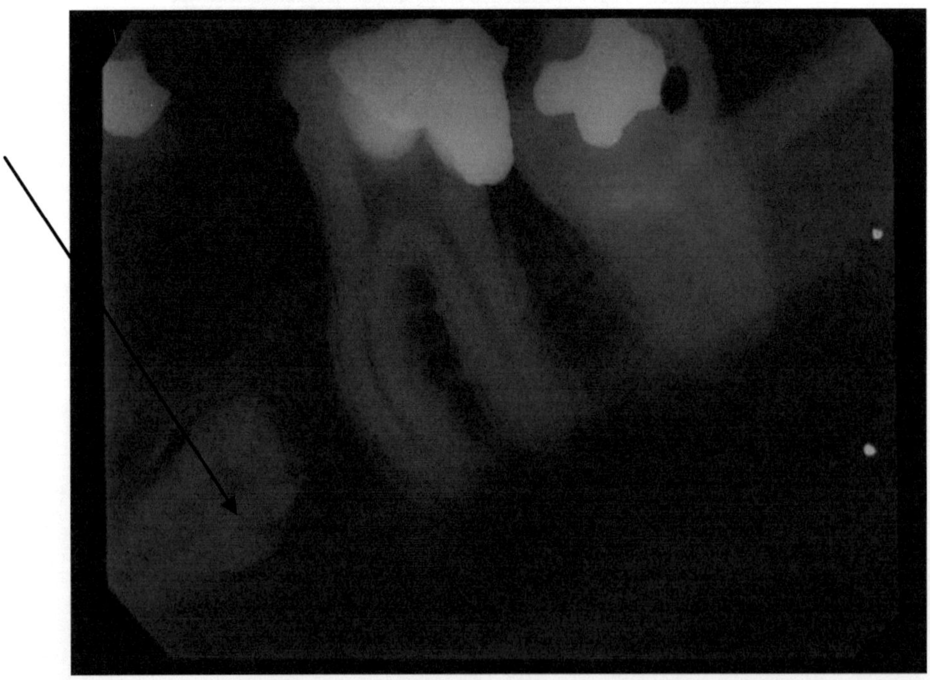

Figure 16.
Periapical radiograph showing a wondering tooth (note the beginning of cystic degeneration around the tooth).

1. Which dentition is shown in the above bitewing radiograph?
2. What is the condition of the patients teeth called?
3. How did you arrive at this diagnosis?
4. What are your differential diagnoses?
5. In this case are the permanent teeth involved?
6. Which dentition is shown in the above periapicals?

   Mixed dentition.

7. What is the condition of the patients teeth called?

   Tooth tissue loss.

8. How did you arrive at this diagnosis?

   Imperfect enamel of all the molar teeth (both primary and secondary dentitions).

9. What are your differential diagnoses?

    1. Amelogenesis imperfect,
    2. Dentinogenesis imperfect,
    3. Dentine dysplasia.

10. In this case are the permanent teeth involved?

    Yes (**Figure 17**) [2].

1. What is your diagnosis?
2. Why have you made this diagnosis?
3. What are your differential diagnosis?
4. Describe the radiograph.
5. Point arrows to all the areas affected by this DDD.
6. What is your diagnosis?

   Oligodontia.

7. Why have you made this diagnosis?

   There are six or more missing teeth.

   Look at the arrows and circles.

   The arrows points to the over-retained deciduous teeth without any permanent successor and also edentulous spaces.

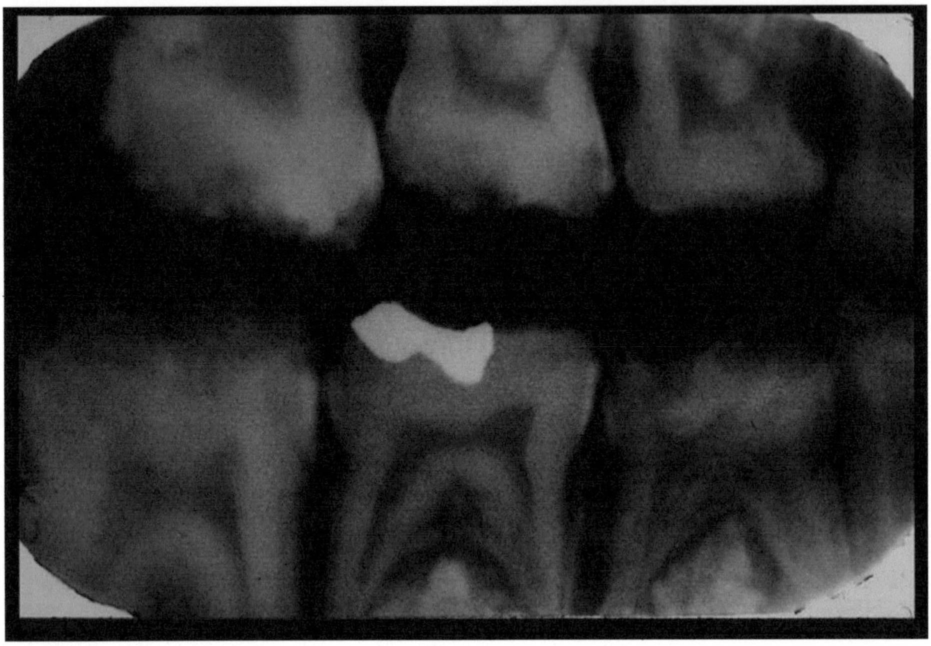

Figure 17.
Bitewing radiograph showing tooth tissue loss in both the upper and lower molar teeth (both the deciduous and permanent dentition are involved).

The circular corticated regions around the third molar attest to the developing status of the third molars, which can also be used as a mark for the determination of the age of this patient.

8. What is your differential diagnosis?

    1. Sporadic hypodontia,

    2. Hypodontia/hypodontia associated with syndrome (i.e., ectodermal dysplasia),

    3. Non-syndromal hypodontia or oligodontia.

9. Describe the radiograph.

    This is the dental panoramic tomogram of a child who is partially edentulous.

    The deciduous teeth pointed to by the arrows are over-retained with the permanent successors absent within the bone.

    The third molars are forming within the bone. Some edentulous spaces are present due to non-development of teeth. The errors in this radiograph are that of severe bowing due to the fact that the patients neck is far too in and down in the machine (**Figure 18**) [2].

1. Describe this radiograph.

2. List the most significant single diagnostic finding.

3. What is your diagnosis?

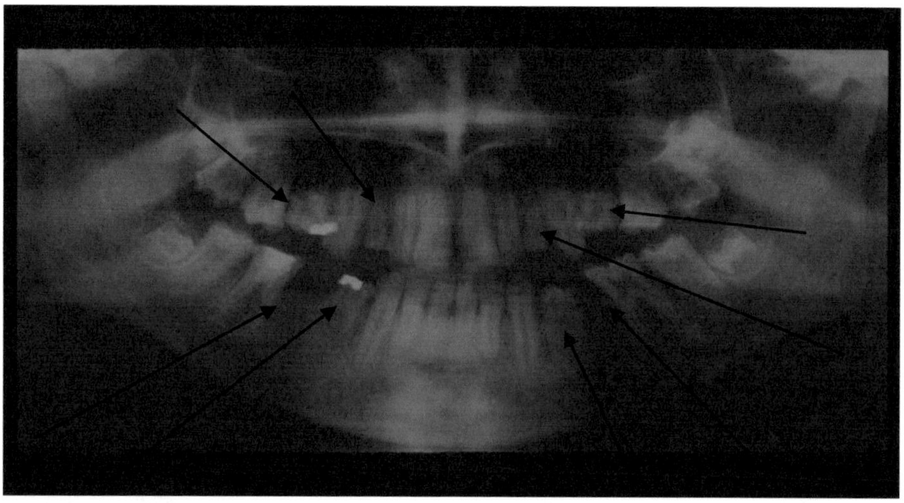

Figure 18.
DPT showing various over-retained deciduous teeth and edentulous regions (areas where no permanent teeth erupted) (see arrows).

4. Could this be related to a syndrome?

5. What is the name of the syndrome?

6. Describe this radiograph.

   The periapical radiograph shows the bulbous roots of teeth #16 and 18, with complete obliteration of the pulp cavity. The retained roots of the tooth #15 have its pulp cavity also obliterated. The edentulous space of tooth #17 is too long but has adequate amount of bone height to receive an implant. The in-standing teeth have no carious lesions or periodontal lesions.

7. List the most significant single diagnostic finding.

   Pulp obliteration.

8. What is your diagnosis?

   Dentine dysplasia or dentinogenesis imperfect.

9. Could this be related to a syndrome?

   Yes.

10. What is the name of the syndrome?

    Osteogenesis imperfecta (**Figure 19**) [2].

1. Describe this radiograph.

2. List the most significant single diagnostic finding.

3. What is your diagnosis?

4. Make a list of differential diagnosis.

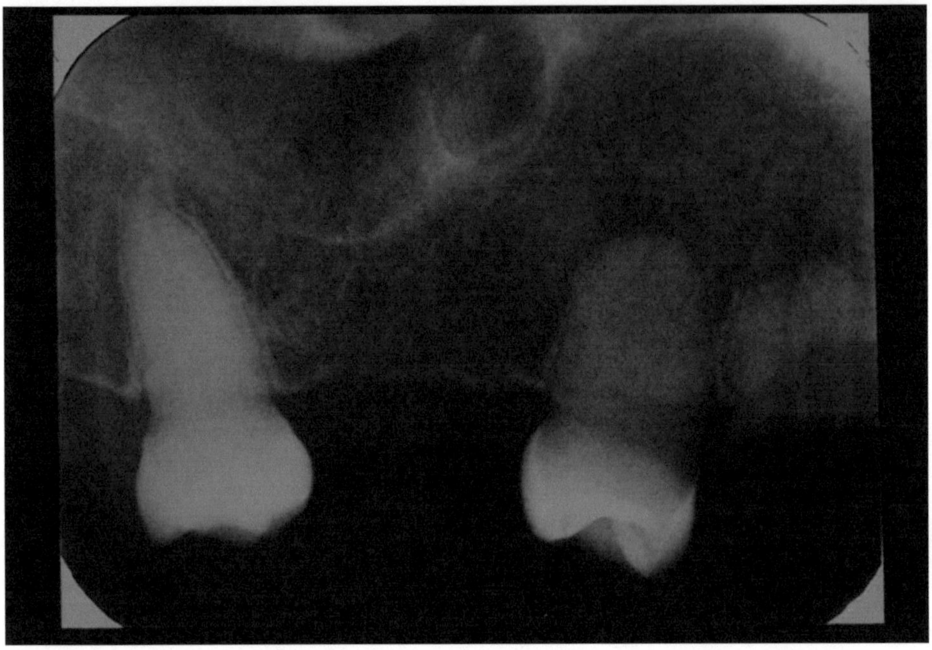

Figure 19.
Periapical radiograph showing molar teeth and retained roots with pulp obliteration.

5. Describe this radiograph.

   This dental periapical radiograph of the anterior teeth shows all the four anterior teeth to have suffered tooth tissue loss. These teeth also have complete obliteration of the pulp cavity.

6. List the most significant single diagnostic finding.

   Tooth tissue loss and complete obliteration of the pulp cavity.

7. What is your diagnosis?

   Dentinogenesis imperfecta.

8. Make a list of differential diagnosis.

   1. Amelogenesis imperfect.

   2. Dentine dysplasia.

9. What makes it not an amelogenesis imperfecta?

   Presence of pulp obliteration (**Figure 20**) [2].

1. Point to the anomalies on this periapical.

2. Describe the radiograph.

3. Point to the anomalies on this periapical

   See the short arrows pointing to the teeth tissue loss and the longer arrows pointing to the obliteration of the pulp cavities.

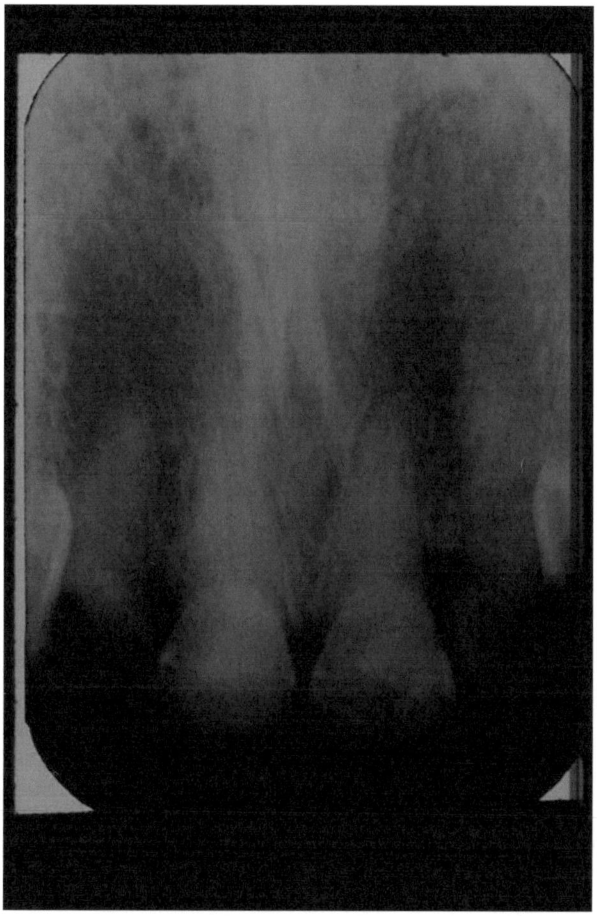

Figure 20.
Periapical radiograph showing tooth tissue loss and pulp obliteration.

4. Describe the radiograph.

   This is a periapical radiograph of the maxillary anterior teeth showing tooth tissue loss of #11, 12, 21, 22 and obliteration of the pulp cavity/canal of all the four incisors. The periodontal membrane space and periapical regions are intact (**Figure 21**) [2].

1. Utilize an arrow to point at all the developmental dental defects.

2. Describe the radiographic findings.

3. What is your diagnosis?

4. How did you arrive at this diagnosis?

5. Name one differential diagnosis.

6. Utilize an arrow to point at all the developmental dental defects.

   See all the arrows.

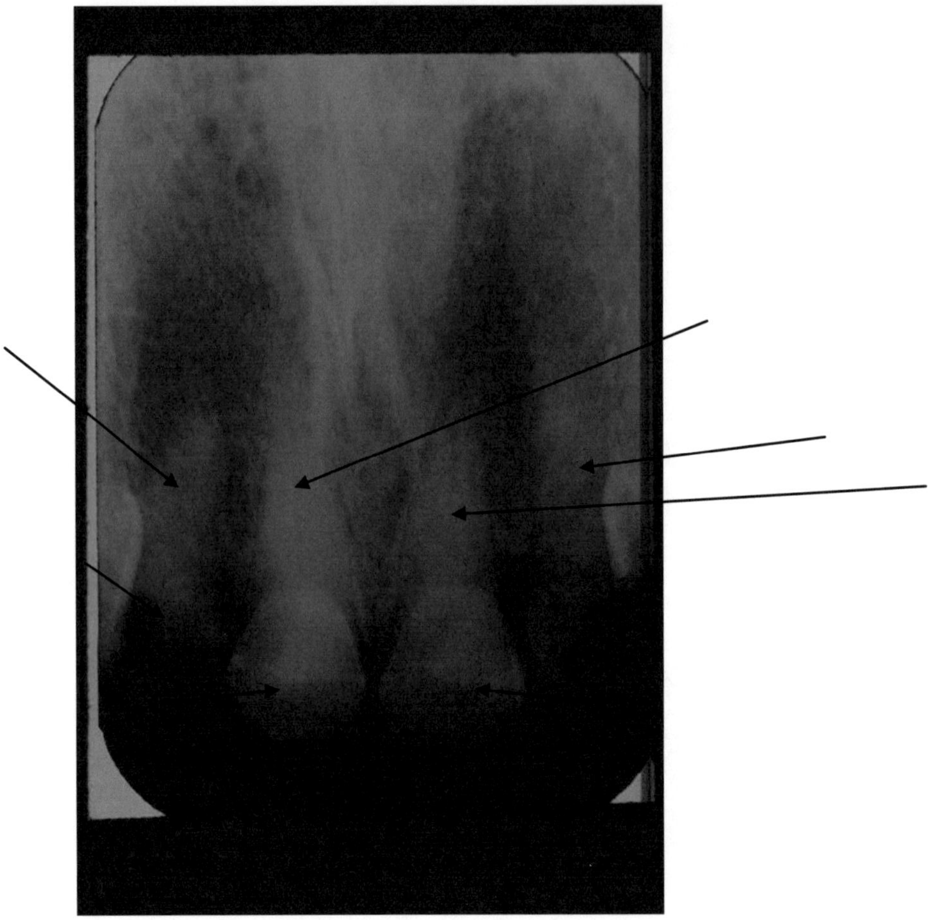

Figure 21.
Periapical radiograph showing tooth tissue loss and pulp obliteration of upper incisors.

7. Describe the radiographic findings.

   Bilaterally is a set of double horizontally impacted third molars, with evidence of pressure effect on the second molars bilaterally with resultant crowing of the anterior teeth. The main issue is that instead of 16 teeth in the mandible, there are a total of 18 teeth. The maxilla is not exempted from these findings except that the bilateral distomolar are microdont and are not putting any pressure on the second molars.

8. What is your diagnosis?

   1. Bilateral germination of the third molars with double horizontally impacted teeth on each side of the mandible.

   2. Bilateral unerupted maxillary microdont third molars.

9. How did you arrive at this diagnosis?

   By counting the number of teeth in the jaw.

10. Name two differential diagnoses.

    1. Fusion.
    2. Concrescence (that is to say, the roots of each of the double teeth could be joined) (**Figure 22**) [2].

1. List two important complications of the surgical removal of all the impacted 3rd molars in the lower jaw.
2. How can you prevent such complications from occurring?
3. List two important complications of the surgical removal of all the impacted third molars in the lower jaw:
    1. Damage to the inferior dental nerve and
    2. Fracture of the mandible (unilateral or bilateral).
4. How can you prevent such complications from occurring?
    1. By surgically fracturing the jaw and dissect out the wisdom teeth (orthognathic surgical removal) and
    2. Removal of the more occlusal third molar and leaving the deeper ones in place (**Figure 23**) [2].

1. What is the most obvious generalized anomaly?
2. List all the possible differential diagnosis based on this generalized anomaly.
3. What is the resultant effect of all these differential diagnosis?
4. If I provide you with a family history of multiple fractures of long bone and hip bones, what would your diagnosis be?
5. What is the most obvious generalized anomaly?

   Obliteration of the pulp cavity/chamber.

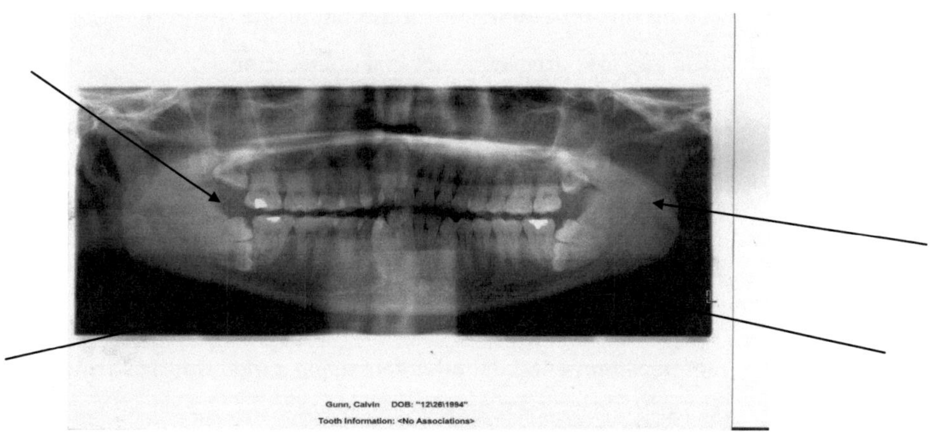

Figure 22.
DPT showing bilateral double third molar teeth, consistent with germination.

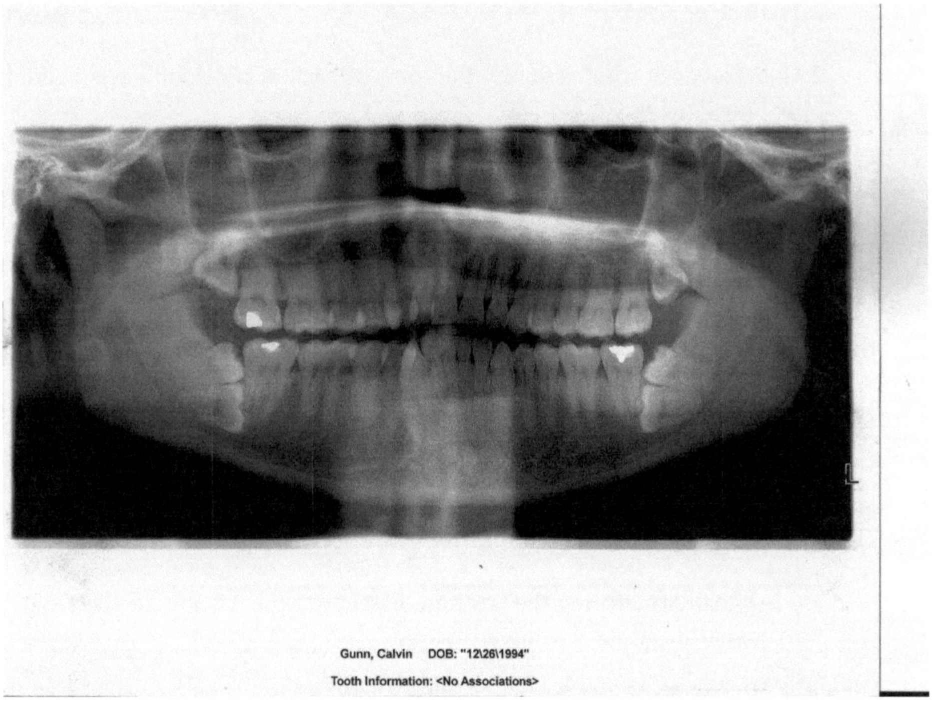

Figure 23.
DPT showing bilateral double third molar teeth, consistent with germination.

6. List all the possible differential diagnosis based on this generalized anomaly:

    1. Dentinogenesis imperfect,

    2. Dentine dysplasia,

    3. Attrition,

    4. Erosion.

7. What is the resultant effect of all these differential diagnoses?

    Tooth/teeth tissue loss and progressive pulpal obliteration.

8. If I provide you with a family history of multiple fractures of long bone and hip bones, what would your diagnosis be?

    Dentinogenesis imperfecta with or without dentine dysplasia in a patient with osteogenesis imperfecta (**Figure 24**) [3].

1. Point to one developmental dental defect using a small sized arrow.

2. Point to one non developmental dental defect using a medium size arrow.

3. What is the non-DDD called________________________

4. Give one differential diagnosis for the non DDD________________________

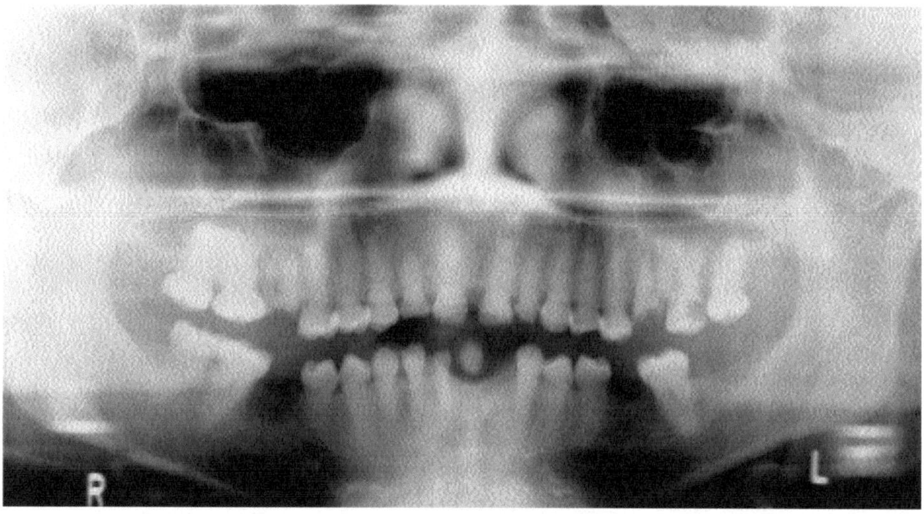

Fig. 2.–Panoramic radiograph showing complete obliteration of the pulp excepting 37 and 47.

Figure 24.
DPT showing obliteration of pulp of all the teeth, a feature consistent with dentinogenesis imperfect in this case of osteogenesis imperfecta.

5. Why is it that in this situation this differential diagnosis will not be considered further?

6. Point to one developmental dental defect using a small sized arrow.

   See arrow.

7. Point to one non-developmental dental defect using a medium sized arrow.

   See arrow.

8. What is the non-DDD called?

   Cervical abrasion.

9. Give one differential diagnosis for the non DDD.

   Cervical burnout.

10. Why in this situation this differential diagnosis will not be considered any further?

    There is no other tooth distal to the tooth affected by the cervical abrasion.

11. What are the three possible differential diagnoses for the DDD that you pointed to with the small-sized arrow?

    1. Fusion,

    2. Germination,

    3. Concrescences.

12. What are they collectively called?

    Double teeth or twinning.

13. The propositus family pedigree shown in Appendix I depicts the familial history of this DDD. On clinical examination of the index case, the number of teeth counted in the mandible is not increased. Provide one definitive diagnosis (**Figure 25**) [2–4].

Fusion.

This is a 37-year-old female. The only tooth ever removed by this patient is the upper first molar on the left side.

1. What is your diagnosis?

2. Can this diagnosis be related to a syndrome?

3. Name one such syndrome.

This is a 37-year-old female. The only tooth ever removed by this patient is the upper first molar on the left side.

1. What is your diagnosis?

   Hypodontia or ologidontia.

2. Can this diagnosis be related to a syndrome?

   Yes?

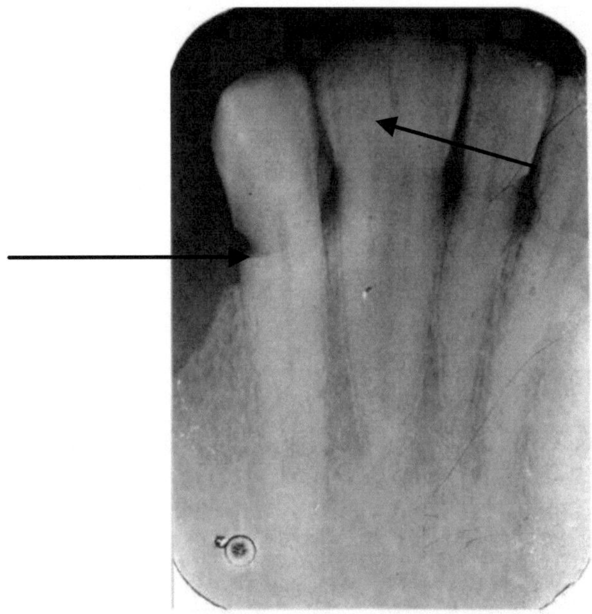

Figure 25.
Periapical radiograph showing twining of lower incisor. Also note the cervical tooth tissue loss of the distal aspect of the canine tooth due to tooth brushing abrasion. The teeth involved in the twining have been protected from the abrasion. (See arrows).

3. Name one such syndrome.

   Ectodermal dysplasia (**Figure 26**) [2–4].

Point at the developmental dental defects in the periapical radiographs shown above.

1. What are they called? ______________________________

2. What other names have they acquired? ____________________

3. In which teeth are they most commonly found?
   ____

4. Can multiple teeth be involved? __________________________

5. Give three (3) differential diagnosis
   ____

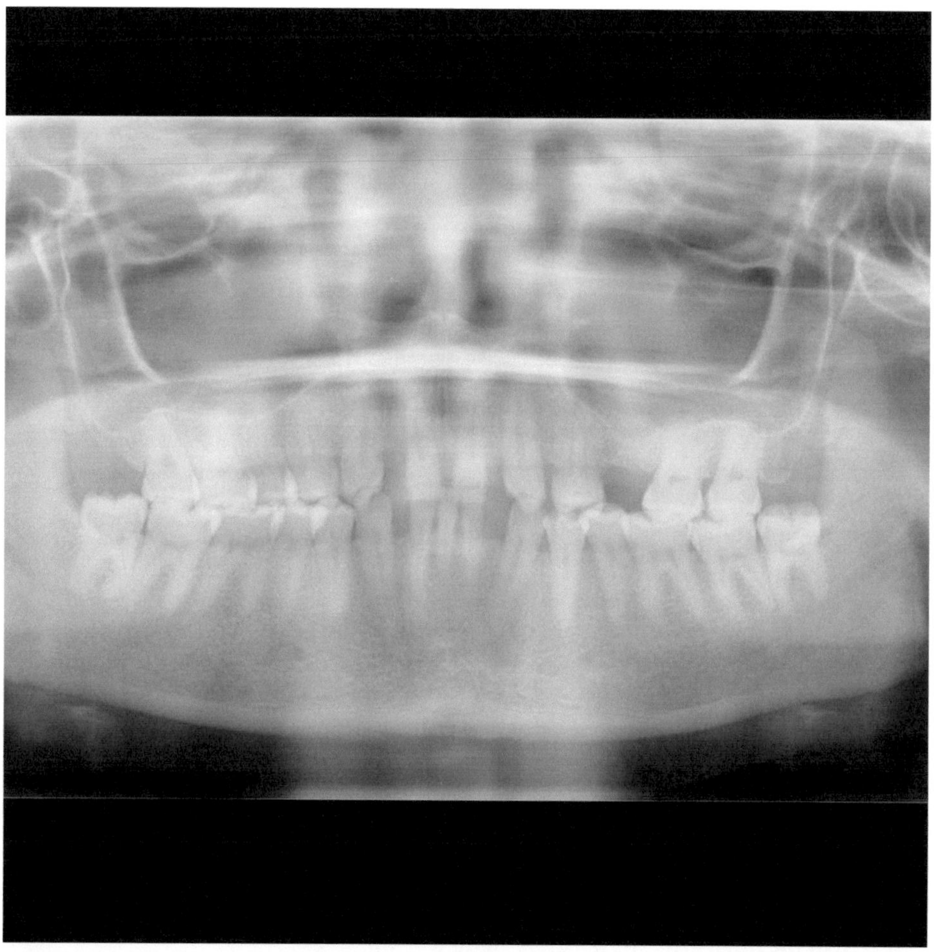

Figure 26.
DPT showing various missing permanent teeth, both in the mandible and maxilla.

6. What problems can this developmental defect pose?

   1. ____________

   2. ____________

7. Is there a role for cone beam CT imaging modalities?

8. What are they called?

   Enamel pearl or ectopic enamel.

9. What other names have they acquired?

   Enamel droplet, enamel globules, enamel nodules, etc. as stated in the introductory section of article on the subject, above.

10. In which teeth are they most commonly found?

    Maxillary and mandibular molars.

11. Can multiple teeth be involved?

    Yes?

12. Give three (3) differential diagnosis

    1. Pulp stone.

    2. Dens exverginatus.

    3. Calculus.

13. What problems can this developmental defect pose?

    1. Can lead to chronic localized or generalized periodontitis,

    2. Can obscure a furcation involvement.

14. Is there a role for cone beam CT Imaging modalities?

    Yes, a confirmatory role.

    Point at the developmental dental defects in the periapical radiographs shown above (**Figure 27**).

1. Make a diagnosis based on this radiograph.

2. Which other names that also constitutes differential diagnosis can you give this condition?

3. What is the clinical significance of this developmental dental defect?

4. What advantage does it have and why is it so?

5. Make a diagnosis based on this radiograph.

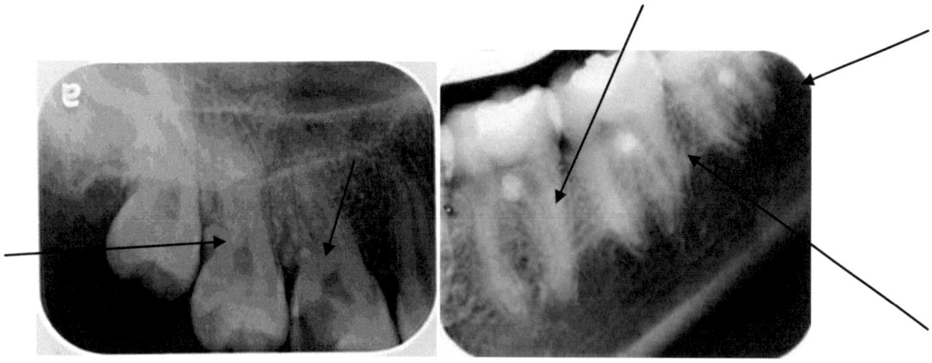

Figure 27.
Periapical radiograph showing multiple enamel pearls (these can be easily misdiagnosed on radiograph as pulp stones. (See arrows).

Concrescence, because the roots appears to be joined, the entire resultant tooth structure is big and the structure has two distinct pulp separated by a tooth tissue with the radiodensity of the dentine.

6. Which other names that also constitutes differential diagnosis can you give this condition?

    1. Fusion,

    2. Germination,

    3. Double teeth,

    4. Twinning.

    In actual fact, double teeth and twinning can be used to express fusion, germination, and concrescence.

7. What is the clinical significance of this developmental dental defect?

    1. Difficulty in confirmatory diagnosis until extraction or CBCT is done.

    2. Difficulty in extraction.

    3. Difficulty in effecting a root canal treatment.

    4. Unnecessary spacing of the teeth.

    5. Likely oro-antral communication following non-surgical extraction.

8. What advantage does it have and why is it so?

    Because it is extremely rare in occurrence and its presentation is very unique, it has a positive role in identification of the deceased, thus giving it a forensic significance and use. It is as such called a *Unique, non coincidental forensic finding* in the antemortem and postmortem correlations and evaluation (**Figure 28**) [2–4].

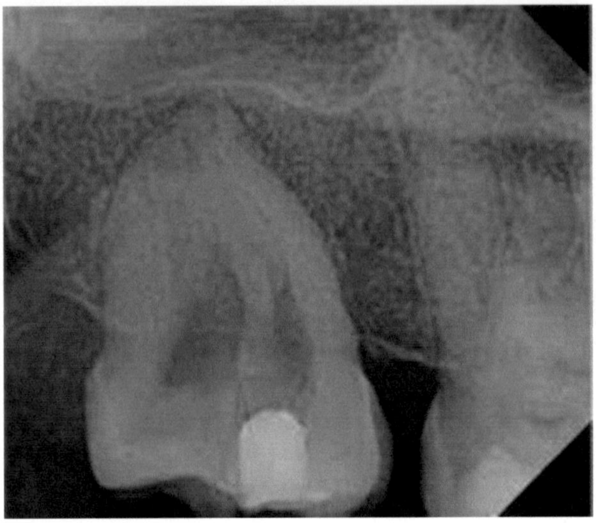

Figure 28.
Periapical radiograph showing concrescence of the maxillary molars (see arrows).

1. Utilize a blue arrow to point at the main developmental dental defect.

2. Utilize a red arrow to point at the third molar.

3. Utilize a green arrow to point at the second molar.

4. Utilize a brown arrow to point at the distomolar.

5. Use these three arrows to deduce an etiology for this condition (at least in this case).

6. Is your deduced etiology consistent with the literature?

7. Utilize a blue arrow to point at the main developmental dental defect.

   Proceed with the blue arrow to point at the main developmental dental defect.

8. Utilize a red arrow to point at the third molar.

   Proceed with the red arrow to point at the third molar.

9. Utilize a green arrow to point at the second molar.

   Proceed with the green arrow to point at the second molar.

10. Utilize a brown arrow to point at the distomolar.

    Proceed with the brown arrow to point at the distomolar.

11. Use these four arrows to deduce an etiology for this condition (at least in this case).

    The mesial root of the second molar seems to be fused with the distal roots of the first molar with an obscured root canal of the joined roots. Since a developing third molar is present and a distomolar is present, a diagnosis of concrescence of the first and second molar teeth can be made.

Diagnosis: Concrescences of the first and second molars. It could, however, be fusion, but it is not germination.

12. Is your deduced etiology consistent with the literature?

    Yes (**Figure 29**) [2–4].

1. This patient has never had a tooth removed before. Point at the DDD.

2. Utilize this radiograph to discuss the diagnosis and clinical significance of the main radiographic feature.

3. Discussion of the diagnosis and clinical significance of the main radiographic feature.

   The main radiographic finding is a larger than normal lower incisor, which has a coronal pit (upper arrow) to simulate two crowns joined together (bifid crown); however, the tooth has one root, which is larger than that of the other incisors (see the lower arrow). The pulp cavity of this large tooth is also larger than the other pulp (see the middle arrow). A count of the teeth shows only the normal number (four incisors). Since this patient has never removed a tooth before, it is reasonable to say that the central and lateral incisors on the left side have fused together during dentinogenesis.

   Diagnosis: Fusion of the central and lateral incisors on the left side of the lower jaw.

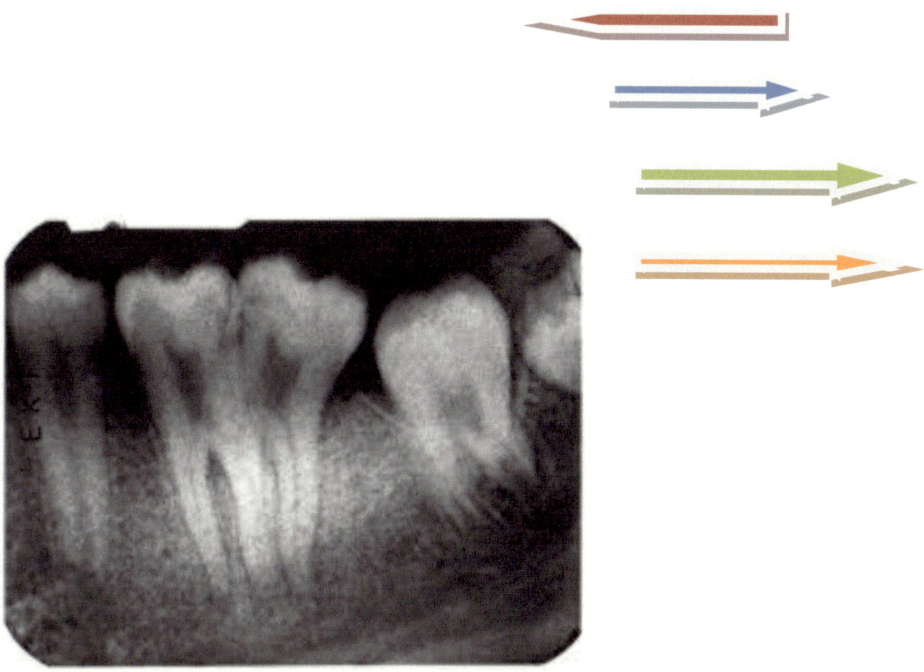

Figure 29.
Periapical radiograph showing germination of the first molar with possible concrescence of the germinated teeth. (See arrows).

Differential diagnosis:

1. Germination,

2. Concrescence (**Figure 30**) [2–4].

1. Describe both the radiographic findings in A and B above.

2. What is your diagnosis?

3. What is the main difference in the two cases?

4. Advice the dentist on the treatment or management.

5. Describe both the radiographic findings in A and B above.

   A and B are periapical radiographs of the upper anterior teeth. Very obvious is the presence of a miniature tooth or tooth-like structure, erupting in the opposite direction (i.e., inverted).

6. What is your diagnosis?

   Inverted mesiodens.

7. What is the main difference in the two cases?

   The mesiodens in B is not only creating pressure effect on the roots of one of the upper centrals, but it is also responsible for the rotation of one of the developing lateral incisors and it is responsible for the creation of the diastema seen.

8. Advice the dentist on the treatment or management.

   Both mesiodens must be removed surgically by raising a flap and skillfully drilling out the surrounding bone before elevation so as not to damage the

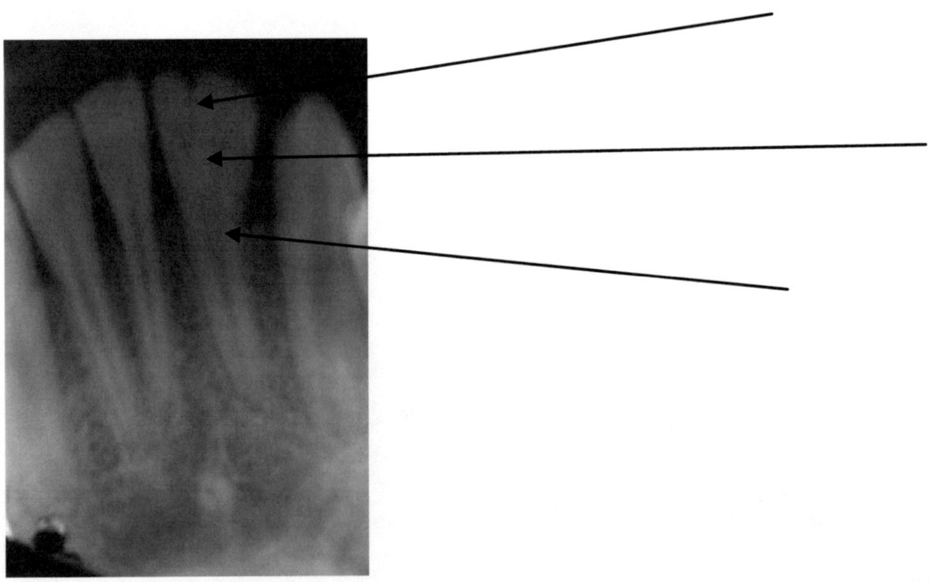

Figure 30.
Periapical radiograph showing double teeth which is consistent with fusion of the lower central and lateral incisors.

roots and crowns of the central incisors. Additionally, the situation in B may warrant endodontic treatment of upper central incisor on the right and also orthodontic treatment to correct anterior crowding and the elimination of the diastema (**Figure 31**).

1. Utilize the three radiographs to arrive at just one diagnosis
____

2. List the radiographic findings that have made you arrive at this diagnosis.

3. What type of developmental dental defect is this? ____________________

4. Point at all the anomalies using multicolored arrows.

5. Utilize the three radiographs to arrive at just one diagnosis.

   This patient has cleiodocranial dysostosis.

6. List the radiographic findings that have made you arrive at this diagnosis.

   1. Extremely short/almost absent clavicle (hypoplasia or aplasia of the clavicle).

   2. Bossing of the forehead (the head actually looks big because of frontal and parietal bossing).

   3. Multiple unerupted supernumerary teeth.

   4. Premature fusion of the coronal suture (brachycephaly).

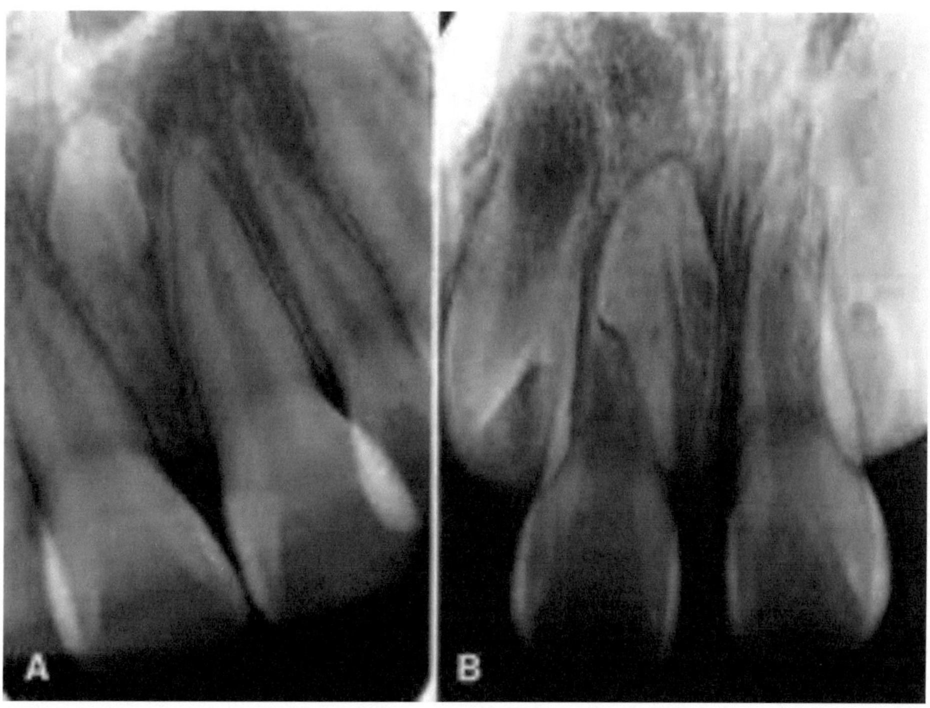

Figure 31.
Periapical radiographs showing inverted mesiodens of the upper jaw.

7. What type of developmental dental defect is this

   Syndrome-associated DDD (**Figure 32**) [2].

The clinical picture above is that of a 27-year old radiographer who presented for the surgical removal of the impacted third molars and also all the four parapremolars (supernumerary teeth) shown.

1. Utilize an arrow to point at the problem already caused by the presence of the parapremolars.

2. Would you consider any form of radiography____________?

3. List the possible radiographic investigations to be done.

   1.____________

   2.____________

   3.____________

4. Utilize an arrow to point at the problem already caused by the presence of the parapremolars.

   See arrow pointing at the carious lesion on the first premolar on the right side.

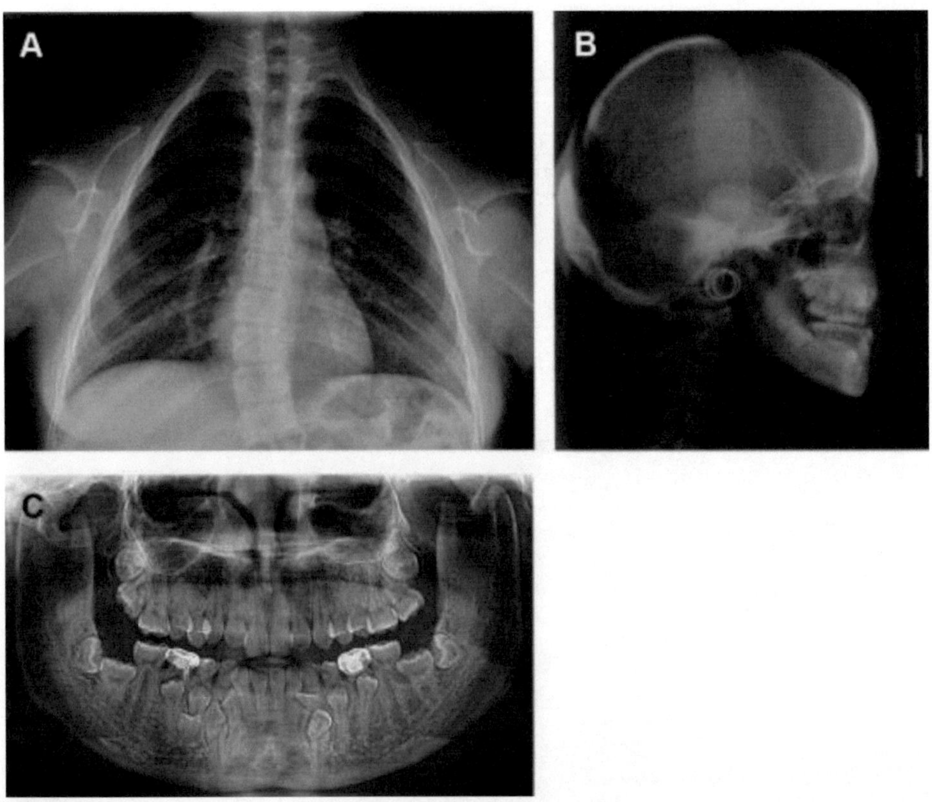

Figure 32.
Chest radiograph, lateral skull view radiograph and DPT showing, absence of clavicle, bossing of the cranial bones and multiple unerupted supernumerary teeth respectively in a patient with cleodocranial dysostosis.

5. Would you consider any form of radiography?

   Yes.

6. List the possible radiographic investigations to be done:

   1. Panoramic radiography,

   2. Periapical imaging,

   3. Bite wing imaging,

   4. Cone beam CT [2–4].

1. Focusing only on the bilateral premolar regions, identify the parapremolars on the radiographs or any other radiographic changes that may bring about a suspicion of something abnormal.

2. Focusing only on the bilateral premolar regions, identify the parapremolars seen clinically on the radiographs or any other radiographic changes that may bring about a suspicion of something abnormal.

   There are no parapremolars seen on this radiograph.

   The following are a list of radiographic changes of suspicion:

   1. Loss of the radiolucency of the mental foramen.

   2. Increased uniformed radiopacification of the crowns of all the presumed normal premolars when compared with all the other teeth in the jaw, without the presence of a radiopaque restoration.

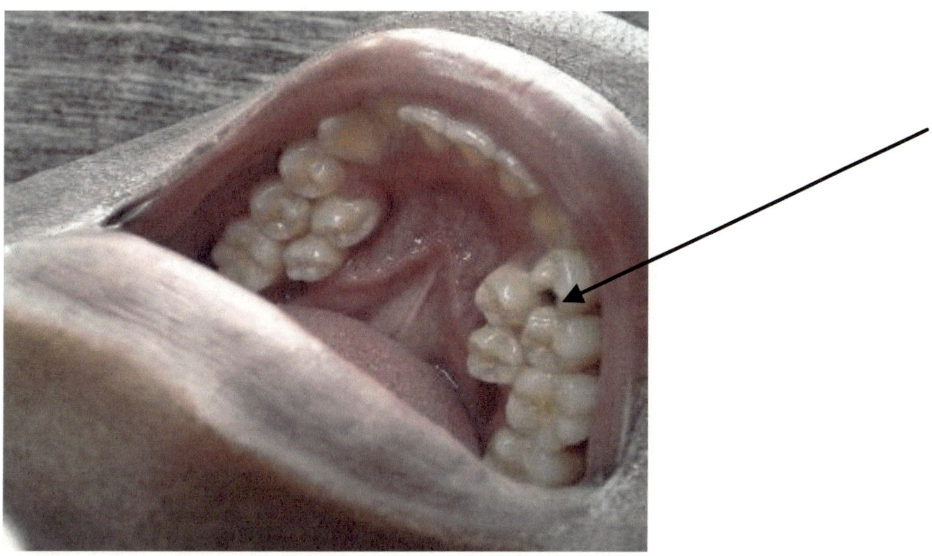

Figure 33.
The clinical picture of a patient showing bilateral doubling of the first and second premolar which is not unlike germination.

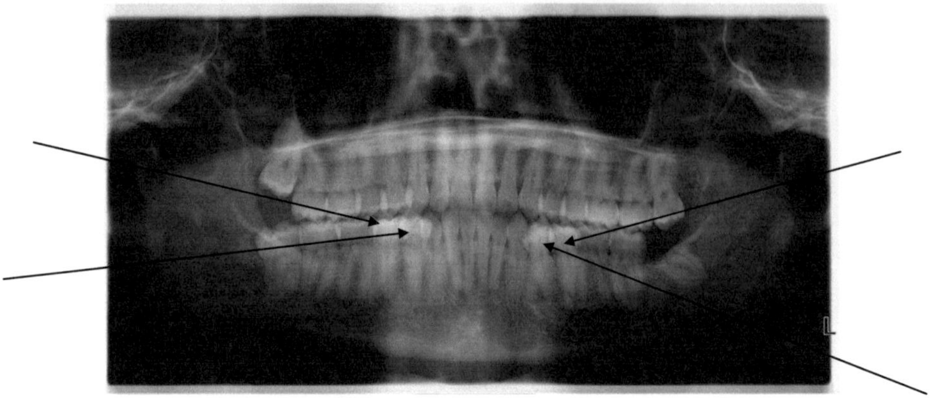

Figure 34.
*DPT of a the patient shown in **Figure 33** above, showing increased radiopacification of the first and second premolar bilaterally as the only radiographic finding to justify the clinical presentation shown in **Figure 33**.*

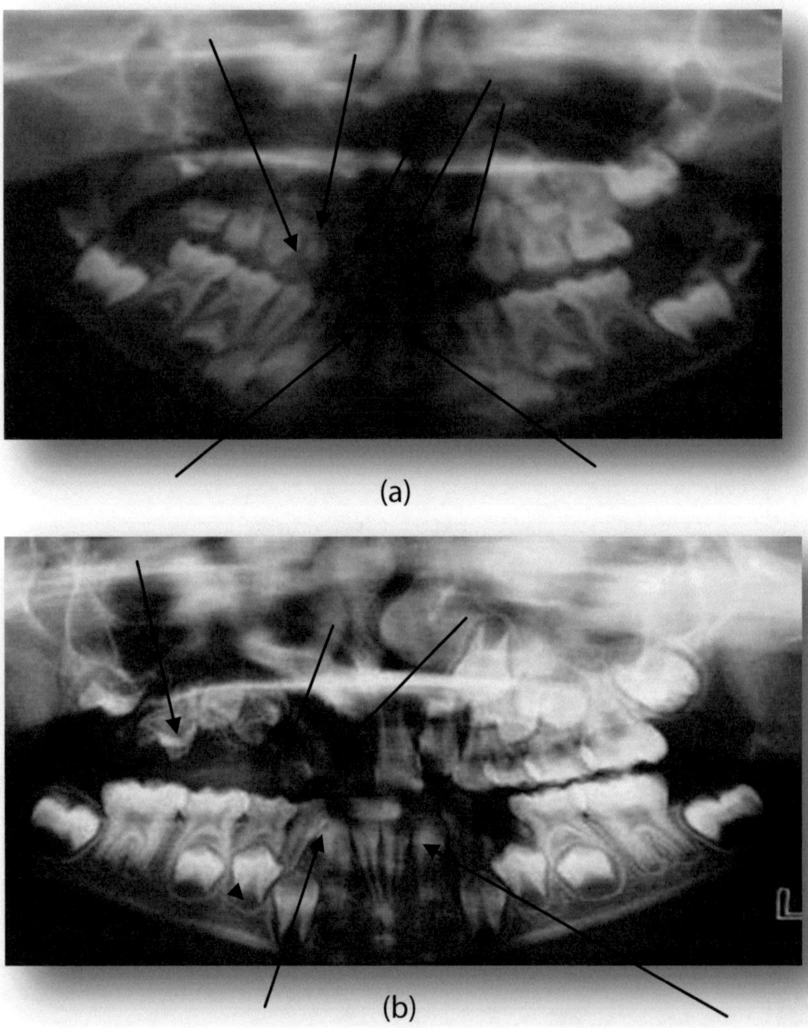

Figure 35.
DPT of a patient with regional odontodysplasia (both DPT'S)

3. The absence of the large carious lesion seen clinically on the first premolar on right side on the radiograph (**Figure 34**) [2–4].

This condition is exceedingly rare in occurrence (**Figure 35a** and **b**). It is a DDD which has no hereditary attribute. There is no sex predilection, but females seem to be more affected by regional odontoplasia. The literature is replete of the clinical, radiological and histological information on regional odontoplasia [5].

Now, read the article below and utilize the information obtained to present a power point presentation on the following: The Investigation of Regional Odontoplasia against the background of the following:

1. Accurate diagnosis of regional odontoplasia.

2. Long-term management and follow-up.

3. Reason for histopathology [1].

3. Conclusion

This book chapter is very significant for the learning of the radiology of developmental dental defects with an aim of demystifying the topic without the need of a lecturer or tutor. By extension, the various areas of the write-up have touched on the use of the radiograph in not only diagnosing the case, but also to understand the basis for the management.

Without much deliberation, this is the way radiology of any topic should be taught and disseminated in online teaching, especially amidst the sudden changes in the modalities of teaching that has been introduced as a result of COVID-19 pandemic. In rounding up let us look at the diverse developmental dental defect that the case in **Figure 36** is depicting.

The dental panoramic tomogram shown in radiographic **Figure 36** is showing a fourth molar (which is a duplication of the third molar), this is not a distomolar. The only possible explanation is that this has occurred as a result of *Germination* of the third molars. What I am trying to emphasis is that despite the fact that this duplication has resulted in the fourth molar tooth on each side, the pathogenesis is actually different from the fourth molar that developed and ascribed as a distomolar!

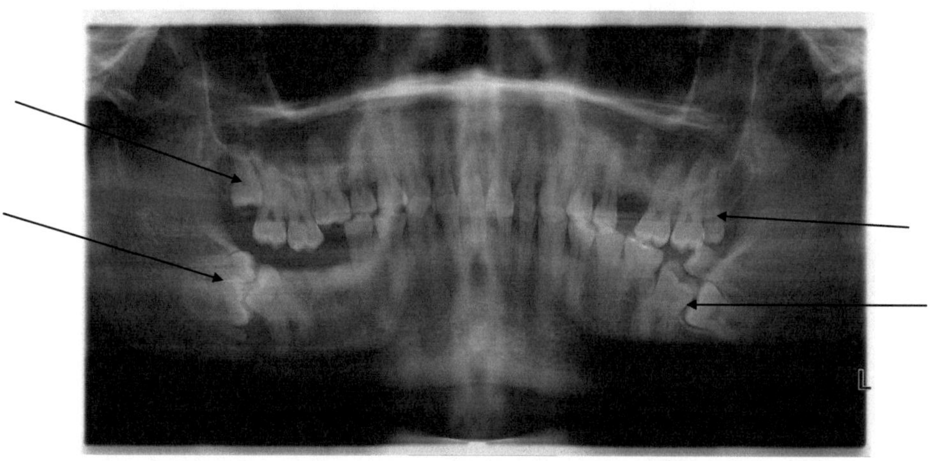

Figure 36.
DPT of a patient showing multiple germination of molar teeth in all the four quadrants of the jaw.

The questions to be asked at this stage are as follows:

1. Why the sizes of each of the fourth molar are smaller than the third molar (that is to say why are the germinated teeth of different sizes)?

2. Why are the fourth molars in the maxilla in different state of eruption from each other and even smaller than the fourth molars in the mandible?

3. Can we make a diagnosis of concrescences with the relationship seen for teeth #28 and 48 and its fourth molar.

4. However, for a postgraduate student to pass and for a distinction undergraduate student we will expect the following diagnosis:

    a. Germination of all the third molars leading to multiple impacted double molars.

    b. Dilaceration of the roots of #47, mesial root.

    c. Concrescence of #28 and 48 and its fourth molar (possible concrescence).

In conclusion, radiology is the key to the diagnosis of most dental defects. It also has a role to play in the suggestion of the etiology and most definitely in the *eventual management* of the particular defect.

A. Appendix

A.1. Appendix I

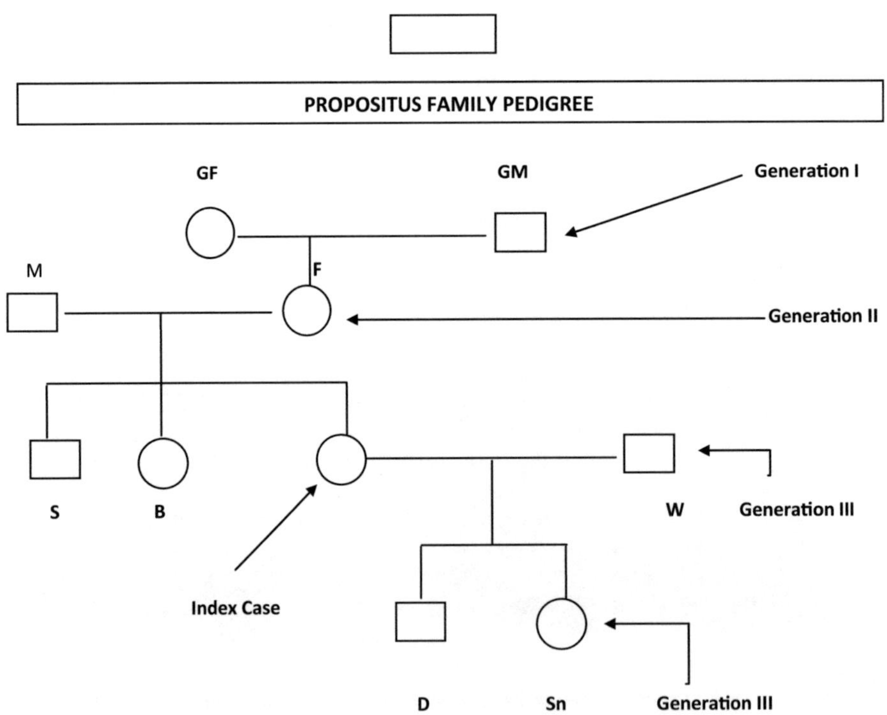

A.1.1. Key

GF: Grandfather
GM: Grandmother
M: Mother
F: Father
S: Sister
B: Brother
W: Wife
D: Daughter
Sn: Son

A.2. Appendix II

Power Point on Regional Odontoplasia: In your power point you must include the * on your first slide and the ** on your last slide.

*Name_______________________________.
*Position_____________________________.
*Institution___________________________.
*Qualifications________________________.
**Audience___________________________.
**Number of people in the audience___________________________.

Author details

Christopher Olubode Ogunsalu[1,2]

1 Faculty of Medical Sciences, Department of Basic Medical Sciences, University of the West Indies, Mona, Jamaica

2 International Postgraduate Medical College, St. James, Jamaica

*Address all correspondence to: chrisogun@yahoo.com

References

[1] Jahanimoghadam F, Pishbin L, Rad M. Clinical, radiographic, and histologic evaluation of regional odontodysplasia: A case report with 5-year follow-up. Journal of Dentistry. 2016;**17**(2):159-163

[2] Whaites E, Drage N. Essentials of Dental Radiography and Radiology. 5th ed

[3] Puri P, Sukia SK, Haque I. Developmental dental anomalies and potential role in establishing identity in postmortem cases: A review. The Medico-Legal Journal. 2019;**87**(1):13-18

[4] Seow WK. Developmental defects of the enamel and dentine: Challenges for basic sciences research and clinical management. Australian Dental Journal. 2014;**59**(Suppl. 1):143-154

[5] Ogunsalu C, Hanchard B. Familial tarda type osteogenesis imperfect with dentinogenesis imperfect type 1. Case report. Australian Dental Journal. 1997; **42**(3):175-177

Chapter 3

Gender-Associated Oral and Periodontal Health Based on Retrospective Panoramic Radiographic Analysis of Alveolar Bone Loss

Ashish Jain, Neeta V. Bhavsar, Amrit Baweja, Aman Bhagat, Anchal Ohri and Vishakha Grover

Abstract

Gender-based heterogeneity in periodontal disease has been witnessed in the recent past with huge mounting evidence. The composite effect of sex-based genetic structure and the sex steroid hormones runs in line with the corresponding gender-related differences in risk for chronic periodontitis. Since estrogens, the predominant sex hormones in women, show immune protective and anti-inflammatory effects in hormonally active premenopausal women, they show better periodontal status compared to age-matched men. Conversely, after menopause with a weakening estrogen signal, women may show an equal or even more serious periodontal status compared to men. Periodontal status of postmenopausal women may be improved by menopausal hormone therapy. Alveolar bone loss, an irreversible sign of past periodontal disease activity can be easily observed on radiographs in an objective manner. Orthopantomographs provide a fairly accurate assessment of the status of alveolar bone in the whole mouth. A cross-sectional retrospective panoramic radiographic analysis has been carried out in a north Indian dental institute to decipher the gender-based distribution of periodontal bone loss. The current chapter shall provide an update on gender-based differences in oral health, underlying mechanisms, differences in patterns and distribution of alveolar bone loss (case study), and potential gender-specific disease protection and management strategies.

Keywords: oral health, periodontal, gender, alveolar bone loss, radiography, panoramic

1. Introduction

Many human diseases, specifically chronic immune-mediated diseases, present differentially in males and females [1]. Differential gene expression and immune system in the human body guided by sex steroid hormones are responsible for the differential physiologic constitution of the two genders [2]. Chronic periodontal disease is an immune-inflammatory disorder affecting teeth and supporting tissues, inducing the destruction of alveolar bone, and ultimately leading to loss of teeth if it remains untreated. As evidence of periodontal infection's influence on overall chronic inflammatory disease states of human body continues to mount from last two decades, a whole new concept of the status of the oral cavity and its impact on systemic health and disease has evolved. Immense research efforts have been directed toward better understanding of the prevention and control of human periodontal diseases that have been warranted in the recent past [3].

Enhanced understanding regarding the causation mechanisms of human periodontal disease in the recent past and the identification and recognition of the potential significant susceptibility factors, which are a part of the causal chain for initiation and progression of periodontal disease, have led to focused research into specific risk factors for periodontal disease. Greater age [4–8], male sex [9, 10], bacterial plaque [4, 8], and smoking [8, 11–13] have been linked with an increased susceptibility to periodontal disease [14].

Epidemiological investigations have explored the role of these risk factors for periodontal disease causation and treatment needs of populations. A risk factor may be anything like environmental exposure, a behavioral aspect, or a constitutional feature which may enhance the chances of occurrence of disease. The term "determinant" is generally used interchangeably with risk factors, but it is more appropriate to limit its usage for the risk factors that cannot be modified, for example, age and sex. Readers are referred to go through many elaborate and exhaustive reviews on these particular aspects to enhance their understanding regarding differential risk and risk factors of periodontal diseases [15]. The current chapter shall provide an update specifically on gender-based differences in oral and periodontal health, underlying mechanisms, differences in patterns and distribution of alveolar bone loss (based on the case study), and potential gender-specific disease protection and management strategies.

2. Periodontal disease

Periodontal diseases primarily comprise the two most common oral inflammatory disorders, that is, gingivitis and periodontitis, which are caused by microbes residing in the subgingival dental plaque. To name a few, primary pathogens like *Porphyromonas gingivalis*, *Aggregatibacter actinomycetemcomitans*, *Tannerella forsythia*, and *Treponema denticola* trigger an immune reaction from the host, including innate, inflammatory, and adaptive components causing major part of the tissue destruction indirectly. Direct damage from the microbial products constitutes a minor part of the total tissue loss [16, 17]. Gingivitis is an inflammation of the gingiva, limited to soft-tissue compartment of the gingival epithelium and connective tissue only and the tooth does not suffer an attachment loss [18]. Periodontitis, on the other hand, is an inflammation of the supporting tissues of the teeth with progressive attachment loss and bone destruction [19, 20].

Many investigations have been conducted in diverse areas worldwide. A variable, yet significant prevalence of the periodontal disease has been noted, which amounts to an enormous disease burden in the domain of public health. The National Institute of Dental and Craniofacial Research refer to periodontal diseases as the leading cause of tooth loss in adults [21]. In 2013, Marcenes et al. ranked periodontitis as the sixth most prevalent condition while estimating the global burden of oral conditions from 1990 to 2010 [22]. Moreover, severe periodontitis is considered as the primary cause of disability-adjusted life years (DALYs) s in the age-group of 35- to 59-year-old. Several studies have reported the prevalence of periodontitis in the United States [23, 24]. The overall prevalence of periodontitis was 66% for all seniors 65 years of age or older with males being predominantly affected [25].

Prevalence of the periodontal disease varies in different regions of the world and a higher prevalence and severity of periodontal disease in Asian countries has been reported [26]. The authors looked into the geographic and economic risk factors, oral health distribution and practices in these vast groups of countries to enhance understanding regarding the oral health care needs and formulating health policy decisions [27]. A study from Pakistan revealed that 63.5% of the subjects had Community periodontal index score ≤ 2 while 34.5% had ≥3. Age, gender, occupation, smoking, diabetes, arthritis, cardiovascular disease, kidney disease, stress, medications, and oral hygiene habits of using tooth powder or tooth brushing were significantly associated with periodontal status [28]. Multiple studies to understand the occurrence, prevalence, and all associated factors have been carried out in many states and across the country in India also [29–34]. A systematic review pointed out that due to lack of homogeneous studies, it is difficult to estimate an overall prevalence rate. A nationwide multicentric prevalence studies initiative is needed to obtain the true prevalence rate of periodontal disease in India so that interventions should be provided for the same to maintain the oral health and quality of life of the affected population [29–34].

2.1 Clinical features of periodontitis

Generally speaking, periodontal disease is a chronic silent disease, which barely has any symptoms at an early stage. Most patients suffering from chronic periodontal disease seek treatment very late by the time the disease has progressed significantly. Redness or bleeding of gums with or without tooth brushing or flossing or biting into hard food, repeat episodes of gingival inflammation, oral malodor or bad breath, and a persistent metallic taste in the mouth. In progressed disease, gingival recession, resulting in loss of gums exposing the roots of teeth, deep pockets between the teeth and the gums mobile teeth, in the later stages, drifting and flaring of incisors, increased spacing between the teeth, tendency to dig between the teeth, packing of food in between teeth, itchy gums, sensitivity to hot and cold foods. Periodontal disease is generally regarded as painless. Patients generally consider only bleeding without pain from gums with or without brushing as an insignificant sign; however, this may be indicative of ongoing disease activity and progression of chronic periodontitis. Poor oral hygiene, soft sticky deposits, that is, dental plaque and hard mineralized subgingival as well as supragingival calculus are frequent findings of periodontal disease [35].

2.2 Periodontal pathogenesis

Periodontitis is a chronic multifactorial disease causing inflammation of the supporting tissues of teeth mediated by the host, which is associated with an imbalance in the existing microbial flora in dental plaque and resulting in a continuous loss of tooth-supporting apparatus [36, 37]. The bacteria in the dental plaque are the essential initiators of the gingival inflammation; however, not all cases suffering from gingivitis progress into periodontitis. This transition is largely determined by the host immune response. Once gingival inflammation is set in, tissue microenvironment changes and causes an alteration in the microbial ecology and also in host response mechanisms against the residing bacteria. This leads to the stimulation of several key molecular and cellular signaling pathways, which ultimately activate host-derived collagenases [matrix metalloproteinases (MMPs)] which are responsible for tissue destruction. Such lytic process cause loss of principal fibers of the periodontal ligament, apical migration of the gingival attachment, and allows apical extension of biofilm and subjacent inflammation along the root surface and further spreads the disease process [36]. It leads to loss of clinical attachment, pocket formation, sometimes gingival recession, and radiographically accompanied bone loss [37, 38]. Gingivitis is a completely reversible disease process and the essential first step to progression to periodontitis, suggests periodontitis can be prevented at its early stage, yet it remains one of the most common causes of tooth loss. Therefore, prevention and early detection of periodontal disease are essential to reduce the damages it implies to the oral and systemic health of the individual.

2.3 Alveolar bone loss in periodontal disease

Alveolar bone loss is a characteristic sign of advanced periodontitis and ongoing bone loss is characteristic of the progression of periodontitis. The prevention of periodontal disease progression and bone loss is a key clinical challenge in periodontal therapy. Bone destruction is an eventual outcome of the host immune and inflammatory response and the dental plaque microbial challenge interplay. However, the underlying mechanism of disruption of the homeostatic balance of bone formation and resorption in favor of bone loss in these clinical situations remains to be understood.

2.3.1 Immunopathogenesis of periodontal bone loss

In chronic periodontal disease, many bioactive microbial molecules from dental plaque incite an immunological response from the resident and immune cells present in gingiva and periodontal tissues [39]. This leads to an influx of multiple cytokines that mediate the biochemical pathways of inflammation, for example, PGE2, IL-1, TNF-alpha and RANK-L, etc., which are responsible for osteoclastogenesis, the primary bone-resorbing process. Thus, the pathologic inflammatory process disrupts the fine balance between protective and destructive processes and leads to initiation of osteoclastic activity [40–45]. "Osteoimmunology" is the science which is dealing with the understanding of the intricacies of this immune-mediated bone destruction [46, 47]. The cellular inflammatory infiltrates of periodontal immunity cells such as T cells, B cells, macrophages, and neutrophils are increased within the gingival connective tissue and a concurrent increase in the inflammatory mediators' production is also evident [48, 49]. RANKL-mediated osteoclastogenesis is the prime mechanism underlying the inflammatory bone resorption in periodontal tissues [43, 50]. Activated T and B lymphocytes in inflamed periodontal tissues are the prime producers of RANKL- [43, 44, 51, 52]. An increase in osteoclast numbers on the alveolar bone crest has been observed in animal studies where antigen-specific lymphocytes are present and which can be suppressed by OPG [51, 53, 54].

Heterogenous populations of gingival fibroblasts are involved in dual actions in the inflammatory process. They are documented to have a protective role to suppress osteoclast formation as they produce OPG in response to LPS and IL-1; however, they may also augment chronic inflammatory processes through IL-6 and IFN production. The known periopathogens *Aggregatibacter actinomycetemcomitans* (*Aa*) and *Porphyromonas gingivalis* (*Pg*) induce the production of RANKL from the resident cells of periodontium viz. osteoblasts and gingival fibroblasts. Recently, it has been shown that an increased RANKL/OPG ratio is associated with periods of tissue destruction and ongoing disease activity. This ratio is further upregulated in patients in the presence of other known risk factors, for example, smokers and diabetics [55]. It has also been reported that the molecular mechanisms of T cell-mediated regulation of osteoclast formation occurs through cross talk signaling between RANKL and IFN-gamma [56].

2.3.2 Patterns and trends of alveolar bone loss

Periodontitis is usually asymptomatic chronic inflammatory condition caused by bacterial aggregation which affects the crest of the alveolar process by reducing the normal height in a vertical and/or a horizontal manner; furthermore, bone loss might be presented in a localized or a generalized form [35]. Bone destruction can be detected using several radiographical techniques that evaluate the quantity of the remaining bone and subsequently estimating the amount of bone loss on a radiograph. Panoramic radiography has a little diagnostic value in the identification of periodontal disease. It is useful to obtain the overall generalized status of bone, rather than very fine or precise details. However, it can be used as a valuable adjunct to conventional diagnostic procedures. It can be recommended as a part of routine dental and periodontal assessment which captures the entire maxilla-mandibular radiographic image on a single film. However, a panoramic radiograph should not be used to replace other intraoral radiographic techniques. Semenoff et al. assessed variations between different dental radiographs for assessment of the interseptal bone crest loss on conventional and digitized periapical, bitewing, and panoramic radiographs. Comparison among them showed that a small reduction in height of the interseptal bone crest observed in panoramic radiographs should be carefully evaluated for overestimation. Moreover, several studies proposed that panoramic radiography might serve as a diagnostic aid in dental health evaluation programs [57].

2.3.3 Bone destruction patterns in periodontal disease

Periodontal disease may affect the bone, altering its morphologic features in addition to reducing the vertical level of the bone height. An understanding of tissue mechanisms causing these alterations is important for effective diagnosis and effective treatment modalities.

I. Goldman and Cohen 1958 [58]: Classified infrabony defects based on the location and number of osseous walls remaining about the pocket as.

- Three osseous walls:
    - Proximal, buccal, and lingual walls
    - Buccal, mesial, and distal walls
    - Lingual, mesial, and distal walls

These trough-like defects are mostly seen in the interdental areas. These may exist as either shallow and wide lesions or deep and narrow ones.

- Two osseous walls:
    - Buccal and lingual walls (crater)
    - Buccal and proximal walls
    - Lingual and proximal walls

Two wall infrabony pockets may also occur in the interdental areas. With the buccal and lingual walls intact, but lost proximal wall, the lesion is termed as an intraosseous interproximal crater.

- One osseous wall:
  - Proximal wall (hemiseptum)
  - Buccal wall
  - Lingual wall

Generally in these lesions, a proximal wall is present with both buccal and lingual walls' resorbed.

- Combination:
  - 3 walls +2 walls
  - 3 walls +2 walls +1 wall
  - 3 walls +1 wall
  - 2 walls +1 wall

They may be seen in a variety of combination forms and can be located on a single or multiple surface of a tooth (**Figure 1**).

II. Karn KW et al. 1983 [59]:

1. When the original topography of the alveolar process is altered by uniform loss of bone from around the teeth and the plan of bone remains perpendicular to the long axis of the tooth: Horizontal bone loss
2. Deformities created by nonuniform loss of bone are based on the following basic terms:
   a. Crater: A crater is formed as a result of loss of alveolar bone and a portion of the contiguous supporting alveolar bone from only one surface of a tooth. They are identified by the mesial, distal, facial, or lingual tooth surface involved. Craters may be confluent if they occur on adjacent proximal surfaces, and termed as two-surface craters (affecting two tooth surfaces), named with two teeth involved.

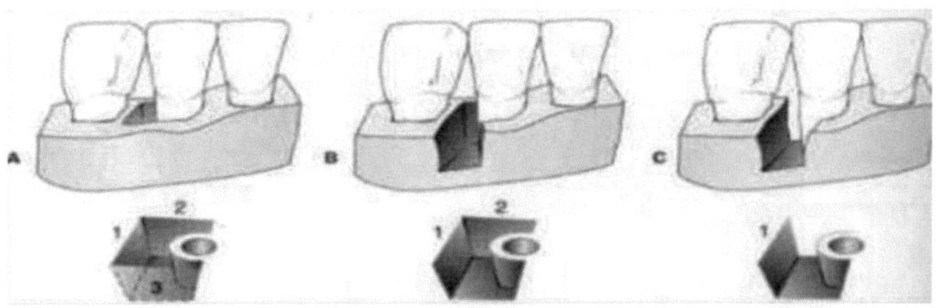

Figure 1.
Showing wall defects.

b. Trench: When bone loss as mentioned for crater affects two or three confluent surfaces of the same tooth, it is known as a trench. Trenches can be similarly identified by the tooth surfaces involved (e.g., mesiofacial and mesio-lingual- distal). There are eight possible types of trenches (MF, ML, DF, DL, MFD, MLD, FML, and FDL).

c. Moat: When bone deformities involves all four surfaces of a tooth. Only the tooth number is necessary to identify it (**Figure 2**).

d. Ramp: When both alveolar bone and its supporting bone are lost to the same degree but that the margins of the deformity are at different levels, it is known as Ramp. These are named for the tooth surface aspect from which the greatest bone loss has occurred and the teeth involved.

e. Plane: It is similar to ramp but the margins of the deformity remain at the same level. It can be considered horizontal bone loss about one tooth or portion of a tooth (**Figure 3**).

f. Cratered ramp: If only the most coronal rim of the deformity were considered, it would represent a ramp. However, a crater is presenting apical to the entire extent of the ramp and hence the term "cratered ramp." It is basically a crater with a portion of its facial and/or lingual wall missing. Cratered ramps are named for the teeth involved, the aspect of the alveolar process from which bone has been lost in the ramp portion and the tooth surfaces involved with the crater (or trench) (**Figure 4**).

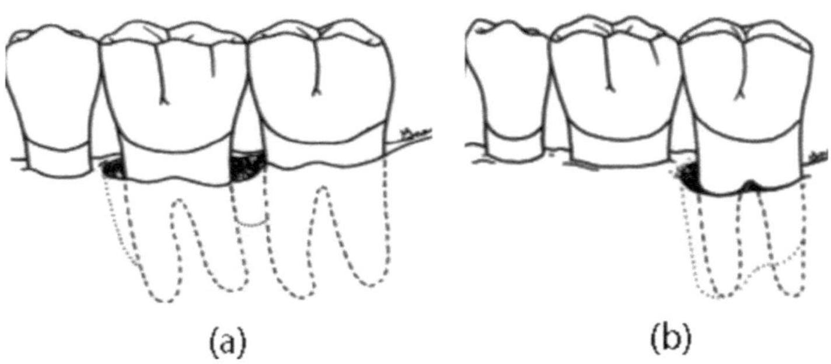

Figure 2.
Showing a moat type of bone defect.

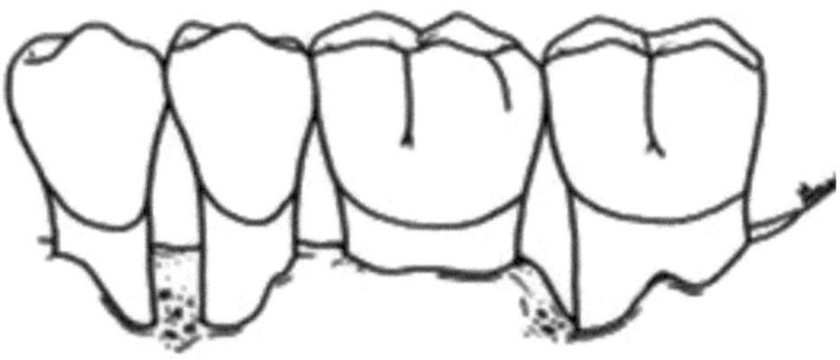

Figure 3.
Showing a plane type of bone defect.

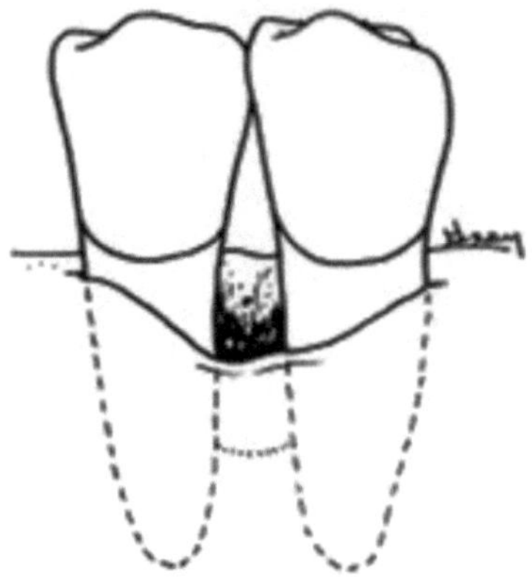

Figure 4.
Showing cratered ramp type of bone defect.

g. Ramp into A Crater or Trench: Its salient characteristic is that it is a ramp in the coronal aspect, but distinctly a crater or trench in the apical portion (**Figure 5**).

h. Furcation invasions: It refers to the involvement of the furcation area of the teeth by any kind of bone loss patterns described above.

III. Prichard JF 1983 [60]: Classified the bone defects as follows:

a. Intrabony defect: It is surrounded by bony walls on three sides and the root of tooth forming the fourth wall. The walls may be at different levels coronally forming combinations with other defects, but only the "inside" of the defect, the part that is apical to all three bony walls, is "within" bone or intrabony. They are also found in the apical region where the base of the arch is usually wider than the crest.

b. Hemiseptum: Periodontitis may affect one tooth and destroy septal bone adjacent to that tooth without affecting the contiguous tooth, thus leaving a hemiseptum of interalveolar bone.

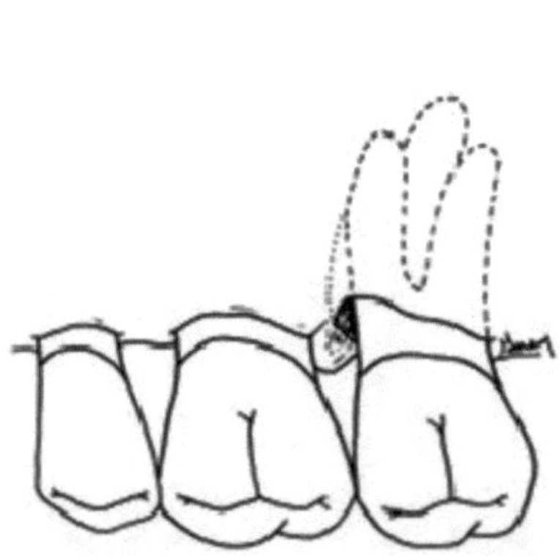

Figure 5.
Showing ramp into a crater type of bone defect.

c. Inconsistent margins: Destruction of marginal bone usually creates what Schluger called an inconsistent margin and on the tooth root the marginal defect may expose a furca. Across the interproximal space, the inconsistent margin may be associated with a crater or a hemiseptum.

d. Crater: A crater is a wide-mouthed cup or bowl-shaped defect in the interalveolar bone, with bone destruction about equal on the roots of the contiguous teeth; the sidewalls of the crater are formed by marginal bone on the vestibular and lingual surfaces.

e. Furca involvement: In the maxilla, defects in the interalveolar bone may be complicated by exposure of a furca and there may be bone destruction in the interradicular area.

2.3.3.1 Progression of periodontal disease

The earlier viewpoint regarding the progression of periodontal disease was that bacterial plaque accumulation universally leads to gingivitis, with subsequent progressive destruction of the supporting tissues of periodontium, with continuous irreversible attachment loss and bone resorption over time. Such conclusions have mostly come from observing cross-sectional populations over long periods of time. Later In order to determine the rate, pattern, and course of bone loss, researchers longitudinally studied subjects with repeated clinical and radiological measurements of patients suffering from periodontitis. Papapanou and coworkers [61] studied over 200 subjects with full-mouth radiographic surveys taken 10 years apart. The findings revealed that the mean annual rate of bone level resorption varied by age. Subjects between the ages of 25 and 65 years exhibited between 0.07 and 0.14 mm/year; whereas subjects over 70 years of age had a significantly higher rate of bone loss (0.28 mm). This particular investigation gave an insight into the trend of alveolar bone loss that it was continuous, slowly progressive, but with a great deal of the variable rate of progression among teeth and subjects. A similar 6-year long study in elderly Chinese subjects also revealed the individual range of bone loss varied dramatically from 0 to 0.53 mm/year [62]. Similar observations had been seen from the previous classically cited study by Löe and coworkers in Sri Lankan tea workers [63], which also reported huge differences in the rate of periodontal destruction among individuals.

Goodson and coworkers [64] challenged the prevalent belief system at that time that oral bone loss proceeded in a gradual fashion. In a series of studies, they examined the individual tooth site for progressive bone loss [65–68]. Among 22 untreated subjects with existing chronic periodontitis and pockets due to bone loss, only 15 subjects witnessed significantly deeper pockets over a time span of 1 year, whereas the other tooth sites rather showed a gain in attachment and reduction in the existing pocket depths. This investigation provided the evidence that alveolar bone destruction associated with periodontal disease was a dynamic condition and exhibited exacerbations and remissions of the disease activity over a period of time. This led to the emergence of "burst model" for periodontal disease progression pattern which had irregular bouts of the disease activity as opposed to continuous slow bone destruction over time. These classic studies utilized conventional manual probing to measure clinical attachment-levels to identify specific sites exhibiting more than 2 mm of progressive attachment loss and merely 5% of tooth sites exhibited progressive attachment loss. Another study [69] revealed 29% of the tooth sites showing progression over a 6-month period in adult patients previously diagnosed with periodontitis, by utilizing a more sensitive electronic probe to measure attachment loss. Modeling of the data over time showed that 76% of tooth sites lost attachment consistent with linear patterns, 12% of tooth sites showed exacerbations and remissions, and 12% revealed bursts of disease activity. Since then, a lot of periodontal disease progression models have come into being based on diverse studies, for example, Socransky, Goodson 1984 [70]. (1) Continuous Models: Slow and continuous, constantly progressive rate of destruction throughout the duration of the disease. (2) Random or episodic burst model: Short bursts of destruction followed by periods of no destruction, random pattern of disease w.r.t. the tooth sites affected. (3) Asynchronous, multiple burst model: periodontal destruction occurs in bursts, around affected teeth during defined periods of life. The chronology of these bursts of disease is asynchronous for individual teeth or groups of teeth. The natural history and progression patterns of intraoral bone loss are yet not clearly and completely understood at this time [71].

3. Risk factors for periodontal disease

Several studies' results indicated d that the tooth loss associated with periodontitis was much higher than the number of persons who suffer such tooth loss [72, 73]. Although a large proportion of the population is susceptible to periodontitis, yet a very small segment of the population witnesses severe forms of periodontitis. Such observations about the differential disease susceptibility led to the emergence of the concept of risk factors impacting the periodontal disease expression [74]. A risk factor is defined as an environmental, behavioral, or biologic factor confirmed by temporal sequence, usually in longitudinal studies, which if present, directly increases the likelihood of a disease occurring, and if absent or removed, reduces the probability of the disease event. Risk factors are considered as a part of the causal chain or expose the host to the causal chain. The most salient feature of a risk factor is its temporal presence before the emergence of the disease itself. Risk factors can be both modifiable and non-modifiable. Once a disease occurs, the removal of a risk factor may not result in a cure [75–77]. Based on whether they can be modified or not and documentation of their strength of association with the consequent disease, these have been classified as different categories as risk factors per se as defined, risk determinants, risk indicators, and risk predictors. Risk indicators are probable or putative risk factors that have been identified in cross-sectional studies but not confirmed through longitudinal studies. Risk predictors/markers, although associated with increased risk for disease, however, have not been clearly known to cause the disease. Risk determinants or background factors are those which are seen to be associated with the disease, but are not modifiable.

The contemporary concept that the rate of progression, age at onset, and severity of periodontal disease in an individual are often determined by systemic risk factors in the host is a recent one, supported by epidemiologic investigations of periodontal disease and the role of an associated multitude of genetic, epigenetic and environmental risk factors.

3.1 Age and gender as a risk determinant for periodontal disease

3.1.1 Age

Epidemiological studies have revealed a higher prevalence of the periodontal disease in elderly people compared to younger age-groups. The evidence demonstrates that both the extent and severity of periodontal disease increase in older individuals. Whether the increased prevalence and the severity in older persons are the outcomes of the lifetime accumulation of local factors such as dental plaque and microbial deposits or an inherent greater chance of susceptibility to periodontal deterioration exists in them remains largely debatable. Aging is associated with an increased incidence of periodontal disease [5, 6]. In a cross-sectional investigation of 1426 individuals aged 25–74 years, age was the most strongly associated risk factor with clinical attachment level with an odds ratio of 1.2 for persons aged 35–44 years and 9.01 for subjects aged 65–74. A stronger association between age and alveolar bone loss was seen in the same body with odds being 2.6 for people aged 35–44 years and 24.08 for age-group 67–74 years. Similar associations were reported in a large military population from the United States (1783 subjects) with an odds ratio of 5.03. Brown et al. reported contradictory findings and found age as not related to attachment loss in older individuals. Ismail et al. found that average attachment loss was greater in older individuals over a period of 28 years, though statistically not significant association, but significant in a multivariate model. Abdellatif and Bart [4] evaluated the relative significance of age and oral hygiene status as determinants of periodontitis and reported the rate of increase of periodontitis with increasing age across all age-groups was much higher for those with poor oral hygiene than those with excellent oral hygiene. They concluded that the effect of the age as a risk factor on periodontal disease progression is minimal when coupled with good oral hygiene [78]. Several studies show that the prevalence and severity of periodontal disease increase with age [79–86]. Papapanou et al. demonstrated that the mean annual rate of bone loss among the initially 70-year-old subjects was 0.28 mm compared to 0.07 on the 25-year-old individuals [86]. The increased severity of periodontal disease and bone loss with age was attributed to the time period, for how long the etiologic factors have been present in contact with the periodontal and is considered to reflect an individual's cumulative risk contact history [87]. More studies carried out in some of the developed countries show changing patterns of periodontal disease progression. These studies have shown that advanced periodontal destruction and bone loss are seldom seen in individuals under the age of 40 [83, 88]. A similar finding has been observed even in the elderly population. Studies among the elderly have shown that advanced periodontal disease affects only a small fraction of this age-group [82, 88]. However, among those with advanced disease, further breakdown does occur with increasing age [89].

Thus, the increased level of periodontal destruction observed with aging is now considered as the result of cumulative destruction rather than a result of increased rates of destruction. Thus aging is not a risk factor per se [76, 79] but enhances the susceptibility of greater incidence, prevalence, extent, and severity of periodontal disease owing to cumulative damage caused by local and other contributing etiologic factors over a period of time.

3.1.2 Gender

Gender has been associated with the diverse occurrence of periodontal disease in population studies and generally, males are known to suffer greater from gum disease than females of comparable age. Males usually exhibit poorer oral hygiene compared to females also. However, when oral hygiene, socioeconomic status, age, is correlated with gender, males are found to be associated with more severe periodontal disease. Females are more hygiene and esthetics conscious and seek dental treatment more often when compared to males. In their life span, there are gingival inflammatory conditions consistent with the physiologic reproductive hormonal fluctuations at different stages, such as puberty, pregnancy, and menopause [78]. Most of the data regarding the effect of female gender on gingival and periodontal tissues come from the clinical manifestations of inflammatory responses during specific periods of reproductive life such as puberty, pregnancy, and menopause, periods of immense alterations of female sex hormones. More gingival inflammatory diseases have been documented in association with sex steroid hormone levels, even without any alteration in the oral hygiene level of the individual. There is recent mounting evidence suggesting alterations in the male periodontium commiserating with androgen level fluctuations, in addition to most studies conducted in premenstrual females [90]. There is largely inconclusive evidence for the role of gender as a discriminating factor, in prevalence, progression, and severity of periodontal disease [3].

Numerous studies reported higher periodontal destruction among males compared to the female population. A high prevalence of periodontal disease of 73.9% was found among Chinese pre-conception women. Self-reported frequent bleeding during tooth brushing and the increased rate of periodontal disease revealed statistically significant association [91, 92]. Shaizu et al. in a systematic review and meta-analyses estimated sex-related differences in the prevalence of periodontitis. They found that sex exhibited a significant association with prevalence, reflecting a 9% difference between males and females (37.4 vs. 28.1%, respectively), although the overall effect of sex in the meta-analysis was comparatively small (d = 0.19; 95% confidence interval, 0.16 and 0.22). They calculated the mean difference in prevalence between males and females to be the same regardless of the severity of disease threshold and after adjustment for other risk factors. They concluded that men appeared at greater risk for destructive periodontal disease than women; however, men do not appear at higher risk for more rapid periodontal destruction than women. Recently, Hass et al. [93] reported almost two-fold higher susceptibility to suffering from periodontitis but similar periodontal status in postmenopausal women not on hormone replacement therapy (HRT) as compared to premenopausal women [94]. The reasons for these sex differences are not clear but can be related to multiple aspects, for example, as a demographic, biological, genetic, or epigenetic [95, 96]. However, the relationship observed between sex and the disease is not apparent and is not considered as strong and consistent [89].

3.1.2.1 Periodontium as a target tissue for sex steroid hormones

Sex steroid hormone receptors are not uniformly distributed but are found concentrated in certain hormone-sensitive tissues known as target tissues. Preferential accumulation and retention of hormones may occur depending upon the number of cytoplasmic and nuclear receptors that bind to particular hormones within the tissue. Many investigations have reported the preferential localization and retention of sex steroids, for example, estrogens [97, 98], androgens [98] and progestins [99] in periodontal tissues as well [90, 100]. The presence of specific hormonal receptors determines the response and regulates gene expression regarding the specific hormone ligand [101].

There are two kinds of estrogen receptors (a and b) which are genetically distinct forms and have differential distribution and functions [102]. Upon binding to a receptor, the activated receptor-steroid hormone complex binds with specific nuclear sites with a strong affinity. The intracytoplasmic or intranuclear activation step, followed by gene activation and transcription of mRNA finally guides the cellular protein synthesis. All sex steroids have effects on cell membranes and thus affect the second messenger systems in addition to regulation of gene transcription [103]. These activities affect neural transmission [104], modify the transport of calcium ions into cells [105], and stimulate the intracellular concentration of polyamines [106]. The periodontium of humans and animals is equipped with all the necessary enzymatic machinery to metabolize sex steroid hormones by common metabolic pathways and increased metabolic activity has been reported in inflamed periodontal tissues [3, 100, 101, 107, 108].

3.1.2.2 Proposed mechanisms for sex-specific hormones effecting periodontal disease pathogenesis

3.1.2.2.1 Periodontal microbiota

The majority of scientific investigations have not been able to identify any remarkable differences in periodontopathogenic bacteria between males and females [109–111]. Kumar et al. (2013) reviewed the effects of gonadal hormones on oral microbiota and documented only a transient alteration in the number and proportions of specific microorganisms during puberty or pregnancy [112]. So, there is not enough support that such minor and transitory relationships can bear a significant effect on susceptibility for periodontal breakdown [113, 114].

3.1.2.2.2 Vasculature

Similar to reproductive system vasculature, the blood vessels of gingiva is also responsive to sex steroid hormones. Many scientific investigations have correlated the increased flow of GCF, coinciding with the periods of fluctuation of sex steroid hormones. A comparison of the amount of gingival crevicular fluid in pregnant women versus postpartum controls has revealed approx. 54% elevation in pregnant females [115]. In a few animal studies, exogenous estrogen and/or progesterone administration has shown a significant increase in the amount of crevicular fluid irrespective of the inflammatory status of the status [116–118]. Both estrogen receptors a and b have effects on blood vascular functions [119].

Several mechanisms have been put forth to explain how the hormone may control the tonicity of the blood vessels by:

1. Inhibiting the calcium ions through the voltage-sensitive calcium channels [120].

2. Influencing the sympathetic transmitters [121, 122], or affecting alpha-adrenoceptor number or affinity [123, 124].

3. Increasing capillary permeability by stimulating the release of various mediators (e.g., adenosine, bradykinin, vasoactive intestinal polypeptide, neurotensin, substance P, various prostaglandins, AMP, ADP, ATP, cAMP, guanosine, thymidine, histamine, cytidine, uridine, acetylcholine, isoproterenol, and glycosaminoglycans) [125]. Some evidence regarding nitric oxide-induced vasodilation, re-endothelialization angiogenesis have also been accounted for such alterations through activation of the estrogen receptor-a [119, 126]. However, progesterone has been known to oppose the actions of estrogen, presumably by reducing estrogen receptor numbers, rather than having any individual effects on vasculature [90, 125].

Resident Cells Estrogen is known to regulate periodontal ligament cell proliferation including fibroblasts, keratinocytes, and promote osteoblastic cell differentiation [127, 128].

3.1.2.2.3 Epithelial cells

Several investigators perceived that estrogens increased epithelial keratinization and stimulated proliferation [129, 130]. Trott noticed a reduction in keratinization of the marginal gingival epithelium in postmenopausal women when plasma estrogens levels were declining [131]. Androgens were perceived to stimulate an increase in epithelial cell number [132, 133].

3.1.2.2.4 Connective tissue cells

The cellular effects of estrogen on collagen synthesis may largely be organ or site-specific [134]. In contrast to testosterone and progesterone, estrogens appear to be stimulatory in gingival fibroblasts derived from either feline or human drug enlarged gingiva [135]. Mariotti reported increased cell proliferation in fibroblasts derived from clinically healthy human gingiva of premenopausal women, with physiological concentrations of estradiol in vitro. They reported a characteristic estrogen-sensitive cellular subpopulation within the whole parent cell population of fibroblasts from premenopausal women [136]. Estradiol also induces a dose-dependent increase in interleukin-6, interleukin-8, and vascular endothelial growth factor in gingival fibroblasts [137]. In periodontal ligament cells, estrogens caused downregulation of lipopolysaccharide-induced cytokines while enhancing the production of osteoprotegerin [138, 139]. Natoli et al. demonstrated the expression of matrix proteins including collagen, elastin, and fibrillin-1, and their regulators as impacted by estrogen [140].

3.1.2.2.5 Bone cells

Sex steroids play a critical for skeletal development and for the maintenance of bone health throughout adult life [141]. The deficiency of estrogen increases osteoclast precursor cells. Estrogen increases osteoprotegerin, upregulates transforming growth factor-beta, an inhibitor of bone resorption that acts directly on osteoclastogenetic cells to decrease activity and increase apoptosis [142–144].

Specifically, increased T-cell production of tumor necrosis may be mediated by estrogen deficiency via a mechanism dependent upon regulatory cytokines, for example, in vivo bone destruction has been shown to involve interleukin-7, probably through its influence on T-cell development and homeostasis [141, 145].

3.1.2.2.6 Immune cells

Straub proposed that sex steroid hormones modulate the immune system via multiple ways: the immune stimulus and antigen-specific immune response; the target cells involved; the microenvironment of the tissue; hormone concentration; the variability of receptor isoforms; and the intracellular metabolism of hormones to either biologically active or inactive forms [146–148].

3.1.2.2.7 Intracellular signaling

Infectious challenge studies have revealed that males produce a significantly higher level of the inflammatory cytokine IL-6 and the acute phase protein LPS-binding protein (LBP) than females, after in vivo endotoxin exposure male-derived macrophages produce higher levels of IL 1b and lower levels of prostaglandin E2 than similarly treated female derived cells on exposure to LPS [147]. Estrogen and progesterone have antagonizing effects on neutrophil chemotaxis [149, 150]. Estrogen has been shown to upregulate nitric oxide synthase expression in neutrophils ex-vivo, with nitric oxide production being the highest [151, 152].

3.1.2.2.8 Adaptive immunity

B cells: documented evidence suggests that estrogen acts as a polyclonal B cell activator and has been shown to alter B lymphocyte function. Estrogen inhibits CD8+ T- cell-mediated suppression of B cells, the accelerated maturation of B cells into plasma cells; or increased amounts of the antibody produced per cell [152]. Similar findings have been demonstrated in animal models [153]. Testosterone has been shown to inhibit immunoglobulin IgG and IgM production of peripheral blood mononuclear cells [154].

T cells: Estrogen displays a biphasic effect on the antigen-stimulated secretion of TNF-α, with inhibition at high concentrations and enhancement at low doses [155]. Pregnancy and periovulatory levels of estrogen enhance IL-10 and IFN-γ response in CD4+ cells in humans and mice [156]. Estrogen inhibits IL-6 cytokine production in T cells. In healthy men and women, the polarization of immune response into Th1 or Th2 cytokines or cellular types is not absolute but the ratio of these components varies according to physiological demand and clinical conditions [157, 158]. Estrogen is known to be a potential physiological regulatory factor for the peripheral development of CD4 + CD25+ Treg cells [159]. Additionally, it was discovered that hormones peripherally activated prohormones and regulated the Th1/Th2 balance [160–163].

3.1.2.2.9 Antigen-presenting cells

(APCs) regulate Th cell differentiation and Th cell functioning under resting and activated conditions of the immune system in both the gender.IL6pathways regulates the homeostasis of the Th cell network in women, while this homeostasis is regulated by IFNγ pathways in men. Physiological homeostasis between Treg, Th17, and Th9 cells in the resting state in the transition to the activation phase and in the return to the resting state [157].

3.1.2.2.10 Immunosenescence-Gender-specific effects

Contemporary studies about the immune system functions have documented that there exists a differential effect on the activities and regulation of T helper (Th) cytokine pathways, which is affected by aging, but not to the same extent in both genders. Different cytokines regulate the development of immune response in humans at different phases, based on gender, for example, early evolution by the positive inter regulation of IFNγ-IL10 and IL6-IL4 in males, and the negative interrelation of IL6-IL10 in females whereas, the late evolution by the positive inter regulation of IFNγ-IL4 in males and by IL6-IFNγ in females. Alterations in these gender-specific cytokines regulatory pathways during aging could adversely affect the success of the immune response [158].

4. Preliminary case study: a retrospective panoramic analysis of distribution patterns of alveolar bone loss in chronic periodontitis patients from North India

A small preliminary investigation designed as a hospital based retrospective study of distribution patterns of alveolar bone loss on panoramic X-rays (OPG) of chronic periodontitis patients from North India was planned to draw an insight regarding the differential role of gender in context of periodontal disease. The aim of this study was to conduct an orthopantomograph radiographic screening in order to determine the overall distribution of alveolar bone loss, patterns (horizontal/vertical), and extent (coronal, middle, and apical thirds of the tooth root) in population by digital measurement analysis based on age and gender of the study participants.

4.1 Materials and methods

Orthopantomographs (OPG X-rays) of a total of 64 patients who visited the Department of Periodontology in the month of February–March, 2020 were recruited from the records, in order to evaluate the interproximal alveolar bone loss and potential explanatory variables including age, gender and number of sites. Panoramic views were obtained using Planmeca 2002 CC Proline with Dimax 3, Panoramic digital X-ray unit (60 KV and 20 mA), 1.2 magnification ratios. The scanned version of OPG X-ray films were analyzed with the help of a publicly available free online image assessment tool viz. Image J. It is a Java-based image processing program developed at the National Institutes of Health and the Laboratory for Optical and Computational Instrumentation (LOCI, University of Wisconsin) [163, 164].

A digital method of estimating alveolar bone height on panoramic radiographs using 3X magnification was employed using constant anatomic landmarks as reference points - CEJ and alveolar crest as shown in **Figures 6** and 7.

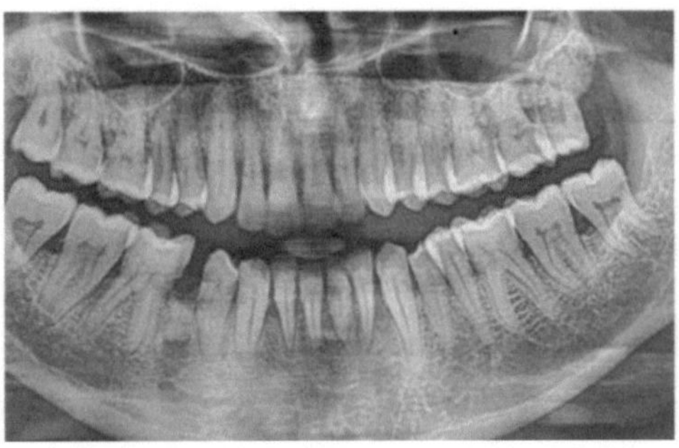

Figure 6.
Digital OPG X-ray image.

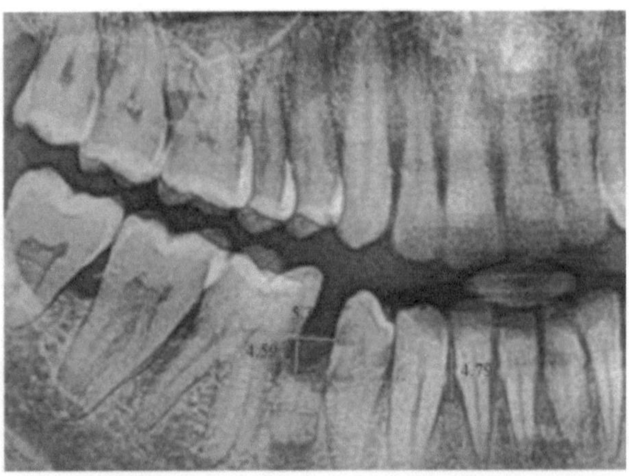

Figure 7.
Method of estimating alveolar bone height on panoramic radiographs using image analysis software.

Bone loss was considered when the distance from the CEJ to the alveolar crest exceeded 2 mm. Radiographic images was interpreted by a single calibrated examiner in order to reduce variability in image assessment and recording of data. Distorted, overlapped, unclear images particularly at the maxillary and mandibular anterior region or patients with orthodontic appliances were excluded for evaluation. Bone loss was estimated digitally by measuring the distance between CEJ and alveolar crest at the interproximal areas minus 2 mm (physiologic high of interseptal alveolar crest) at sites with reduced normal level of interseptal bone. The data so collected was put to appropriate descriptive and inferential statistics. Student, s T test and Mann Whitney test was used to intercept the differences in the mean of normal and skewed data parameters for different categories resp. Further, odds ratio was calculated to predict the future bone loss trends for patients with existing periodontal bone loss based on the no. of sites involved in bone loss.

4.2 Results

The collected OPG X-rays were categorized according to age and gender based on the accompanying clinical history recording and it was observed that there were OPGs from 30 females and 34 males and 11 subjects were below 30 years of age and 53 were above 30 years of age (**Table 1**).

Table 2 demonstrates the mean age and the distribution of bone loss patterns in total study population based on different defined categories of the bone loss providing mean no. of bone loss sites, along with the observed range in each category. As the study population was chronic periodontitis patients, all radiographic images showed evidence of bone loss at one or more than one site. Overall, 17 sites of bone loss were observed as an average no. of bone loss sites in the total population. Similarly, a mean value of 9.69 and 7.50 was observed for horizontal and vertical kind of bone loss sites in all population. The no. of bone loss sites extended to coronal, middle third and apical third of the root surface revealed a mean score of 3.11, 11.45, and 2.52 per individual, respectively (**Table 1**).

Tables 3 and **4** reveals comparative analysis of gender and age based distribution of total no. of bone loss sites in the total study population in current study. According to the gender, there was not observed any statistically significant difference in the total no. of bone loss sites, whereas there existed significant difference in the total no. of bone loss sites as per age.

Tables 5 and **6** reveals genderwise distribution of no. of bone loss site based on categories and its comparatives analysis, respectively. None of the categories revealed statistically significant difference in the no. of bone loss sites between males and females. Similarly, **Tables 7** and **8** reveals agewise distribution of no. of bone loss site based on categories and its comparatives analysis, respectively. Statistically significant difference in the no. of bone loss sites between males and

No. of subjects	Category	Frequency	Percent	Valid percent	Cumulative percent
64	Females	30	46.9	46.9	46.9
	Males	34	53.1	53.1	100.0
	<=30 years	11	17.2	17.2	17.2
	>30 years	53	82.8	82.8	100.0

Table 1.
Distribution of study participants based on categories.

S. No	Clinical Parameters	No. of subjects	Minimum	Maximum	Mean	Std. Deviation	Median	Inter quartile range
1	Age	64	17	84	41.67	11.982	—	—
2	Total No. of sites	64	4	29	17.03	5.768	—	—
3	No. of Sites with horizontal bone Loss	64	0	26	9.69	5.377	9.00	5–13.75
4	No. of Sites with vertical bone loss	64	0	22	7.50	5.507	7.00	3.25–10.00
5	Coronal 3rd	64	0	18	3.11	4.303	1.00	0.00–4.75
6	Middle 3rd	64	0	26	11.45	7.322	12.00	4.25–17.75
7	Apical 3rd	64	0	23	2.52	4.922	0.00	0.00–2.00

Table 2.
Distribution of study parameters in total study population based on different categories.

Sex	Mean	N	Std. deviation	Std. error mean	Sig. (2-tailed)
M	17.03	34	5.060	.868	0.998
F	17.03	30	6.568	1.199	

Table 3.
Comparative analysis of gender based distribution of total No. of bone loss sites in study population.

Age-groups	Mean	N	Std. deviation	Std. error mean	Sig. (2-tailed)
<=30 years	12.91	11	6.789	2.047	0.008**
>30 years	17.89	53	5.206	0.715	

Table 4.
Comparative analysis of age-based distribution of total No. of bone loss sites in study population.

females in the category of subjects with bone loss extending to middle third of the root, whereas none of the categories revealed statistically significant difference in the no. of bone loss sites between subjects above and below 30 years of age.

Further, a risk estimate analysis based on both age and gender as risk factors was carried out for prediction of future susceptibility of bone loss by calculating Odds ratio s, which revealed age of the individual as a significant risk determinant for the same (**Tables 9** and **10**).

4.3 Discussion

Gender has been implicated as a risk factor for many human diseases particularly rooted in chronic diseases, where disease pathogenesis is impacted significantly by immune mechanisms of the body including periodontal disease [165, 166]. The findings from the present case study revealed the presence of bone loss in all study participants which is indicative of the fact that periodontal bone loss is the hallmark of chronic periodontal disease. On average, 17 sites with bone loss were found to be

Category of patient		No. of patients	Median	Std. deviation	Interquartile range	
M	No. of sites with horizontal bone loss	34	9.00	5.132	5.00	13.25
	No. of sites with vertical bone loss	34	7.50	5.710	4.00	10.00
	Coronal 3rd	34	1.00	4.351	0.00	5.00
	Middle 3rd	34	12.00	6.881	6.25	16.00
	Apical 3rd	34	.00	4.931	0.00	2.25
	Sex	34	1.00	0.000	1.00	1.00
F	No. of sites with horizontal bone loss	30	9.50	5.637	5.00	14.00
	No. of sites with vertical bone loss	30	6.50	5.078	3.00	10.25
	Coronal 3rd	30	1.00	4.321	0.00	4.50
	Middle 3rd	30	11.67	7.906	4.00	18.25
	Apical 3rd	30	2.43	4.994	0.00	2.50

Table 5.
Genderwise distribution of No. of bone loss site based on categories.

	No. of sites with horizontal bone loss	No. of sites with vertical bone loss	Coronal 3rd	Middle 3rd	Apical 3rd
Mann-Whitney U	453.000	458.000	503.000	488.000	495.000
Wilcoxon W	1048.000	923.000	1098.000	1083.000	960.000
Z	−0.769	−0.702	−0.100	−0.297	−0.230
Asymp. Sig. (2-tailed)	0.442	0.483	0.920	0.767	0.818
a. Grouping variable: Sex					

Table 6.
Comparative analysis of genderwise distribution of No. of bone loss site based on categories.

present across the study population. Horizontal bone loss was more prevalent than the vertical bone loss, which is again in sync with the existing knowledge regarding the periodontal bone loss patterns. Most patients suffered from moderate periodontitis in terms of the severity of bone loss as maximum sites in population revealed bone loss extending up to the middle third of the root surface. With the new 2017 World Workshop on the Classification of Periodontal and Peri-Implant Diseases and Condition as a reference, the majority study population falls under the Stage III periodontitis category based on the residual bone level criteria for categorization [167]. Further, there was observed no statistically significant difference in the total number of bone loss sites based on gender, but there existed a significant difference in the total number of bone loss sites as per age in the study population. A statistically significant difference in the number of bone loss sites between males and females in the category of subjects with bone loss extending to the middle third of the root are also revealed, but neither of the other two categories based on age nor all categories based on gender witnessed any statistically significant differences in terms of the number of bone loss sites varied according to the severity of the bone loss.

Category of patient		No. of patients	Median	Std. deviation	Interquartile range	
<=30 years	No. of sites with horizontal bone loss	11	5.00	4.657	4.00	13.00
	No. of sites with vertical bone loss	11	4.00	6.496	0.00	8.00
	Coronal 3rd	11	5.00	3.828	.00	7.00
	Middle 3rd	11	4.00	8.201	0.00	14.00
	Apical 3rd	11	0.00	4.771	0.00	2.00
>30 years	No. of sites with horizontal bone loss	53	10.00	5.375	6.00	14.00
	No. of sites with vertical bone loss	53	7.00	5.170	4.00	10.00
	Coronal 3rd	53	0.00	4.383	0.00	4.00
	Middle 3rd	53	13.00	6.739	8.00	18.00
	Apical 3rd	53	0.00	4.984	0.00	3.50

Table 7.
Agewise distribution of No. of bone loss site based on categories.

	No. of sites with horizontal bone loss	No. of sites with vertical bone loss	Coronal 3rd	Middle 3rd	Apical 3rd
Mann-Whitney U	187.500	211.000	211.500	159.000	248.000
Wilcoxon W	253.500	277.000	1642.500	225.000	314.000
Z	−1.856	−1.437	−1.514	−2.362	−0.881
Asymp. Sig. (2-tailed)	0.064	0.151	0.130	0.018*	0.378
a. Grouping variable: Age-groups					

Table 8.
Comparative analysis of agewise distribution of No. of bone loss site based on categories.

Previous literature has also reported that there was no significant sex difference. Gender is inherently a very complex risk factor that may play a role through diverse mechanisms as discussed in earlier sections. Premenopausal women exhibit the lower prevalence of periodontitis as compared with men and on contrary, after menopause, with a weakening estrogen signal, women may show equal or even greater periodontal destruction as compared to age matched men [168]. Wulandari et al. reported no difference in periodontal severity between perimenopausal and postmenopausal women, however, emphasized the role of the bacterial plaque regarding periodontal disease severity in perimenopausal and postmenopausal women in a cross-sectional investigation in 63 subjects, aged 45–59 years, in East Jakarta [169]. Paramashivaiah et al. examined 104 postmenopausal women, age-group ranging from 35 to 60 years, and reported radiographic alveolar bone loss correlated with clinical indicators including attachment loss. Most females had periodontitis and low serum 17-β estradiol and calcium levels [170]. Lee et al. indicated an association between hormone replacement therapy (HRT) and periodontal disease, after adjusting for various potential confounders for periodontal diseases. The authors showed that the HRT+ group was less likely to develop periodontal diseases

			M	F		Asymp. Sig. (2-sided)
Total sites 13	>13	Count	26	0.559	47	0.559
		% within Sex	76.50%	70.00%	73.40%	
	<=13	Count	8	9	17	
		% within Sex	23.50%	30.00%	26.60%	
Total		Count	34	30	64	
		% within Sex	100.00%	100.00%	100.00%	
Risk Estimate						
		Value	95% Confidence interval			
			Lower		Upper	
Odds ratio for total sites 13 (>13 / <=13)		1.393	0.458		4.237	
For cohort SEX = M		1.176	0.668		2.07	
For cohort SEX = F		0.844	0.487		1.462	
No. of valid cases		64				

Table 9.
Risk estimate of bone loss based on gender as a risk determinant.

			Age-groups		Total	Asymp. Sig. (2-sided)
			>30 years	<=30 years		
Total sites 13	>13	Count	42	5	47	0.021*
		% within age-groups	79.2%	45.5%	73.4%	
	<=13	Count	11	6	17	
		% within age-groups	20.8%	54.5%	26.6%	
Total		Count	53	11	64	
		% within age-groups	100.0%	100.0%	100.0%	
Risk estimate						
		Value	95% Confidence interval			
			Lower		Upper	
Odds ratio for total sites 13 (>13/<=13)		4.582	1.176		17.849	
For cohort age-groups = > 30 years		1.381	0.959		1.989	
For cohort age-groups = <= 30 years		0.301	0.106		0.861	
No. of valid cases		64				

Table 10.
Risk estimate of bone loss based on age as a risk determinant.

than the HRT- group upon analysis of 45 and 74 years old menopausal women [171]. Another study by Pizzo et al. in 91 Italian menopausal women (50 ~ 62 years) reported similar periodontal pocket depths between the group who underwent HRT and who did not, but the group without HRT had a higher level of dental plaque [172]. López-Marcos et al. [173] studied in 210 Spanish menopausal women aged 40–58 years that the estrogen patch group showed a reduction in periodontal pocket depth. People with a longer menopausal period and lower bone mass more evidently witnessed the effects of esterogen deficiency [174, 175]. The authors recommend that the studies aimed at a clear delineation of the role of gender as a risk factor should rather be more meticulously designed in terms of studying the role of gender in differential age-groups, larger study samples, and well-designed investigations as females undergo specific periods of hormonal fluctuations according to the stage of their reproductive life cycle.

A study was conducted by Wouters et al. in 1989 in 733 randomly selected dentate individuals aged 20 years and above using periapical radiographs with interproximal intrabony periodontal defect depth and width of at least 5 and 10 mm, respectively, to determine the relationship between the prevalence of interproximal periodontal intrabony defect and age. It was reported that the prevalence increased with age and was higher in men than in women [168]. However, the significantly lower prevalence of interproximal periodontal intrabony defect in women than in men does not support the studies of Nielsen et al. [176], in which no significant sex differences were reported [177]. The present study findings still need to compare with caution as it differed in the X-ray images taken as reference was OPGs of the study subjects. So the differences in study settings, design and tools may also be responsible for the observed heterogeneity in study results.

A higher incidence of bone loss in adult patients (24–30 years old) is a fact, that periodontitis is an age dependent disease the incidence and severity of bone loss and attachment loss increase with age (16) as a result of longer exposure to local factors as age grows older. The present study revealed a nonsignificantly higher prevalence of bone loss among females than males, and the authors attributed these findings to a higher prevalence of aggressive periodontitis among females rather than males [178].

Khateeb et al. carried out an investigation in a total of 190 female patients (mean age, 22.4 ± 2.46 years) and Patients' age was found to be a good predictor for alveolar bone loss and number of periapical lesions ($P \leq 0.05$) [179]. Another study from China revealed that 40–59-year-old patients with chronic periodontitis had severe bone loss. And a lesser degree of alveolar bone loss was seen in males than females [179]. Menopause in females and smoking in both genders may have affected the level of bone loss. Male smokers experienced a greater degree of bone loss (41.67 ± 5.76%) than male non-smokers (32.95 ± 4.31%). A 42.23 ± 6.34% bone loss was found in menopausal females versus 31.35 ± 3.62% in non-menopausal females [180].

Bansal M et al. (2015) [181], in a cross-sectional prevalence study among hospital-based Indian population, assessed the prevalence of the periodontal disease. They stated that healthy periodontium was found in 19 (3.9%) subjects with the highest percentage in the 15–19 years age-groups and after 44 years no person had healthy teeth. Also, advanced stages were more prevalent in older age-groups, deep pockets occurring in 87 (17.90%) subjects that increased as the age advanced up to 45–54. According to them, males were more affected with moderate and severe periodontitis as compared to females. Bokhari et al. (2015) [28], reported that subjects aged 40 years and above were four times more likely to have periodontitis using Community Periodontal Index (CPI) methods. Marya, CM, et al. (2020) [182], in a cross sectional study assessed if there are any gender differences in oral health-related quality of life (OHRQoL) among the elderly population of Haryana. Genderwise, no significant association was found with different parameters of periodontitis. They found a significant association of OHRQoL with the main factor causing periodontal problems, that is, mobile teeth and no comparable difference was observed in the OHRQoL among males and females. They suggested one needs to target the geriatric population as a whole for planning and implementing public oral health strategies.

5. Clinical relevance of understanding the specific effects of gender on periodontal disease

Despite the extensive evidence from the recent past has recognized gender as an important factor in the regulation of immune responses, sex differences are still very much understudied and poorly understood in scientific research with females being under-represented in clinical disease trials. Specific exploration of sex-specific biomarkers should be considered for both the genders. Studies of multifactorial diseases demonstrate differential susceptibilities between genders encounter confounding variables, such as lifestyle, socioeconomic status, environmental exposures, and genetic polymorphisms. Hence, novel experimental models with gender differences shall be developed to understand disease pathogenesis based on gender [183, 184].

Effie Ioannidou in 2017 developed the methodological and analytical framework with the recognition of sex/gender as important determinants of disease pathogenesis. The authors aimed to present relevant sex biologic evidence to understand the plausibility of the epidemiologic data. In periodontitis pathogenesis, sex dimorphism has been implicated in the disease etiology. With the clear distinction between sex and gender, gender oral health disparities have been explained by socioeconomic factors, cultural attitudes as well as access to preventive and regular care. Economic inequality and hardship for women have resulted in limited access to oral care in some parts of the world. As a result, gender emerged as a complex socioeconomic and behavioral factor influencing oral health outcomes [185].

With the expanding knowledge regarding gender as a risk factor, we must intend to perform specific gender-based periodontal research to find better insight into the mechanisms of disease pathogenesis and mediators, so that specific gender-based tools for periodontal diagnosis, risk assessment, predictive medicine, and disease management strategies can be developed to provide optimized periodontal health care solutions to our patients.

6. Conclusion

Our current knowledge and understanding of the specific role of gender in the context of periodontal health status remain limited and need further elucidation. The combined effect of sex-specific genetic architecture and the circulating levels of sex steroid hormones may account for variation in risk for chronic periodontitis, with men exhibiting greater susceptibility than women. The preliminary case study presented here revealed age as a significantly associated factor, with the total number of bone loss sites and with the bone loss site extended up to a middle third of tooth root (moderate to severe periodontitis cases), but could not delineate gender, the primary factor being explored as a clear-cut risk factor, owing to the lack of statistical strength and study limitations as the small-sized sample, retrospective study design. This shall not obviate the need to explore this factor as a cause of concern as contemporary models of periodontal pathogenesis; differences in susceptibility, and progression of destructive periodontal disease are attributed to the individual and collective biologic and modifiable risk factors. With this framework of information, gender as a risk factor for periodontal disease needs to decipher in detail its underlying mechanisms by conducting longitudinal well-controlled, designed, and characterized studies. Such investigations to further explore the role of gender in the prevalence, progression, and severity of chronic periodontal disease are warranted in the future so that novel strategies for risk assessment, disease identification, and individualized therapeutic approaches can be developed for optimized patient care based on gender.

Author details

Ashish Jain[1], Neeta V. Bhavsar[2], Amrit Baweja[3], Aman Bhagat[3], Anchal Ohri[1] and Vishakha Grover[1*]

1 Department of Periodontology and Oral Implantology, Dr. H.S.J. Institute of Dental Sciences, Panjab University, Chandigarh, India

2 Department of Periodontology and Oral Implantology, Government Dental College and Hospital, Ahmedabad, India

3 Dr. H.S.J. Institute of Dental sciences, Panjab University, Chandigarh, India

*Address all correspondence to: vishakha_grover@rediffmail.com

References

[1] Alam N, Mishra P, Chandrasekaran SC. Gender basis of periodontal diseases. IJBAMR. 2012;**2**(1):128-135

[2] Mcclleland EE, Smith JM. Gender specific differences in the immune response to infection. Archivum Immunologiae et Therapiae Experimentalis (Warsz). 2011;**59**:203-213

[3] Grover V, Jain A, Kapoor A, Malhotra R, Chahal GS. The gender bender effect in periodontal immune response. Endocrine, Metabolic & Immune Disorders Drug Targets. 2016;**16**:12-20

[4] Abdellatif HM, Burt BA. An epidemiological investigation into the relative importance of age and oral hygiene status as determinants of periodontitis. Journal of Dental Research. 1987;**66**(1):13-18

[5] Grossi SG, Genco EE, Machtei AW, et al. Assessment of risk for periodontal disease. I. Risk indicators for attachment loss. Journal of Periodontology. 1994;**65**(3):260-267

[6] Grossi SG, Genco RJ, Machtei EE, et al. Assessment of risk for periodontal disease. II. Risk indicators for alveolar bone loss. Journal of Periodontology. Intech Open; 1995;**66**(1):23-29

[7] Marshall-day CD, Stephens RG, Quigley LFJ. Periodontal disease: prevalence and incidence. Journal of Periodontology. 1955;**26**(3):185-203

[8] Norderyd O, Hugoson A. Risk of severe periodontal disease in a Swedish adult population. A cross-sectional study. Journal of Clinical Periodontology. 1998;**25**(12):1022-1028

[9] Brown LF, Beck JD, Rozier RG. Incidence of attachment loss in community-dwelling older adults. Journal of Periodontology. 1994;**65**(4): 31623

[10] Haber J, Wattles J, Crowley M, Mandell R, Joshipura K, Kent RL. Evidence for cigarette smoking as a major risk for periodontitis. Journal of Periodontology. 1993;**64**(1):16-23

[11] Bergström J. Cigarette smoking as risk factor in chronic periodontal disease. Community Dentistry and Oral Epidemiology. 1989;**17**(5):245-247

[12] Haffajee AD, Socransky SS. Relationship of cigarette smoking to attachment level profiles. Journal of Clinical Periodontology. 2001;**28**(4):28395

[13] Martinez-Canut P, Lorca A, Magán R. Smoking and periodontal disease severity. Journal of Clinical Periodontology. 1995;**22**(10):743-749

[14] Ragghianti MS, Greghi SLA, Lauris JRP, Santana ACP, Passanezzi E. Influence of age, sex, plaque and smoking on periodontal conditions in a population from Bauru, Brazil. Journal of Applied Oral Science. 2004;**12**(4):273-279

[15] Hatem AE. In: Manakil J, editor. Epidemiology and Risk Factors of Periodontal Disease, Periodontal Diseases—A Clinician's Guide. Intech Open; 2012. ISBN: 978-953-307-818-2

[16] Nora S, Loreto A, Denisse B, Nicolás D, Jocelyn GS, Rolando V, et al. Host response mechanisms in periodontal diseases. Journal of Applied Oral Science. 2015;**23**(3):329-355

[17] Bendre MS, Montague DC, Peery T, Akel NS, Gaddy D, Suva LJ. Interleukin-8 stimulation of osteoclastogenesis and bone resorption is a mechanism for the increased osteolysis of metastatic bone disease. Bone. 2003;**33**:28-37. [PubMed: 12919697]

[18] Newman MG, Takei HH, Klokkevold PR, editors. Carranza's Clinical Periodontology. St Louis: Saunders/ Elsevier; 2006. pp. 110-132

[19] Flemmig TF. Periodontitis. Annals of Periodontology. 1999;**4**:32-38. [PubMed: 10863373]

[20] Ali C, Alpdogan K, Hatice H, Van Dyke TE. Inflammatory and immune pathways in the pathogenesis of periodontal disease, 2014. Periodontology 2000. 2000;**64**(1): 57-80. DOI: 10.1111/prd.12002

[21] NIDCR. Periodontal Disease. 2014. Available from: https://www.nidcr.nih.gov/DataStatistics/ByPopulation/Adults/

[22] Marcenes W, Kassebaum NJ, Bernabe E, Flaxman A, Naghavi M, Lopez A, et al. Global burden of oral conditions in 1990-2010: A systematic analysis. J Dent Res. United States. 2013;**92**(7):592-597

[23] Eke PI, Dye BA, Wei L, Slade GD, Thornton-Evans GO, Borgnakke WS, et al. Update on prevalence of periodontitis in adults in the United States: NHANES 2009 to 2012. Journal of Periodontology United States. 2015;**86**(5):611-622

[24] Eke PI, Wei L, Borgnakke WS, Thornton-Evans G, Zhang X, Lu H, et al. Periodontitis prevalence in adults >/= 65 years of age, in the USA. Periodontology 2000. Journal of International Society of Preventive and Community Dentistry. 2016;**72**(1):76-95

[25] Helmi MF, Hui Huang J, Goodson M, Hasturk H, Tavares M, Natto ZS. Prevalence of periodontitis and alveolar bone loss in a patient population at Harvard School of Dental Medicine. BMC Oral Health. 2019;**19**:254. DOI: 10.1186/s12903-019-0925-z

[26] Abdul-Kadir R. Periodontal profile of 15- to 19-year-old west Malaysian secondary school students. The Journal of Nihon University School of Dentistry. 1994;**36**:34-39

[27] Corbet EF, Zee KY, Lo EC. Periodontal diseases in Asia and Oceania. Periodontology 2000. 2002;**29**:122-152

[28] Bokhari SA, Suhail AM, Malik AR, Imran MF. Periodontal disease status and associated risk factors in patients attending a dental teaching Hospital in Rawalpindi, Pakistan. Journal of Indian Society of Periodontology. 2015;**19**:678-682

[29] Shaju JP, Zade RM, Das M. Prevalence of periodontitis in the Indian population: A literature review. Journal of Indian Society of Periodontology. 2011;**15**(1):29-34. DOI: 10.4103/0972-124X.82261

[30] Ramoji Rao MV, Katari PK, Vegi L, Bypureddy TT, Prabhakara Rao KS, Tejaswi KS. Prevalence of periodontal diseases among rural population of Mustabad, Krishna District. Journal of International Society of Preventive and Community Dentistry. 2016;**6**(Suppl 1):S59-S63. DOI: 10.4103/2231-0762.181169

[31] Shewale AH, Gattani DR, Bhatia N, Mahajan R, Saravanan S. Prevalence of periodontal disease in the general population of India-A systematic review [Internet]. 2016 [cited 20 June 2020];**10**(6):ZE04-ZE09

[32] Chandra A, Yadav OP, Narula S, Dutta A. Epidemiology of periodontal diseases in Indian population since last decade. 2016;**6**(2):91-96

[33] Bansal M, Mittal N, Singh TB. Assessment of the prevalence of periodontal diseases and treatment needs: A hospital-based study. Journal of Indian Society of Periodontology. Journal of International Society of Preventive & Community Dentistry; 2015;**19**(2):211-215. DOI: 10.4103/0972-124X.145810

[34] Batra M, Tangade P, Gupta D. Assessment of periodontal health among the rural population of Moradabad, India. Journal of Indian Association Public Health Dentistry. 2014;**12**:28-32

[35] Newman MG, Takei HH, Klokkevold PR, Carranza FA. Carranza's Clinical Periodontology. St. Louis, Missouri: Elsevier/Saunders; 2015

[36] Papapanou PN, Sanz M, Buduneli N, Dietrich T, Feres M, Fine DH, et al. Periodontitis: Consensus report of workgroup 2 of the 2017 world workshop on the classification of periodontal and peri-implant diseases and conditions. Journal of Periodontology. 2018;**89**(Suppl. 1):S173-S182. DOI: 10.1002/JPER.17-0721

[37] Tonetti MS, Greenwell H, Kornman KS. Staging and grading of periodontitis: Framework and proposal of a new classification and case definition. Journal of Periodontology. 2018;**89**(Suppl. 1):S159-S172. DOI: 10.1002/JPER.18-0006

[38] Muñoz C, Jose L. Pathogenesis of Periodontal Disease. Intech Open; 2019. DOI: 10.5772/intechopen.86548

[39] Nanci A, Bosshardt DD. Structure of periodontal tissues in health and disease. Periodontology 2000. 2006;**40**(1):11-28

[40] Oates TW, Cochran DL. Bone cell interactions and regulation by inflammatory mediators. Current Opinion in Periodontology. 1996;**3**:34-44

[41] Cauley LKM, Nohutcu RM. Mediators of periodontal osseous destruction and remodeling: Principles and implications for diagnosis and therapy. Journal of Periodontology. 2002;**73**(11):1377-1391

[42] Teitelbaum SL. Osteoclasts: What do they do and how do they do it? The American Journal of Pathology. 2007;**170**(2):427-435

[43] Yasuda H, Shima N, Nakagawaetal N. Osteoclast differentiation factor is a ligand for osteoprotegerin / osteoclastogenesis inhibitory factor and is identical to TRANCE/RANKL. Proceedings of the National Academy of Sciences of the United States of America. 1998;**95**(7):3597-3360

[44] Nagasawa T, Kiji M, Yashiroetal R. Roles of receptor activator of nuclear factor-κB ligand (RANKL) and osteoprotegerin in periodontal health and disease. Periodontology 2000. 2007;**43**(1):65-84

[45] MacDonald BR. Parathyroid hormone, prostaglandins and boneresorption. World Review of Nutrition and Dietetics. 1986;**47**:163-201

[46] Gruber R. Cell biology of osteo-immunology. Wiener Medizinische Wochenschrift. 2010;**160**:438-445

[47] Ohlrich EJ, Cullinan MP, Seymour GJ. The immunopathogenesis of periodontal disease. Australian Dental Journal. 2009;**54**(1):S2-S10

[48] Di Benedetto A et al. Periodontal disease: linking the primary inflammation to bone loss. Clinical and Developmental Immunology. 2013;**2013**:503754. DOI: 10.1155/2013/503754

[49] Yucel-Lindberg T, Bage T. Inflammatory mediators in the pathogenesis of periodontitis. Expert Reviews in Molecular Medicine. 2013;**15**:7

[50] Liu D, Xu JK, Figliomenietal L. Expression of RANKL and OPG mRNA in periodontal disease: Possible involvement in bone destruction. International Journal of Molecular Medicine. 2003;**11**(1):17-21

[51] Taubman MA, Valverde P, Han X, Kawai T. Immune response: the key to bone resorption in periodontal disease. Journal of Periodontology. 2005;**76**(11):2033-2041

[52] Udagawa N, Takahashi N, Jimi E, et al. Osteoblasts/stromal cells stimulate osteoclast activation through expression of osteoclast differentiation factor/RANKL but not macrophage colony-stimulating factor: Receptor activator of NF-kappa B ligand. Bone. 1999;**25**(5):517-523

[53] Jin Q , Cirelli JA, Parketal CH. RANKL inhibition through osteoprotegerin blocks bone loss in experimental periodontitis. Journal of Periodontology. 2007;**78**(70):1300-1308

[54] Kawai T, Matsuyama T, Hosokawa Y, et al. B and T lymphocytes are the primary sources of RANKL in the bone resorptive lesion of periodontal disease. The American Journal of Pathology. 2006;**169**(3):987-998

[55] Belibasakis GN, Bostanci N. The RANKL-OPG system in clinical periodontology. Journal of Clinical Periodontology. 2012;**39**(3):239-248

[56] Hienz SA, Paliwal S, Ivanovski S. Mechanisms of bone resorption in periodontitis. Journal of Immunology Research. 2015;**2015**:615486. 10 p. DOI: 10.1155/2015/615486

[57] Semenoff L, Semenoff TDV, Pedro F, Volpato L, Machado M, Borges A, et al. Are panoramic radiographs reliable to diagnose mild alveolar bone resorption? ISRN Dentistry. 2011;**2011**:363578. DOI: 10.5402/2011/363578

[58] Goldman HM, Cohen DW. The infrabony pocket: Classification and treatment. The Journal of Periodontology. 1958;**29**:272-291. DOI: 10.1902/jop.1958.29.4.272

[59] Karn KW, Shockett HP, Moffitt WC, Gray JL. Topographic classification of deformities of the alveolar process. Journal of Periodontology. 1984;**55**(6):336-340. DOI: 10.1902/jop.1984.55.6.336

[60] Prichard JF. The diagnosis and management of vertical bony defects. Journal of Periodontology. 1983;**54**: 29-35. DOI: 10.1902/jop.1983.54.1.29

[61] Papapanau PN, Wennstrom JL. A 10 year retrospective study of periodontal disease progression. Clinical characteristics of subjects with pronounced and minimal disease development. Journal of Clinical Periodontology. 1990;**17**:78-84

[62] Baelum V, Wen-Min L, Dahlen G, Fejerskov O, Xia C. Six year progression of destructive periodontal disease in two subgroups of elderely chinese. Journal of Periodontology. 1993;**64**:891-899

[63] Löe H, ÅNerud Å, Boysen H, Smith M. The natural history of periodontal disease in man. Journal of Periodontal Research. 1978;**13**:550-562. DOI: 10.1111/j.1600-0765.1978.tb00209.x

[64] Goodson JM, Tanner AC, Haffajee AD, Sornberger GC, Socransky SS. Patterns of progression and regression of advanced destructive periodontal disease. Journal of Clinical Periodontology. Nov 1982;**9**(6):472-481

[65] Socransky SS, ACR T, Haffajee AD, Hillman JD, Goodson JM. Present Status of Studies on the Microbial Etiology of Periodontal Diseases. Washington DC: American Society of Microbiology; 1982

[66] Socransky SS, Haffajee AD. The bacterial etiology of destructive periodontal disease: Current concepts. Journal of Periodontology. 1992;**63**:322-331. DOI: 10.1902/jop.1992.63.4s.322

[67] Haffajee AD, Socransky SS, Goodson JM. Clinical parameters as predictors of destructive periodontal

disease activity. Journal of Clinical Periodontology. 1983;**10**(3):257-265. DOI: 10.1111/j.1600-051x.1983.tb01274.x

[68] Haffajee AD, Socransky SS, Dzink JL, Taubman MA, Ebersole JL, Smith DJ. Clinical, microbiological and immunological features of subjects with destructive periodontal diseases. Journal of Clinical Periodontology. 1988;**15**(4):240-246. DOI: 10.1111/j.1600-051x.1988.tb01577.x

[69] Jeffcoat MK, Reddy MS. Progression of probing attachment loss in adult periodontitis. Journal of Periodontology. 1991;**62**:185-189. DOI: 10.1902/jop.1991.62.3.185

[70] Socransky SS, Haffaje AD, Goodson JM, Lindhe J. New concepts of destructive periodontal disease. Journal of Clinical Periodontology. 1984;**11**:21-32. DOI: 10.1111/j.1600-051X.1984.tb01305.x

[71] Jeffcoat MK. Oral Bone Loss and Systemic Osteoporosis: Weighing the risk benefit ratio of treatment. Philadelphia, PA,USA: Univeristy of Pennsylvania School of Dental Medicine;

[72] Scherp HW. Current concepts in periodontal disease research: Epidemiological contributions. Journal of the American Dental Association (1939). 1964;**68**:667-675

[73] Brown LJ, Löe H. Prevalence, extent, severity and progression of periodontal disease. Periodontology 2000. 1993;**2**:57-71

[74] Timmerman MF, van der Weijden GA. Risk factors for periodontitis. International Journal of Dental Hygiene. 2006;**4**:2-7

[75] Beck JD. Risk revisited. Community Dentistry and Oral Epidemiology. 1998;**26**:220-225

[76] Van Dyke TE, Sheilesh D. Risk factors for periodontitis. Journal of the International Academy of Periodontology. 2005;**7**:3-7

[77] Mehta A. Risk factors associated with periodontal diseases and their clinical considerations. International Journal of Contemporary Dental and Medical Reviews. 2015;**2015**. Article ID: 040115. DOI: 10.15713/ins.ijcdmr.31

[78] Nagarathna DV. Risk factors in periodontal disease progression. Indian Journal of Dental Education. 2013;**6**(4):195-209

[79] RGenco RJ. Current view of risk factors for periodontal diseases. Journal of Periodontology. 1996;**10**:1041-1049

[80] Axelsson P, Lindhe J. Effect of controlled oral hygiene procedures on caries and periodontal disease in adults. Journal of Clinical Periodontology. 1978;**5**(2):133-151

[81] Baelum V, Wen-Min L, Fejerskov O, Xia C. Tooth mortality and periodontal conditions in 60-80-year-old Chinese. Scandinavian Journal of Dental Research. 1998;**96**(2):99-107

[82] Beck JD, Koch GG, Rozier RG, Tudor GE. Prevalence and risk indicators for periodontal attachment loss in a population of older community-dwelling blacks and whites. Journal of Periodontology. 1990;**61**(8):521-528

[83] Hugoson A, Laurell L, Lundgren D. Frequency distribution of individuals aged 20-70 years according to severity of periodontal disease experience in 1973 and 1983. Journal of Clinical Periodontology. 1992;**19**(4):227-232

[84] Locker D, Leake JL. Periodontal attachment loss in independently living older adults in Ontario, Canada. Journal of Public Health Dentistry. 1993;**53**(1):6-11

[85] Mack F, Mojon P, Budtz-Jørgensen E, et al. Caries and periodontal disease of the elderly in Pomerania, Germany: Results of the study of health in Pomerania. Gerodontology. 2004;**21**(1):27-36

[86] Papapanou PN, Wennstrom JL. Radiographic and clinical assessments of destructive periodontal disease. Journal of Clinical Periodontology. 1989;**16**(9):609-612

[87] Loe H, Anerud A, Boysen H, Morrison E. Natural history of periodontal disease in man. Rapid, moderate and no loss of attachment in Sri Lankan laborers 14 to 46 years of age. Journal of Clinical Periodontology. 1986;**13**(5):431-445

[88] Miller PD Jr. Root coverage with the free gingival graft. Factors associated with incomplete coverage. Journal of Periodontology. 1987;**58**(10):674-681

[89] AlJehani Y. Risk factors of periodontal disease: Review of the literature. International journal of dentistry. 2014;**2014**:182513. DOI: 10.1155/2014/182513

[90] Mariotti A, Mawhinny M. Endocrinology of sex steroid hormones and cell dynamics in the periodontium. Periodontology 2000. 2013;**11**:69-88

[91] Jiang H, Su Y, Xiong X, et al. Prevalence and risk factors of periodontal disease among pre-conception Chinese women. *Reproductive Health*. 2016;**13**(1):141. Published 2016 Dec 1. DOI: 10.1186/s12978-016-0256-3

[92] Nesbitt MJ, Reynolds MA, Shiau H, et al. Association of periodontitis and metabolic syndrome in the Baltimore longitudinal study of aging. Aging Clinical and Experimental Research. 2010;**22**:238-242

[93] Haas AN, Wagner MC, Oppermann RV, Rösing CK, Albandar JM, Susin C. Risk factors for the progression of periodontal attachment loss: A 5-year population-based study in South Brazil. Journal of Clinical Periodontology. 2014;**41**:215-223. DOI: 10.1111/jcpe.12213

[94] Ozcaka O, Bicakci N, Pussinen P, Sorsa T, Kose T, Buduneli N. Smoking and matrix metallo proteinases, neutrophil elastase and myeloperoxidase in chronic periodontitis. Oral Diseases. 2011;**17**(1):68-76

[95] Slade GD, Spencer AJ. Periodontal attachment loss among adults aged 60+ in South Australia. Community Dentistry and Oral Epidemiology. 1995;**23**(4):237-242

[96] Albandar JM, Kingman A. Gingival recession, gingival bleeding, and dental calculus in adults 30 years of age and older in the United States, 1988-1994. Journal of Periodontology. 1999;**70**(1):30-43

[97] Vittek J, Hernandez MR, Wenk EJ, Rappaport SC, Southren AL. Specific estrogen receptors in human gingiva. The Journal of Clinical Endocrinology and Metabolism. 1982;**54**:608-612

[98] Vittek J, Hernandez MR, Wenk EJ, Rappaport SC, Southren AL. Binding of 3H-methyltrienolone (3H-R1881) to androgen receptors in human gingiva. Journal of Periodontal Research. 1985;**20**:41-46

[99] Weaker FJ, Sheridan PJ, Aufdemorte TB, Gages GA, Triplett RG. Nuclear uptake of progesterone in oral and laryngeal tissues. Experimental and Clinical Endocrinology. 1988;**7**:177-180

[100] El Attar TM, Hugoson A. The in vitro conversion of female sex steroid, oestrone, in normal and inflamed human gingiva. Archives of Oral Biology. 1974;**19**:425-429

[101] Mariotti A. Sex steroid hormones and cell dynamics in the periodontium.

Critical Reviews in Oral Biology and Medicine. 1994;**5**:27-53

[102] Nilsson S, Gustafsson JA. Estrogen receptors: Therapies targeted to receptor subtypes. Clinical Pharmacology and Therapeutics. 2011;**89**:44-55

[103] Ordonez-Moran P, Munoz A. Nuclear receptors: Genomic and nongenomic effects converge. Cell Cycle. 2009;**8**:1675-1680

[104] Lan NC, Chen JS, Belelli D, Pritchett DB, Seeburg PH, Gee KW. A steroid recognition site is functionally coupled to an expressed GABA (a)-benzodiazepine receptor. European Journal of Pharmacology. 1990;**188**:403-406

[105] Blackmore PF, Beebe SJ, Danforth DR, Alexander N. Progesterone and 17 alpha- hydroxyprogesterone. Novel stimulators of calcium influx in human sperm. The Journal of Biological Chemistry. 1990;**265**:1376-1380

[106] Koenig H, Fan CC, Goldstone AD, Lu CY, Trout JJ. Polyamines mediate androgenic stimulation of calcium fluxes and membrane transport in rat heart myocytes. Circulation Research. 1989;**64**:415-426

[107] Ojanotko-Harri A. Metabolism of progesterone by healthy and inflamed human gingiva in vitro. Journal of Steroid Biochemistry. 1985;**23**:1031-1035

[108] Vittek J, Rappaport SC, Gordon GG, Munnangi PR, Southren AL. Concentration of circulating hormones and metabolism of androgens by human gingiva. Journal of Periodontology. 1979;**50**:254-264

[109] Reynolds MA, Dawson DR, Novak KF, Ebersole JL, Gunsolley JC, Branch-Mays GTL, et al. Effects of caloric restriction on inflammatory periodontal disease. Nutrition. 2009;**25**:88-97

[110] Lafaurie GI, Contreras A, Baron A, Botero J, MayorgaFayad I, Jaramillo A, et al. Demographic, clinical, and microbial aspects of chronic and aggressive periodontitis in Colombia: A multicenter study. Journal of Periodontology. 2007;**78**(4):629-639

[111] Schenkein HA, Burmeister JA, Koertge TE, Brooks CN, Best AM, Moore LV, et al. The influence of race and gender on periodontal microflora. Journal of Periodontology. 1993;**64**:292296

[112] Kumar PS. Sex and the subgingival microbiome: Do female sex steroids affect periodontal bacteria? Periodontology 2000. 2013;**61**:103-124

[113] Kornman KS, Loesche WJ. Effects of estradiol and progesterone on Bacteroides melaninogenicus and Bacteroides gingivalis. Infection and Immunity. 1982;**35**:256-263

[114] Jensen J, Liljemark W, Bloomquist C. The effect of female sex hormones on subgingival plaque. Journal of Periodontology. 1981;**52**:599602

[115] Hugoson A. Gingivitis in pregnant women. A longitudinal clinical study. Odontologisk Revy. 1971;**22**:65-84

[116] Hugoson A, Lindhe J. Gingival tissue regeneration in female dogs treated with sex hormones histological observations. Odontologisk Revy. 1971;**22**:237-249

[117] Lindhe J, Attstrom R, Bjorn AL. Influence of sex hormones on gingival exudation in dogs with chronic gingivitis. Journal of Periodontal Research. 1968;**3**:279-283

[118] Lindhe J, Attstrom R, Bjorn AL. Influence of sex hormones on gingival exudation in gingivitis-free female dogs. Journal of Periodontal Research. 1968;**3**:273-278

[119] Arnal JF, Fontaine C, Billon-Gales A, Favre J, Laurell H, Lenfant F, et al. Estrogen receptors and endothelium. Arteriosclerosis, Thrombosis, and Vascular Biology. 2010;**30**:1506-1512

[120] Stice SL, Ford SP, Rosazza JP, Van Orden DE. Interaction of 4-hydroxylated estradiol and potential-sensitive Ca2+ channels in altering uterine blood flow during the estrous cycle and early pregnancy in gilts. Biology of Reproduction. 1987;**36**:369-375

[121] Bengtsson B. Estrogen induced inhibition of 3H-noradrenaline release in the uterus and portal vein of the rat. Acta Physiologica Scandinavica. 1978;**104**:287-298

[122] Hamlet MA, Rorie DK, Tyce GM. Effects of estradiol on release and disposition of norepinephrine from nerve endings. The American Journal of Physiology. 1980;**239**:450-456

[123] Colucci WS, Gimbrone MA Jr, McLaughlin MK, Halpern W, Alexander RW. Increased vascular catecholamine sensitivity and alpha-adrenergic receptor affinity in female and estrogen treated male rats. Circulation Research. 1982;**50**:805-811

[124] Hoffman BB, Lavin TN, Lefkowitz RJ, Ruffolo RR Jr. Alpha adrenergic receptor subtypes in rabbit uterus: Mediation of myometrial contraction and regulation by estrogens. The Journal of Pharmacology and Experimental Therapeutics. 1981;**219**:290-295

[125] Magness RR, Rosenfeld CR. In: Alexander NJ, d_Arcangues C, editors. Steroid Hormones Uterine Bleeding. Washington, DC: AAAS Press; 1992. pp. 107-120

[126] Losordo DW, Isner JM. Estrogen and angiogenesis: A review. Arteriosclerosis, Thrombosis, and Vascular Biology. 2001;**21**:6-12

[127] Mariotti A. The extracellular matrix of the periodontium: dynamic and interactive tissues. Periodontology 2000. 1993;**3**:39-63

[128] Mamalis A, Markopoulou C, Lagou A, Vrotsos I. Oestrogen regulates proliferation,osteoblasticdifferentiation, collagen synthesis and periostin gene expression in human periodontal ligament cells through oestrogen receptor beta. Archives of Oral Biology. 2011;**5**:446-455

[129] Richman MJ, Abarbanel AR. Effects of estradiol, testoterone, diethylstilbesteriol and several of their derivatives upon the human oral mucous membrane. Journal of the American Dental Association (1939). 1943;**30**:913-923

[130] Ziskin DE, Blackberg SN, Slanetz CA. Effects of subcutaneous injections of estrogenic and gonadotropic hormones on gums and oral mucous membranes of normal and castrated rhesus monkeys. Journal of Dental Research. 1935;**15**:407-428

[131] Trott JR. A histological investigation into the keratinisation found in human gingiva. British Dental Journal. 1957;**103**:421-427

[132] Shklar G, Chauncey HH, Shapiro S. The effect of testosterone on the periodontium of normal and hypophysectomized rats. Journal of Periodontology. 1967;**38**:203-210

[133] Ziskin DE. Effects of male sex hormone on gingivae and oral mucous membranes. Journal of Dental Research. 1941;**20**:419-423

[134] Canalis E, Raisz LG. Effect of sex steroids on bone collagen synthesis in vitro. Calcified Tissue Research. 1978;**25**:105-110

[135] Fukuda H. Experimental studies on the effect of sex hormones on the proliferation of cells derived from the

gingival tissue in culture. Shika Gakuho. 1971;**71**:1214-1232

[136] Mariotti AJ. Estrogen and extracellular matrix influence human gingival fibroblast proliferation and protein production. Journal of Periodontology. 2005;**76**:1391-1397

[137] Yokoyama M, Hinode D, Masuda K, Yoshioka M, Grenier D. Effect of female sex hormones on campylobacter rectus and human gingival fibroblasts. Oral Microbiology and Immunology. 2005;**20**:239-243

[138] Shu L, Guan SM, Fu SM, Guo T, Cao M, Ding Y. Estrogen modulates cytokine expression in human periodontal ligament cells. Journal of Dental Research. 2008;**87**:142-147

[139] Zhou Y, Fu Y, Li JP, Qi LY. The role of estrogen in osteogenetic cytokine expression in human periodontal ligament cells. The International Journal of Periodontics & Restorative Dentistry. 2009;**29**:507-513

[140] Natoli AK, Medley TL, Ahimastos AA, Drew BG, Thearle DJ, Dilley RJ, et al. Sex steroids modulate human aortic smooth muscle cell matrix protein deposition and matrix metalloproteinase expression. Hypertension. 2005;**46**:1129-1134

[141] Shiau HJ, Aichelmann-Reidym E, Reynolds MA. Influence of sex steroids on inflammation and bone metabolism. Periodontology 2000. 2014;**64**:81-94

[142] Ammann P, Rizzoli R, Bonjour JP, Bourrin S, Meyer JM, Vassalli P, et al. Transgenic mice expressing soluble tumor necrosis factor-receptor are protected against bone loss caused by estrogen deficiency. The Journal of Clinical Investigation. 1999;**99**:1699-1703

[143] Kimble RB, Bain S, Pacifici R. The functional block of TNF but not of IL-6 prevents bone loss in ovariectomized mice. Journal of Bone and Mineral Research. 1997;**12**:935-941

[144] Ralston SH. Analysis of gene expression in human bone biopsies by polymerase chain reaction: Evidence for enhanced cytokine expression in postmenopausal osteoporosis. Journal of Bone and Mineral Research. 1994;**9**:883-890

[145] Roggia C, Gao Y, Cenci S, Weitzmann MN, Toraldo G, Isaia G, et al. Up-regulation of TNF-producing T cells in the bone marrow: A key mechanism by which estrogen deficiency induces bone loss in vivo. Proc. Natl. Acad. Sci. USA. 2001;**98**:13960-13965

[146] Straub RH. The complex role of estrogens in inflammation. Endocrine Reviews. 2007;**28**:21-574

[147] Marriott I, Bost KL, Huet-Hudson YM. Sexual dimorphism in expression of receptors for bacterial lipopolysaccharides in murine macrophages: A possible mechanism for gender-based differences in endotoxic shock susceptibility. Journal of Reproductive Immunology. 2006;**71**:12-27

[148] Frisancho-Kiss S, Davis SE, Nyland JF, Frisancho JA, Cihakova D, Barrett MA, et al. Cutting edge: Crossregulation by TLR4 and T cell Ig mucin- 3 determines sex differences in inflammatory heart disease. Journal of Immunology. 2007;**178**:6710-6714

[149] Miller AP, Feng W, Xing D, Weathington NM, Blalock JE, Chen YF, et al. Estrogen modulates inflammatory mediator expression and neutrophil chemotaxis in injured arteries. Circulation. 2004;**110**:1664-1649

[150] Miyagi M, Aoyama H, Morishita M, Iwamoto Y. Effects of sex hormones on chemotaxis of human peripheral polymorphonuclear leukocytes and

monocytes. Journal of Periodontology. 1992;**63**:28-32

[151] Garcia-Duran M, de Frutos T, Dıaz-Recasens J, GarcíaGálvez G, Jiménez A, Montón M, et al. Estrogen stimulates neuronal nitric oxide synthase protein expression in human neutrophils. Circulation Research. 1999;**85**:1020-1026

[152] Stefano GB, Peter D. Cell surface estrogen receptors coupled to cNOS mediate immune and vascular tissue regulation: Therapeutic implications. Medical Science Monitor. 2001;**7**:1066-1074

[153] Verthelyi D. Sex hormones as immunomodulators in health and disease. International Immuno-pharmacology. 2001;**1**:983-993

[154] Latham KA, Zamora A, Drought H, Subramanian S, Matejuk A, Offner H, et al. Estradiol treatment redirects the isotype of the autoantibody response and prevents the development of autoimmune arthritis. Journal of Immunology. 2003;**171**:5820-5827

[155] Correale J, Arias M, Gilmore W. Steroid hormone regulation of cytokine secretion by proteolipid protein-specific CD4+ T cell clones isolated from multiple sclerosis patients and normal control subjects. Journal of Immunology. 1998;**161**:3365-3374

[156] Gilmore W, Weiner LP, Correale J. Effect of estradiol on cytokine secretion by proteolipid protein-specific T cell clones isolated from multiple sclerosis patients and normal control subjects. Journal of Immunology. 1997;**158**:446-451

[157] Mosmann TR, Schumacher JH, Street NF, Budd R, O'Garra A, Fong TA, et al. Diversity of cytokine synthesis and function of mouse CD4+ T cells. Immunological Reviews. 1991;**123**: 209-229

[158] Berghella AM, Contasta I, Del Beato T, Pellegrini P. The discovery of how gender influences age immunological mechanisms in health and disease, and the identification of ageing gender-specific biomarkers, could lead to specifically tailored treatment and ultimately improve therapeutic success rates. Immunity & Ageing. 2012:9-24

[159] Tai P, Wang JH, Song X, Yan J, Kang Y, Zhao L, et al. Induction of regulatory T cells by physiological level estrogen. Journal of Cellular Physiology. 2008;**214**:456-464

[160] Rook GA, Hernandez-Pando R, Lightman SL. Hormones, peripherally activated prohormones and regulation of the Th1/Th2 balance. Immunology Today. 1994;**15**:301-303

[161] McCarthy M. The "gender gap" in autoimmune disease. Lancet. 2000;**356**:1088

[162] Beageley KW, Gockel CM. Regulation of innate and adaptive immunity by the female sex hormones oestradiol and progesterone. FEMS ImmunolMed. Microbiol. 2003;**38**:13-22

[163] Schneider CA, Rasband WS, Eliceiri KW. NIH image to ImageJ: 25 years of image analysis. Nature Methods. 2012;**9**(7):671-675. DOI: 10.1038/nmeth.2089. PMC 5554542. PMID 22930834

[164] Collins TJ. ImageJ for microscopy. BioTechniques. 2007;**43**(1 Suppl): 25-30. DOI: 10.2144/000112517. PMID 17936939

[165] Furuta M, Shimazaki Y, Takeshita T, Shibata Y, Akifusa S, Eshima N, et al. Gender differences in the association between metabolic syndrome and periodontal disease: The Hisayama study. Journal of Clinical Periodontology. 2013;**40**:743-752. DOI: 10.1111/jcpe.12119

[166] Schulze A, Busse M. Gender differences in periodontal status and oral hygiene of non-diabetic and type 2 diabetic patients. *The Open Dentistry Journal*. 2016;**10**:287-297. Published 2016 Jun 9. DOI: 10.2174/1874210601610010287

[167] Caton J, Armitage G, Berglundh T, et al. A new classification scheme for periodontal and peri-implant diseases and conditions – Introduction and key changes from the 1999 classification. *Journal of Clinical Periodontology*, Suppl 20. 2018;**45**:S1-S8. DOI: 10.1111/jcpe.12935

[168] Wouters FR, Satonen LE, Helldën LB, Frithiof L. Prevalence of interproximal periodontal intrabony defects in an adult population in Sweden. Journal of Clinical Periodontology. 1989;**16**(3):144-149

[169] Wulandari P, Masulili SLC, Kusdhany LS, Tadjoedin FM, Puspitadewi SR, Baziad A. Differences in periodontal severity between perimenopausal and postmenopausal women with chronic periodontitis. Pesqui. Bras. Odontopediatria Clín. Integr. [Internet]. 2019;**19**:e5091

[170] Paramashivaiah R, Padmanabhan S, Dwarakanath CD, Ramesh AV. Periodontal status of postmenopausal women with osteoporosis. World Journal of Dentistry. 2011;**2**(4):297-301

[171] Lee Y, Kim I, Song J, Hwang KG, Choi B, Hwang SS. The relationship between hormone replacement therapy and periodontal disease in postmenopausal women: a cross-sectional study the Korea National Health and Nutrition Examination Survey from 2007 to 2012. BMC Oral health. 2019;**19**(1):151. Published 2019 Jul 15. DOI: 10.1186/s12903-019-0839-9

[172] Pizzo G, Guiglia R, Licata ME, Pizzo I, Davis JM, Giuliana G. Effect of hormone replacement therapy (HRT) on periodontal status of postmenopausal women. Medical Science Monitor. 2011;**17**(4):PH23-PH27

[173] López-Marcos JF, García-Valle S, García-Iglesias AA. Periodontal aspects in menopausal women undergoing hormone replacement therapy. Medicina Oral, Patología Oral y Cirugía Bucal. 2005;**10**(2):132-141

[174] Singh A, Sharma RK, Siwach RC, Tewari S, Narula SC. Association of bone mineral density with periodontal status in postmenopausal women. Journal of Investigative and Clinical Dentistry. 2014;**5**(4):275-282

[175] Richa RY, Puranik MP, Shrivastava A. Association between osteoporosis and periodontal disease among postmenopausal Indian women. Journal of Investigative and Clinical Dentistry. 2017;**8**(3). DOI: 10.1111/jicd.12223

[176] Nielsen IM, Glavind L, Karhing T. Interproximal periodontal intrabony defects. Journal of Clinical Periodontology. 1980;**7**(3):187-198

[177] Vandana KL, Nazam L, Pavagouda G, Kumar N. Radiographic evaluation of periodontal osseous defects-A retrospective study. Saudi Journal of Oral and Dental Research. 2017;**2**(1):18-21

[178] Zardawia FM, Aboud AN, Khursheed DA. A retrospective panoramic study for alveolar bone loss among young adults in Sulaimani City, Iraq. The Sulaimani Dental Journal. 2014;**1**:94-98

[179] Alwaeli HA, Al-Khateeb SN, Al-Sadi A. Long-term clinical effect of adjunctive antimicrobial photodynamic therapy in periodontal treatment: A randomized clinical trial. Lasers in Medical Science. 2015;**30**(2):801-807. DOI: 10.1007/s10103-013-1426-y

[180] Zhao H, Li C, Lin L, Pan Y, Wang H, Zhao J, et al. Assessment of alveolar bone status in middle aged Chinese (40-59 Years) with chronic periodontitis—using CBCT. PLoSONE. 2015;**10**(10):e0139553. DOI: 10.1371/journal.pone.0139553

[181] Bansal M, Mittal N, Singh TB. Assessment of the prevalence of periodontal diseases and treatment needs: A hospital-based study. Journal of Indian Society of Periodontology; 2015;**19**(2):211-215

[182] Marya CM, Grover HS, Tandon S, Taneja P, Gupta A, Marya V. Gender-wise comparison of oral health-related quality of life and its relationship with periodontal status among the Indian elderly. Journal of Indian Society of Periodontology; 2015;**24**(1):72-79

[183] Whitacre CC, Reingold SC, O'Looney PA. A gender gap in autoimmunity. Science. 1999;**283**: 1277-1278

[184] Jeffrey JY, Matthew J, Ruddy H, Conti R, Boonanantanasarn K, Gaffen SL. The interleukin-17 receptor plays a gender dependent role in host protection against *Porphyromonas gingivalis*-induced periodontal bone loss. Infection and Immunity. 2008:4206-4213

[185] Ioannidou E. The sex and gender intersection in chronic periodontitis. Frontiers in Public Health. 2017;**5**:189. DOI: 10.3389/fpubh.2017.00189

Section 2

Endodontics and Restorative Dentistry

Chapter 4

Regenerative Endodontic Procedure in Immature Permanent Teeth

Meshal G. Al-shammari

Abstract

This literature review will aim to recapitulate the different factors involved in the endodontic regenerative procedure, with a focus on different bacterial disinfecting techniques, intra-canal dressings and expected treatment outcomes. The electronic databases searched were EMBASE, MEDLINE and PUBMED. Articles included were limited to the English language from the year 1988 to May 2019. A hand search of the literature was also performed for articles dating back to 1958. No clear guidelines were available regarding follow-up and expected treatment outcomes in terms of success, survival (acceptable) or treatment failure. However, calcium hydroxide as an intra-canal medicament was found to be the best treatment modality in comparison to antibiotic paste for intra-canal dressing.

Keywords: regeneration, endodontics, dentistry, necrotic pulp

1. Introduction

It is widely recognised that full maturation of the root apex of permanent tooth is expected to occur three years after the time of eruption. During this period, an immature tooth may encounter situations such as traumatic injury, extensive caries and dental anomalies to the developing dentition, which in turn may lead to pulpal necrosis. This will hinder root maturation and will cause premature loss of the permanent dentition.

Necrotic immature teeth exhibit challenges for cleaning and shaping due to the presence of wide pulp canals, thin fragile walls and blunt root apices. In addition, it is difficult to obturate such a wide canals with large open apices to obtain hermetic apical seals.

At first, necrotic immature teeth were treated by calcium hydroxide apexification [1], which requires multiple visits to a clinic in order to change the calcium hydroxide dressing until a hard apical barrier is formed. However, long-term calcium hydroxide dressings will negatively affect the root canal dentine flexural strength and will make the tooth more susceptible to fracture [2, 4]. The apexification procedure was later modified by introducing an artificial hard barrier, Mineral Trioxide Aggregate (MTA) [3]. MTA apexification can be done in one or two sessions and provides a more reliable apical bacteria-tight seal. It also is biocompatible with periapical tissues and promotes hard tissue barrier formation [4]. However, MTA apexification does not induce root maturogensis, leaving the immature tooth with thin root walls that are susceptible to fracture. On the contrary, regenerative endodontic procedures can help stimulate the formation of a new pulp/dentin complex in the pulp canal space, which will put the tooth in a more favourable physiological status [5].

Regenerative endodontic procedure (REP) is a biologically based treatment that aims to heal periapical periodontitis and substitutes the damaged structure including dentin, cementum, and cells of pulp/dentin complex in order to continue the tooth-growing process. Although the histological characteristics of dentin/pulp tissues are not yet clear, radiographic evaluation has revealed a resolution of periapical lesions, an increase in root length to complete apical root formation, and a thickening of canal walls.

The idea of revitalization of lost tissues in the empty root canal was discussed first by Nyggard Ostby in 1961 [5]. He suggested that introducing a blood clot into the sterilized pulp canal would stimulate new tissue formation and heal the periapical pathosis. His hypothesis was based on the significance of blood clots in the healing of fractured bones [6].

In the histologic analysis, Ostby [5] noted connective tissue ingrowth inside the pulp canal, with scattered islands of mineralized tissue implanted into the newly formed connective tissue. In addition, the signs and symptoms of the necrotic teeth had disappeared and the apical radiolucency had healed. Although no odontoblasts were observed in the histological analysis and unwanted cells (cementoblast) were present, the presence of fibroblast and newly formed tissues was the foundation for regenerative endodontic treatment.

In 1971, Ostby and Hjortdal [7], published a case series of regenerative treatments, but they used antibiotics in the disinfection protocol. They observed an increase in root length, healing of periapical lesions, and a resolution of signs and symptoms.

The contemporary REP was first published in 2001 by Iwaya et al. [8]. In this case, the author reported on a necrotic immature premolar treated with sodium hypochlorite (NaOCl) and hydrogen peroxide (H_2O_2), then dressed with a double-antibiotic paste (DAP), which consist of metronidazole and ciprofloxacin **Figure 1**. This treatment protocol resulted in the resolution of inflammatory signs and symptoms, full root maturation and response to cold test. The second case by Banchs and Trope in 2004 [9] used NaOCl and chlorohexidine (CHX) to disinfect the canal

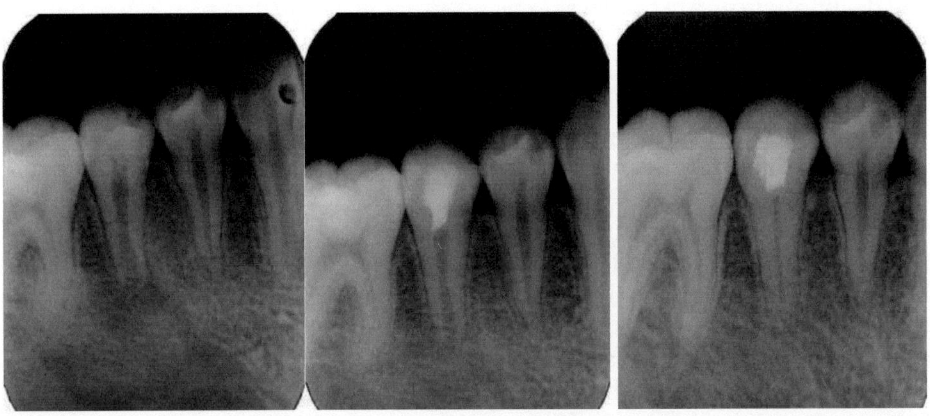

Figure 1.
On the left side, pre-operative radiograph of lower right 2nd premolar with open apex, incomplete root formation and periapical radiolucency. In the middle, radiograph taken after five months of calcium hydroxide dressing. On the right side, 35 months after treatment completion revealing complete root formation increase in root width and length [8].

chemically and employed a Triple Antibiotic Paste (TAP) containing metronidazole, ciprofloxacin, and minocycline, and observed the same result of Iwaya et al. [8].

These two cases established the fundamentals for the recent regenerative case reports. The fundamentals were the removal of bacteria and disinfecting the root canal; establishment of a scaffold; the introduction the stem cells for new tissue formation; and having a coronal bacterial tight seal to prevent recontamination of the root canal system.

Several terms had been used in case reports to describe the ingrowth of new tissue inside the root canal. These are revascularization, revitalization and regeneration. Revascularization is defined as the re-establishment of vascular supply to the already-present pulp of the immature tooth [10]. Revitalization is defined as the ingrowth of tissue that may differ from the initial original tissue [11]. Endodontic regeneration is defined as the replacement of lost or damaged structures including dentine, root structures and cells from pulp/dentin complex, by another structure [12].

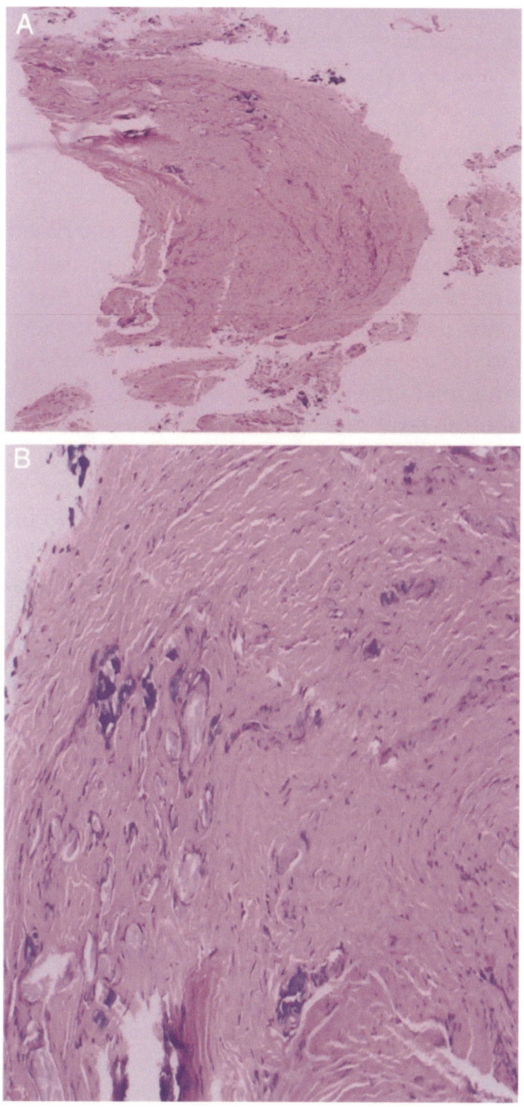

Figure 2.
(A) Pulp like connective tissue generated in human tooth after Regenerative Endodontic Therapy. (B) Higher magnification of the soft tissue showing the presence of collagen fibers, cells, and blood vessels in this tissue [13].

Lately, there have been two histological case reports of teeth extracted after having endodontic regenerative treatment [13, 14]. These studies gave a clearer idea of what was happening inside the canal after regeneration.

In the first histological case report [13], the tooth became painful and symptomatic 14 months after receiving regenerative treatment. When the pulp was extirpated and examined histologically, the author found a vital loose pulp-like connective tissue **Figure 2**.

In the second histological report [14], three and a half weeks after regenerative treatment was completed, the tooth had a complicated crown root fracture that left the remaining tooth structure beyond restoration. After extracting the tooth, the pulp canal content was examined histologically; the author reported the content of the pulp canal as a loose connective tissue, similar to pulp tissue, but histologically proven to be not pulpal tissue.

The histological findings of these two case reports did not provide sufficient evidence to represent all teeth that had undergone an endodontic regenerative procedure. However, the available findings suggest that tissue regeneration is occurring inside the root canal. Accordingly, endodontic regenerative procedure is the most relevant term to describe the type of tissue grows in the pulp canal.

2. Case selection

The regenerative endodontic procedure is a biologically based procedure in which good case selection will have an impact on the outcomes. The recent recommendations of the American Association of Endodontists (AAE) suggest that the regenerative endodontic procedure should be carried out in teeth with necrotic pulp and immature roots, and that the root canal space should not be utilized to retain a coronal restoration in the future. In other words, the selected tooth should have enough coronal tooth structure that it will need a post to retain the coronal core [15].

It would appear that the aetiology of pulp necrosis does not play a role in case selection here; many regenerative endodontic case studies did include necrotic immature teeth with different aetiologies, whether the pulp necrosis was caused by a caries lesion [16], was secondary to trauma [17] or due to dental anomalies [9].

In view of the fact that root canal space will be occupied by a blood clot and a bacterially tight hard barrier, teeth with insufficient remaining tooth structure are not recommended to be selected, since this would require further retentive means (post). In addition, in some cases, if the tooth structure loss is massive, isolation might become problematic. Patient and/or parental cooperation is necessary, as the treatment requires multiple visits and regular monitoring and follow-up appointments. Furthermore, the consent form must be signed.

The chances of success for teeth with immature root apices to be re-vascularized are significantly higher than for teeth with fully or nearly fully formed root apices. This could be attributed to the better ingrowth of vasculatures and stem cells flow in the pulp canal.

A study by Kling et al. [18] on re-implanted teeth noticed that teeth with apical foramen diameters of 1 mm or less had no chance of re-vascularization. In different circumstances, teeth with apical foramen diameters ranging from (1.1 mm - 5.0 mm) had spontaneously vascularized 18% of the time. They noticed also that when extra-oral time was under 45 minutes re-vascularization significantly increased; 39% of the teeth re-vascularized with shorter periods, compared to 11% only with longer periods ($P < 0.05$).

In addition, blood samples taken from incomplete root apices showed levels of CD 73 and CD 105 (Mesenchymal stem cell markers) almost 600 times higher than in samples obtained from the circulating blood stream, indicating the higher availability of stem cells in the apical dental papilla of immature roots [19].

Lovelace et al. did not obtain samples from mature roots for comparison. This could have produced similar results. However, the findings are supported by another study that apical papilla of the immature root apices represent a superior reliable source of stem cells that possess high surviving and cells turn over levels [20].

Immature roots with periapical pathosis of endodontic origin can undergo the regenerative endodontic procedure. Many published case reports have revealed potential root maturation in non-vital immature permanent teeth with the presence of periapical lesion or apical abscess [8, 9, 21, 22] that produced a complete resolution of the apical radiolucency in addition to a successful root maturation.

There are three possible explanations for this. The first is that immature roots with open apices allow easy communication between the root canal pulp and the periapical area. This may allow infection and inflammatory cells to reach the apex quickly while the pulp tissue is partially vital. In addition, the stem cells in the pulp and periapical papilla could survive the infection due to the high vascularity. Thus, the stem cells still can differentiate and allow root maturation in spite of the ongoing infection. The second explanation is that in young patients, the majority of the jawbone is cancellous and the bony trabeculations are larger. Therefore, resorption and periapical radiolucency may be formed in a short period and not all of the pulp tissues had turned necrotic [20]. Finally, the periapical radiolucency could be related to the apical dental papilla, where a radiolucent shadow of the dental papilla is expected and not necessarily to periapical pathology.

As a general statement, regenerative endodontic procedures should be performed if the patient is not allergic to any of the antibiotics or the medicament or irrigation agents that are usually used in sterilizing and dressing the canal in this procedure. In addition, patients should be classified as American Society of Anaesthesiologist (ASA) I or ASA II physical status. ASA I means that the patient is healthy and is a non-smoker, with no or minimal alcohol consumption. ASA II defined as with a mild disturbance without any significant functional limitations, for example if a person is fit and well but a smoker or social alcohol consumer. In addition, pregnancy, controlled Diabetes mellitus, and obesity (BMI over 30 and less than 40) all fall into ASA II classification.

This requirement is to ensure better tissue healing and a favourable response toward a stem cells differentiation, and thus continuation of root maturation without complication.

3. Endodontic regeneration in an infected root canal

Given the proper environment, many body tissues are programmed to regenerate new cells in order to compensate for lost ones; dental pulp tissue is no an exception. One of the most critical factors for regeneration is a bacteria-free root canal to allow stem cells to continue to regenerate and grow the root further into its full maturation without any damage.

Sterilizing an infected root canal can be sometimes quite challenging since roughly 20 different bacterial species can be found in an infected root canal with chronic apical periodontitis [23]. In addition, the root canal anatomy can provide a good sanctuary for the microbiota to thrive, containing places antimicrobial agents have difficulty reaching, for example accessory canals, isthmuses and fins.

Teeth can be subjected to many conditions in which lead to bacterial contamination of the root canal. The most prevalent are caries lesions, traumatic injuries and dental anomalies. Caries lesions can cause pulp exposure in teeth with immature apex, often in the permanent first molars. Permanent first molars erupt at an early age (6 to 7 years old), often when children are not sufficiently skilled in maintaining adequate oral hygiene on their own. This explains why caries is more prevalent in children who live in families of low socioeconomic status that have the inadequate oral hygiene and/or poor dietary habits that lead to early dental caries [24].

3.1 Sequelae of pulpal infection in immature root canal

Caries exposure related to vital pulp can present clinically with mild to moderate symptoms. In this case, vital pulp therapy like pulp capping [25] or pulpotomy [26, 27] using calcium hydroxide [$Ca(OH)_2$] or Mineral Trioxide Aggregate (MTA) would allow full root maturation. In spite of this treatment approach, usually the pulp goes necrotic and presents with asymptomatic or symptomatic apical periodontitis.

Periapical radiolucency of the dental follicle in immature teeth makes it hard to diagnose periapical periodontitis from dental radiographs. For this reason, apical periodontitis should be confirmed with clinical examinations such as cold tests, percussion, palpation, swelling and the presence of sinus tract. Once the pulp is confirmed to be necrotic in an immature tooth, a regenerative procedure may allow normal root maturation.

3.2 Dental anomalies that contribute to pathogenesis of pulp in immature teeth

Among congenital tooth anomalies, dens evaginatus is the most prevalent anomaly that causes early pulp devitalization and subsequent pulp necrosis in immature teeth [9, 28]. Dens evaginatus is a developmental anomaly causes a formation of accessory cusp (tubercle) project in the tooth surface. This tubercle consists of enamel, dentin and pulp tissues. With normal physiological tooth wear, the pulp gets exposed, leading to asymptomatic pulp necrosis in immature teeth [29]. Nevertheless, pulp exposure can be avoided if the tubercle is discovered early. Simple occlusal adjustment and topical fluoride application increases the enamel hydroxyapatite which contributes to enamel remineralization. Another treatment option would be the use of flowable composite resin sealant or in the case of pinpoint pulp exposure shallow pulpotomy using layer of tri calcium silicate cement (MTA, Biodentine®) or calcium hydroxide would be a conservative solution in case of dens evaginatus and thus avoid early pulp devitalization. Dens invaginatus is described as the folding of enamel into dentine which increases the risk of caries development and pulpal involvement. However, pulpal exposure can be avoided by simple preventive measures such as a fissure sealant.

4. Endodontic regeneration in traumatized teeth

Many studies have revealed some situations in which an immature root may regenerate pulpal tissue and dentine after trauma spontaneously. Kling et al. [30] monitored 154 replanted avulsed teeth (72 were immature teeth) radiographically for pulp revascularization.

In all mature teeth with apical foramen width 1 mm and smaller, revascularization did not occur, while 18% of the immature teeth (apical foramen width larger than 1.1 mm) revealed signs of revascularization. Instead, all teeth that did not respond to pulp revascularization revealed signs of periapical lesions and/or external resorption. Post-operative systemic antibiotics did not have any effect on the probability of pulp/dentine revascularization in replanted avulsed teeth in this study. The same result regarding post-operative systemic antibiotic use after avulsed teeth replantation was found in a later study by Andereason et al. [31]. Two types of hard tissue formation were found in teeth with revascularized pulp. There was either normal root maturation in both length and thickness of the root, or radiopaque material separated from the root and continued to grow with alveolar bone, while the tooth length arrested [32].

4.1 Effect of extra oral time of avulsed tooth on spontaneous regeneration

Extra-alveolar time can be defined as the time that the avulsed tooth spends out of its original socket. Andersson et al. [32] Found that extra-alveolar time of avulsed teeth was less than 45 minutes, the probability of revascularization was 39%, compared to 11% in teeth with extra-alveolar time more than 45 minutes. 60 minutes of extra-alveolar time can cause necrosis of the Periodontal Ligament (PDL) membrane and cells, which leads to external root resorption and the inhibition of further root development. When avulsed teeth are implanted immediately or within 15 minutes, no resorption was noted. In addition to this, after 15 minutes, replanted avulsed teeth revealed some root resorption but not in a progressive pattern [32]. Extra-alveolar time of less than 45 minutes shows better root formation and less inflammatory resorption when compared to times longer than 45 minutes. There was no significant difference in regeneration and subsequent root formation between different extra-alveolar storage media (dry medium, wet media [saliva, tab water, etc.], and combination medium [dry then wet]) for the avulsed tooth. Although it is not significant, a dry extra-alveolar time of less than 45 minutes led to more frequent root formation and completion [33].

For avulsed teeth kept in a wet storage media (saliva, tap water, etc.), the survival of the pulp is significantly greater when it is kept for less than 5 minutes. This is because only part of the pulp that communicates with the storage medium is the pulpal tissue in the apical foramen; the body of the root protects the rest of the pulp. However, if the apical foramen were to be contaminated with bacteria due a longer duration of storage, the vascularization process as a whole would be jeopardised [31].

The extent of root maturation is related to the pulp revascularization; in healing pulp, more root maturation is found compared to necrotic pulp. Immature roots with large apical foramen had more tendencies toward pulpal tissue regeneration; large apical foramen facilitates the flow of apical papilla stem cells into root canal easier than a mature, narrow apical foramen.

4.2 Factors that could contribute to REP in traumatized teeth

A factor that had a strong correlation with pulp regeneration in avulsed teeth is the length of the pulp canal (the distance between the apical foramen and pulp chamber). Since pulp regeneration may be arrested by infection process, the longer the distance to be regenerated, the more chances there are of an infection occurring, and thus less chance for the pulp to regenerate [34]. The correlation between the length of the pulp canal and the probabilities of pulp revascularization has also been found in another study of revascularization of auto-transplanted 370 premolars [35].

Partial or arrested root formation is generally followed by bone ingrowth and formation of internal PDL tissues. Hertwig's epithelial root sheath (HERS) is presumed to prevent the invasion of bone and PDL derived cells inside the canal and thus reduce disturbance to root development. This presumption is explained by a partial or total loss of HERS being accompanied by partial or arrested root development. In case of pulpal necrosis, root development and maturation may occur because HERS can tolerate trauma to avulsed tooth and damage by extra-alveolar time [33].

The predominant root resorption found in replanted avulsed teeth is external replacement resorption (Ankylosis), followed by inflammatory root resorption and finally, external inflammatory surface resorption. Inflammatory root resorption is most common in immature roots, while replacement resorption (ankyloses) is found more in mature roots [36]. Although bone remodelling is higher in young adolescents, rate of resorption in general is not affected by age. However, if the HERS and PDL are viable, age would not make a difference in the rate of resorption. In addition, Root Canal Treatment within the first three weeks (usually the third week) after tooth replantation can reduce the rate of resorption [32].

5. Follow up

In follow-up visits, clinical and radiographic outcomes should be evaluated. Clinical evaluation includes absence of pain on percussion and palpation, no presence of soft tissue swelling and disappearing of sinus tract if present before treatment. The tooth response to sensibility tests (cold and EPT) should be recorded, but the absence of response does not indicate treatment failure. Radiographic evaluation includes: resolution of pre-treatment periapical radiolucency if it was present, further root length maturation and an increase in canal wall thickness.

There is no standard follow-up protocol after endodontic regenerative procedures as of yet. Nevertheless, in the published endodontic regenerative case reports, the follow-up ranged from 6 months [37] up to 60 months [38] after completing treatment. The European Society of Endodontology recommends follow-up and recall appointments every 3, 6, 12, 18 and 24 months, with annual recall after the follow-up period for the next 5 years [39].

In most endodontic regenerative cases, enhancement or resolution of periapical lesion is expected in the first 6 months. Wiggler et al. [40] endorse a recall every three months in the first year after completion of treatment and then every six months, unless symptoms developed.

6. Conclusions

In conclusion, regenerative endodontic procedure is a non-invasive treatment that restores the dentin/pulp complex in necrotic immature teeth, and is now an essential part of the endodontic speciality. In many case reports it shows a promising potential for saving necrotic immature teeth and helping the continuation of root maturation. Unlike conventional MTA or calcium hydroxide apexification, it tends to promote further root development and increases root canal wall thickness, which will improve the overall survival of the tooth.

Author details

Meshal G. Al-shammari
Magrabi Dental Centers, Riyadh, Kingdom of Saudi Arabia

*Address all correspondence to: meshal.alshammari@outlook.com

References

[1] *Treatment of non-vital permanent incisors with calcium hydroxide. I. Follow-up of periapical repair and apical closure of immature roots.* **Cvek, M.** 1, 1972, Odontol Revy, Vol. 23, pp. 27-44.

[2] *Prognosis of luxated non-vital maxillary incisors treated with calcium hydroxide and filled with gutta-percha. A retrospective clinical study.* **Cvek, M.** 2, 1992, Endod Dent Traumatol, Vol. 8, pp. 45-55.

[3] *Clinical applications of Mineral Trioxide Aggregate.* **Torabinejad, M. and N. Chivian.** 3, 1999, J Endod, Vol. 25, pp. 197-205.

[4] *Mineral Trioxide Aggregate: a comperhensive literature review-part II: leakage and biocompatibility investigatios.* **Torabinejad, M. and M. Parirokh.** 36, 2010, J Endod, Vol. 2, pp. 190-202.

[5] *the role of the blood clot in endodontic therapy. An experimental histologic study.* **Ostby, B.N.** 1961, Acta Odontol Scand, Vol. 19, pp. 324-353.

[6] **Weinmann, J.** Bone and bones. *Fundamentals of bone biology.* 1955, pp. 18-139.

[7] *Tissue formation in the root canal following pulp removal.* **Nygaard-Ostby, B. and O. Hjortdal.** 5, 1971, Scand J Dent Res, Vol. 79, pp. 333-349.

[8] *Revascularization of an immature permanent tooth with apical periodontitis and sinus tract.* **Iwaya, S.I., M. Ikawa, and M. Kubota.** 4, 2001, Dent Traumatol, Vol. 17, pp. 185-187.

[9] *Revascularization of immature permanent teeth with apical periodontitis: new treatment protocol?* **Banchs, F. and M. Trope.** 4, 2004, J Endod, Vol. 30, pp. 196-200.

[10] **Andreasen, F.M.** Root Fractures. *Textbook and color atlas of traumatic injuries to the teeth.* 1994, pp. 297-314.

[11] *Histologic characterization of regenerated tissues in canal space after the revitalization/revascularization procedure of immature dog teeth with apical periodontitis.* **Wang, X., et al.** 1, 2010, J Endod, Vol. 36, pp. 56-63.

[12] *Regenerative endodontics: a review of current status and a call for action.* **Murray, P.E., F. Garcia-Godoy, and K.M. Hargreaves.** 4, 2007, J Endod, Vol. 33, pp. 377-90.

[13] *A clinical and histological report of a tooth with an open apex treated with regenerative endodontics using platelet-rich plasma.* **Torabinejad, M. and H. Faras.** 6, 2012, J Endod, Vol. 38, pp. 864-8.

[14] *Histologic observation of a human immature permanent tooth with irreversible pulpitis after revascularization/regeneration procedure.* **Shimizu, E., et al.** 9, 2012, J Endod, Vol. 38, pp. 1293-7.

[15] **Endodontics, American Association of.** *AAE Clinical Considerations for a Regenerative Procedure.* 2016.

[16] *Regenerative endodontic treatment (revascularization) for necrotic immature permanent molars: a review and report of two cases with a new biomaterial.* **Nosrat, A., A. Seifi, and S. Asgary.** 4, 2011, J Endod, Vol. 37, pp. 562-7.

[17] *Revascularization of necrotic pulp of immature teeth with apical periodontitis.* **Petrino, J.A.** 3, 2007, Northwest Dent, Vol. 86, pp. 33-5.

[18] *Rate and predictability of pulp revascularization in therapeutically reimplanted permanent incisors.* **Kling, M., M. Cvek, and I. Mejare.** 3, 1986, Endod Dent Traumatol, Vol. 2, pp. 83-9.

[19] *Evaluation of the delivery of mesenchymal stem cells into the root canal*

space of necrotic immature teeth after clinical regenerative endodontic procedure. **Lovelace, T.W., et al.** 2, 2011, J Endod, Vol. 37, pp. 133-8.

[20] *The hidden treasure in apical papilla: the potential role in pulp/dentin regeneration and bioroot engineering.* **Huang, G.T., et al.** 6, 2008, J Endod, Vol. 34, pp. 645-51.

[21] *Immature teeth with periradicular periodontitis or abscess undergoing apexogenesis: a paradigm shift.* **Chueh, L.H. and G.T. Huang.** 12, 2006, J Endod, Vol. 32, pp. 1205-13.

[22] *Regenerative treatment of an immature, traumatized tooth with apical periodontitis: report of a case.* **Cotti, E., M. Mereu, and D. Lusso.** 5, 2008, J Endod, Vol. 34, pp. 611-6.

[23] *Root canal microbiota of teeth with chronic apical periodontitis.* **Rocas, I.N. and J.F. Siqueira, Jr.** 11, 2008, J Clin Microbiol, Vol. 46, pp. 3599-606.

[24] *Determinants of early childhood caries in low-income African American young children.* **Ismail, A.I., et al.** 4, 2008, Pediatr Dent, Vol. 30, pp. 289-96.

[25] *Direct pulp capping with mineral trioxide aggregate: an observational study.* **Bogen, G., J.S. Kim, and L.K. Bakland.** 3, 2008, J Am Dent Assoc, Vol. 139, pp. 305-15.

[26] *Comparison of mineral trioxide aggregate and calcium hydroxide as pulpotomy agents in young permanent teeth (apexogenesis).* **El-Meligy, O.A. and D.R. Avery.** 5, 2006, Pediatr Dent, Vol. 28, pp. 399-404.

[27] *Mineral trioxide aggregate pulpotomies: a case series outcomes assessment.* **Witherspoon, D.E., J.C. Small, and G.Z. Harris.** 5, 2006, J Am Dent Assoc, Vol. 137, pp. 610-8.

[28] *Challenges in regenerative endodontics: a case series.* **Petrino, J.A., et al.** 3, 2010, J Endod, Vol. 36, pp. 536-41.

[29] *Dens evaginatus: literature review, pathophysiology, and comprehensive treatment regimen.* **Levitan, M.E. and V.T. Himel.** 1, 2006, J Endod, Vol. 32, pp. 1-9.

[30] *Rate and Predictability of Pulp Revascularization in Therapeutically Reimplanted Teeth.* **Kling, M., I. Mejare, and M. Cvek.** 4, 1983, Journal of Dental Research, Vol. 62, pp. 486-486.

[31] *Replantation of 400 avulsed permanent incisors. 2. Factors related to pulpal healing.* **Andreasen, J.O., et al.** 2, 1995, Endod Dent Traumatol, Vol. 11, pp. 59-68.

[32] *Avulsed human teeth replanted within 15 minutes--a long-term clinical follow-up study.* **Andersson, L. and I. Bodin.** 1, 1990, Endod Dent Traumatol, Vol. 6, pp. 37-42.

[33] *Replantation of 400 avulsed permanent incisors. 3. Factors related to root growth.* **Andreasen, J.O., M.K. Borum, and F.M. Andreasen.** 2, 1995, Endod Dent Traumatol, Vol. 11, pp. 69-75.

[34] *Pulp revascularization in reimplanted immature monkey incisors--predictability and the effect of antibiotic systemic prophylaxis.* **Cvek, M., et al.** 4, 1990, Endod Dent Traumatol, Vol. 6, pp. 157-69.

[35] *A long-term study of 370 autotransplanted premolars. Part II. Tooth survival and pulp healing subsequent to transplantation.* **Andreasen, J.O., et al.** 1, 1990, Eur J Orthod, Vol. 12, pp. 14-24.

[36] *Replantation of 400 avulsed permanent incisors. 1. Diagnosis of healing complications.* **Andreasen, J.O., et al.** 2, 1995, Endod Dent Traumatol, Vol. 11, pp. 51-8.

[37] *Mahidol study 1: comparison of radiographic and survival outcomes of immature teeth treated with either regenerative endodontic or apexification methods: a retrospective study.* **Jeeruphan, T., et al.** 10, 2012, J Endod, Vol. 38, pp. 1330-6.

[38] *Biologically based treatment of immature permanent teeth with pulpal necrosis: a case series.* **Jung, I.Y., S.J. Lee, and K.M. Hargreaves.** 7, 2008, J Endod, Vol. 34, pp. 876-87.

[39] *European Society of Endodontology position statement: Revitalization procedures.* **Galler, K.M., et al.** 8, 2016, Int Endod J, Vol. 49, pp. 717-23.

[40] *Revascularization: a treatment for permanent teeth with necrotic pulp and incomplete root development.* **Wigler, R., et al.** 3, 2013, J Endod, Vol. 39, pp. 319-26.

Chapter 5

Regeneration of Dentin Using Stem Cells Present in the Pulp

Toshiyuki Kawakami, Kiyofumi Takabatake, Hotaka Kawai, Keisuke Nakano, Hidetsugu Tsujigiwa and Hitoshi Nagatsuka

Abstract

Dentin is one of the major hard tissues of the teeth. Dentin is similar to bone in texture, but it is different from bone tissue histologically. It is formed by odontoblasts; however, these cells are present in a limited area in the human body and are not found anywhere other than the dental pulp. It is difficult to collect and proliferate mature odontoblasts for regenerative medicine. However, odontoblast are necessary for regenerating dentin. It is known that odontoblasts differentiate from mesenchymal stem cells in the dental pulp during tooth development. Dentin can be generated using the stem cells present in the pulp. Many stem cells are recruited from the bone marrow to the teeth, and it is possible that the stem cells present in the pulp are also supplied from the bone marrow. Herein, we explain the mechanism of stem cell supply to the teeth and the possibility of dentin regeneration by specific cell differentiation induction methods.

Keywords: dental pulp cell, odontoblast, bone marrow-derived cell, mesenchymal stem cell, differentiation induction

1. Introduction

Stem cells have the special property of differentiating into different types of cells. In the human body, stem cells are present in organs with a high regenerative and proliferative ability. Bone marrow is an organ that supplies blood cells throughout the body. The bone marrow is also rich in stem cells. The special nature of stem cells in the bone marrow is that they can migrate to all tissues throughout the body. Bone marrow-derived cells (BMDCs) that appear in peripheral tissues have the characteristics of stem cells and show multiple differentiation. Recently, many researchers have shown that BMDCs may differentiate into a variety of organs, including skeletal muscle, hepatocytes, neurons, myocardium, mucosal epithelial cells, and blood vessels [1, 2]. This is an important fact because such cells can be used to regenerate organs for treating various diseases [3]. The local supply and delivery of BMDCs has been extensively studied for treating ischemic diseases, including peripheral tissue ischemia and myocardial infarction, and has been attempted as a therapeutic tool [4, 5].

In previous studies, we used bone marrow transplant animal models in which bone marrow cells were transplanted from green fluorescent protein (GFP) transgenic mice to investigate the ability of BMDCs to be distributed and differentiated in the bones and teeth. GFP-positive cells were observed diffusely in the pulp and periodontal ligament of mouse incisors, Langerhans cells in the oral epithelium, stromal fibroblasts, blood vessels, and osteoclasts in the tooth area [6]. Tissue stem cell differentiation is triggered by a variety of stimuli. We have shown previously that orthodontic mechanical stress and artificial inflammation stimulate the cells of the periodontium and dental pulp to express various cell differentiation factors. The osteoblast marker alkaline phosphatase (ALP), runt-related transcription factor 2 (Runx2), which induces osteoblast differentiation, and heat shock proteins (HSPs), which are involved in homeostasis and cell differentiation, may be strongly expressed in cells exposed to injurious stimuli [7–12]. Moreover, periodontal tissue and dental pulp respond to mechanical stresses and inflammation, causing periodontal tissue remodeling and expression of cell differentiation-related factors [13]. Furthermore, orthodontic mechanical stress on the periodontium causes activation of hard tissue-forming cells in the pulp tissue [10, 11]. This indicates the potential of dental pulp stem cells to differentiate into hard tissue-forming cells upon stimulation. Moreover, mechanical stress and inflammation on the periodontal tissue affect the local recruitment of BMDCs [13, 14].

Recently, dental pulp has been proposed as a promising source of pluripotent mesenchymal stem cells for use in a variety of clinical applications. We isolated stem cells from the pulp, which is rich in BMDCs. The isolation and culture of dental pulp cells is an important factor. We attempted to establish cells that induce dentin-like hard tissue from the cells present in rat dental pulp and succeeded in establishing cells that resemble odontoblasts under *in vitro* conditions. These cells were named as the tooth matrix-forming GFP rat-derived cells (TGCs). The TGCs were maintained in cultures over 80 passages without showing any changes in morphology or properties. Physiological dentin has a characteristic structure, which is derived from the cell polarity of odontoblasts. However, the TGCs form dentin-like hard tissue under *in vivo* conditions but do not lead to the induction of polarized odontoblasts. Conversely, the geometric structure of biomaterials is considered important for inducing cell differentiation and tissue formation. Focusing on the importance of the geometry of artificial biomaterials in inducing cell differentiation and hard tissue formation, we have already succeeded in developing new honeycomb tricalcium phosphate (TCP) structures with holes of various diameters. We used the honeycomb TCP as a scaffold to induce TGCs into odontoblasts for the purpose of inducing odontoblasts with cell polarity [15].

2. Recruitment of BMDCs to periodontal tissue and dental pulp

Caries are a major cause of pulpitis. When the tooth crown is destroyed by caries, the pulp cavity is perforated. High proliferative activity of the pulpal tissue results in chronic inflammatory hyperplasia [16]. Granulation tissue grows from the pulp and forms periodontal polyps that can grow from inside the pulp cavity to outside the pulp. Experimental histopathological studies have long been performed on periodontal polyps, including histological analysis and treatment [17–20]. However, there is a lack of knowledge about the origin of the cells present in the pulp. As a result, using an experimental system of GFP mouse bone marrow transplantation, this study revealed that the cells were derived from bone marrow mesenchymal cells. Our research group used an experimental system of GFP bone marrow transplanted mice to study the migration and differentiation of cells in different parts of the oral cavity and teeth. Muraoka et al. showed that the BMDCs migrate to periodontal tissue and differentiate into periodontal ligament cells, such as macrophages and osteoclasts [21]. Tomida et al. showed the pluripotency of BMDCs, which migrated to periodontium, after the application of orthodontic mechanical stress loading [13]. Kaneko et al. also reported the differentiation of BMDCs into cell components of periodontal tissue [14]. In our study, the method suggested by Osuga et al. [22] was used for the formation of granulation tissue through chronic inflammation in the dental pulp of GFP bone marrow transplanted mice [16]. Observations by micro-computed tomography (m-CT) [23, 24], histopathology, and immunohistochemistry were followed over time. Immunohistochemistry revealed notable results. Oka et al. used rats to observe periodontal tissue reactions in the tooth roots associated with dental pulp perforation [17]. In a similar study, Imaizumi et al. examined the spread of inflammatory lesions in the periodontal ligament [18]. Other experiments have shown the formation of inflammatory lesions in the pulp because of perforation of the pulp cavity, examining the types of cells that appear with inflammation and the evolution of the inflammatory state [19, 20]. A detailed histopathological examination by Nakamura et al. showed continuous granulation tissue growth in the pulp [25]. Thus, periodontal polyps are considered suitable for observing cell dynamics in the regeneration and repair of dental pulp tissue. The focus of previous studies was on histopathological examination, and the origin of the cellular components of pulp granulation tissue was not mentioned. Recently, it has been widely reported that mesenchymal stem cells derived from bone marrow migrate to various organs and play a role in tissue formation. To histologically examine the *in vivo* recruitment of bone marrow-derived undifferentiated mesenchymal cells, these cells need to be marked. GFP transgenic mice express GFP in all cells of the body. Therefore, in wild-type mice transplanted with GFP mouse bone marrow, it is possible to trace BMDCs using GFP as a marker [26, 27]. We used an experimental system using GFP bone marrow transplanted mice to perforate the pulp cavity of the maxillary left first molar and induce pulpitis. With the development of pulpitis, the origin of the cellular components involved in the growth of periodontal polyps was investigated.

The periodontal polyp model used in our experiment was based on Osuga's method [22]. Anesthetized GFP bone marrow transplanted mice were secured to the plate, and a hole was made in the crown of the maxillary left first molar using a dental cutting device. Thereafter, the pulp was histologically observed over time for 2 weeks, 1 month, 3 months, and 6 months.

At 2 weeks, granulation tissue proliferation with neutrophil infiltration occurred just below the pulpal perforation. Round to short oval cells appeared around the granulation tissue. The granulation tissue was composed of fibroblast-like cells, capillaries, and chronic inflammatory cells (**Figure 1**). Immunohistochemical examination of GFP revealed that GFP-positive cells made up the majority of the small oval cells that emerged around the granulation tissue. A small number of fibroblasts also showed a GFP-positive reaction (**Figure 1-d**).

At 1 month, the granulation tissue that proliferated in the pulp cavity increased. The number of short oval cells increased around the granulation tissue, and the number of fibroblasts and capillaries, which are the cellular components that make up the granulation tissue, also increased (**Figure 2**). Compared to the tissue at 2 weeks, the total number of GFP-positive cells increased. Most of the GFP-positive reactions occurred in small oval cells. However, the number of positive reactions in fibroblasts also increased (**Figure 2-d**).

At 3 months, the number of fibroblasts in the granulation tissue increased the most, and collagen fiber proliferation was also apparent. The number of capillaries also increased the most. Conversely, the number of small oval cells decreased (**Figure 3**). The number of GFP-positive cells in the tissue was the highest, with positive reactions occurring in small oval cells and fibroblasts (**Figure 3-d**).

At 6 months, the continuous growth of granulation tissue resulted in an increase in mature fibroblasts and collagen fibers. However, inflammatory cells, capillaries,

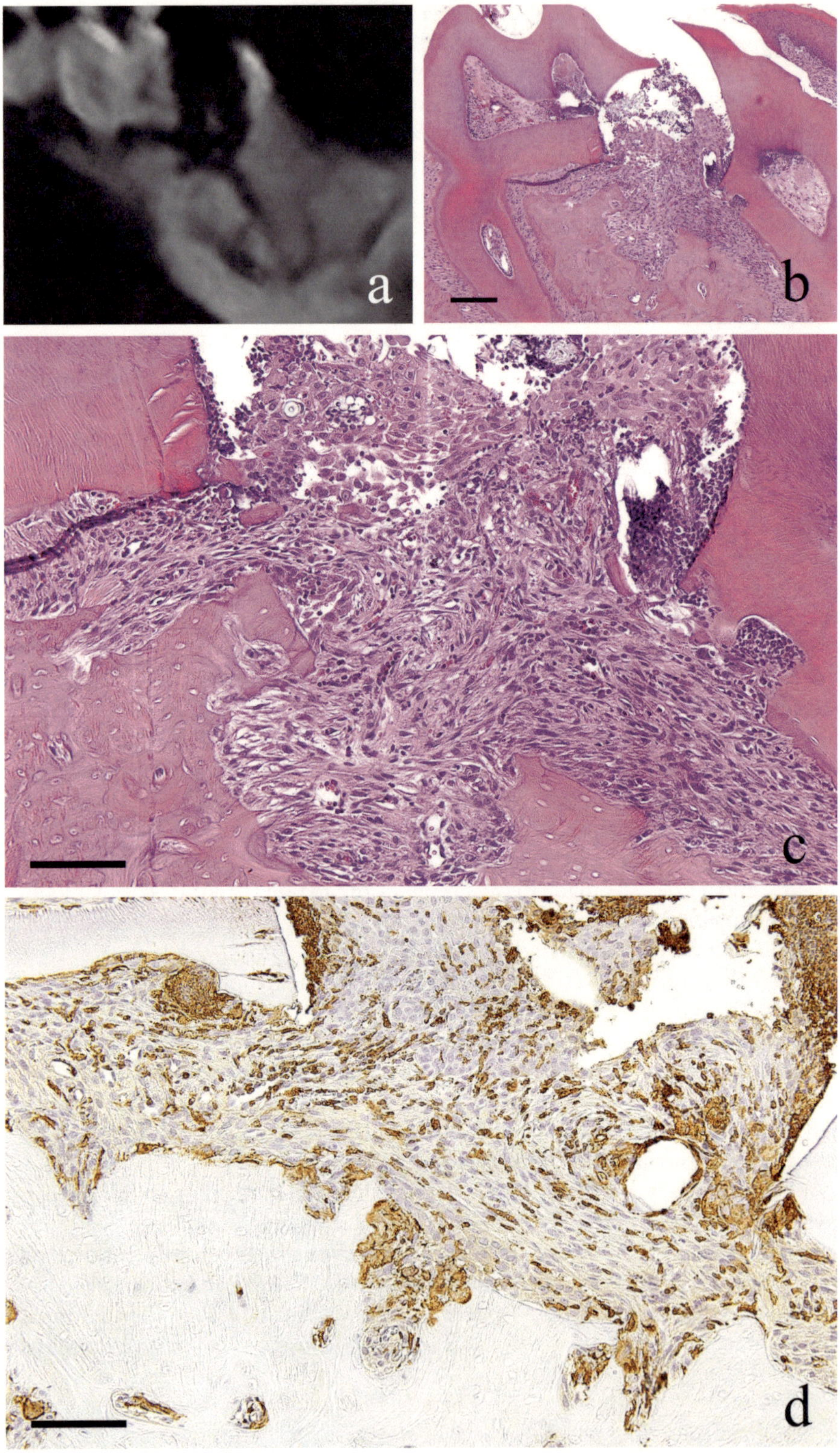

Figure 1.
2-week-specimen. a: m_CT image; b: Histopathological view of the same part of a, Scale bar = 200 μm; c: Enlarged view of b, Scale bar = 100 μm; d: IHC for GFP, Scale bar = 100 μm.

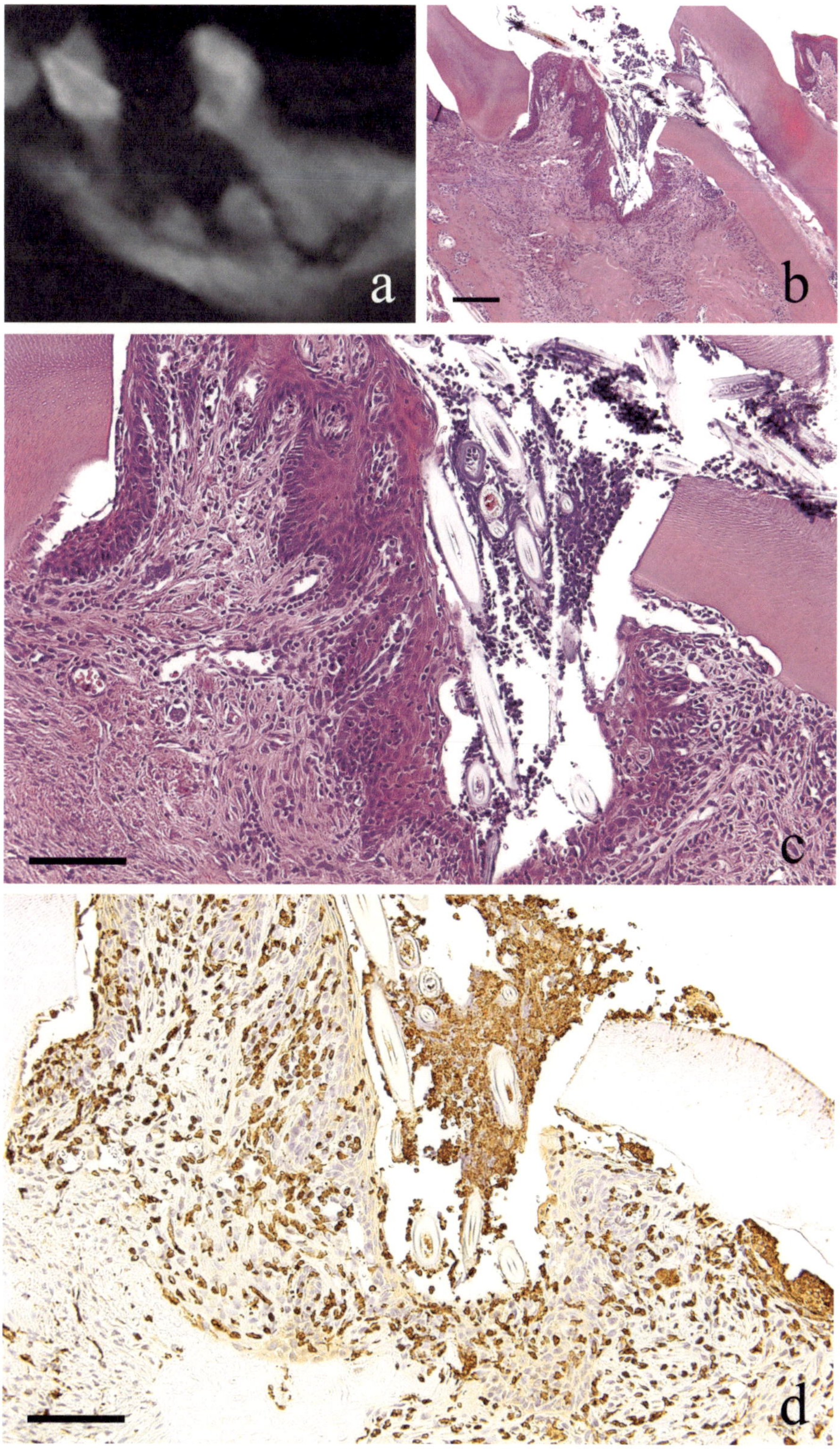

Figure 2.
1-month-specimen. A: m_CT image; b: Histopathological view of the same part of a, scale bar = 200 μm; c: Enlarged view of b, scale bar = 100 μm; d: IHC for GFP, scale bar = 100 μm.

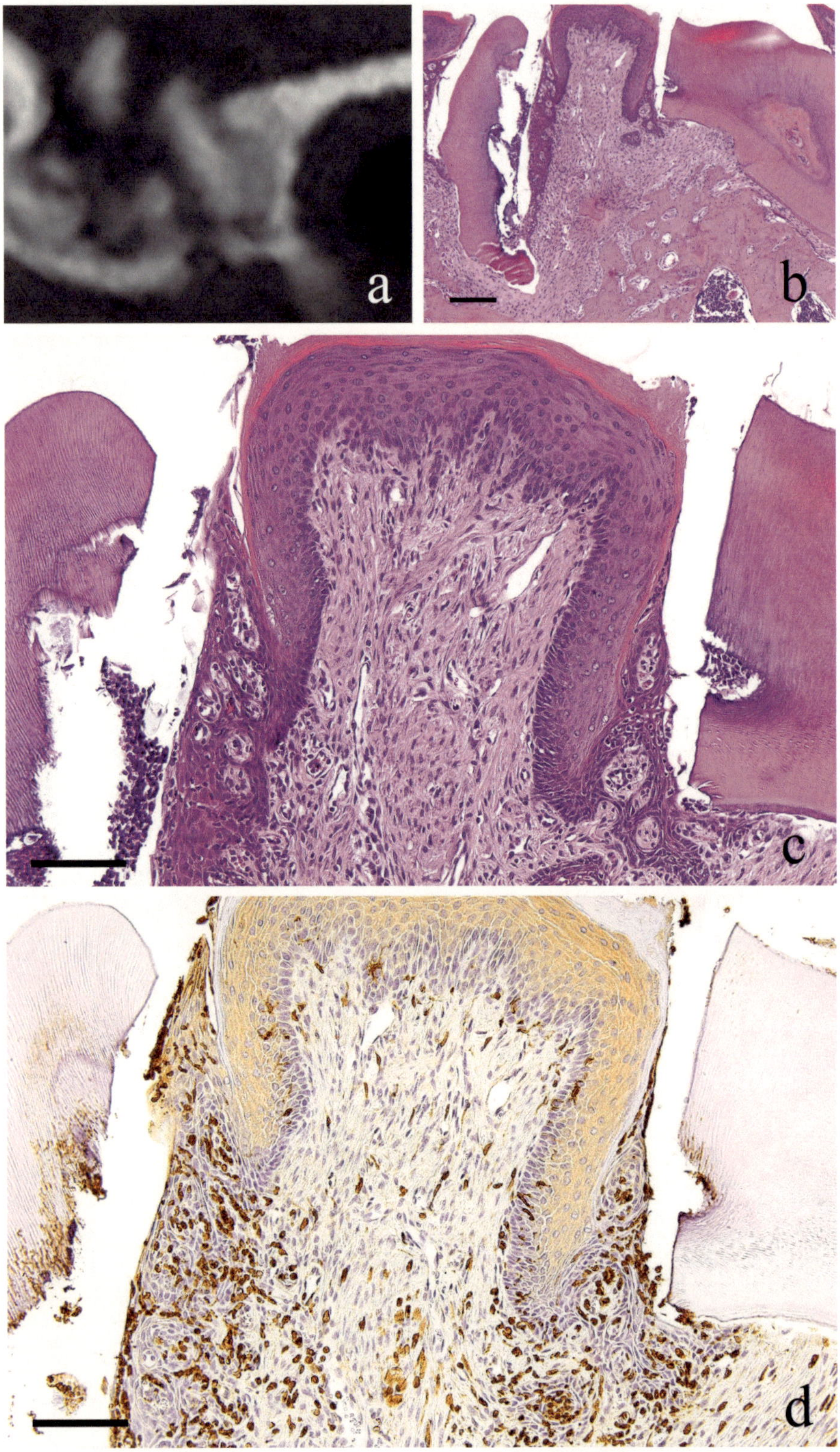

Figure 3.
3-month-specimen. A: m_CT image; b: Histopathological view of the same part of a, scale bar = 200 μm; c: Enlarged view of b, scale bar = 100 μm; d: IHC for GFP, scale bar = 100 μm.

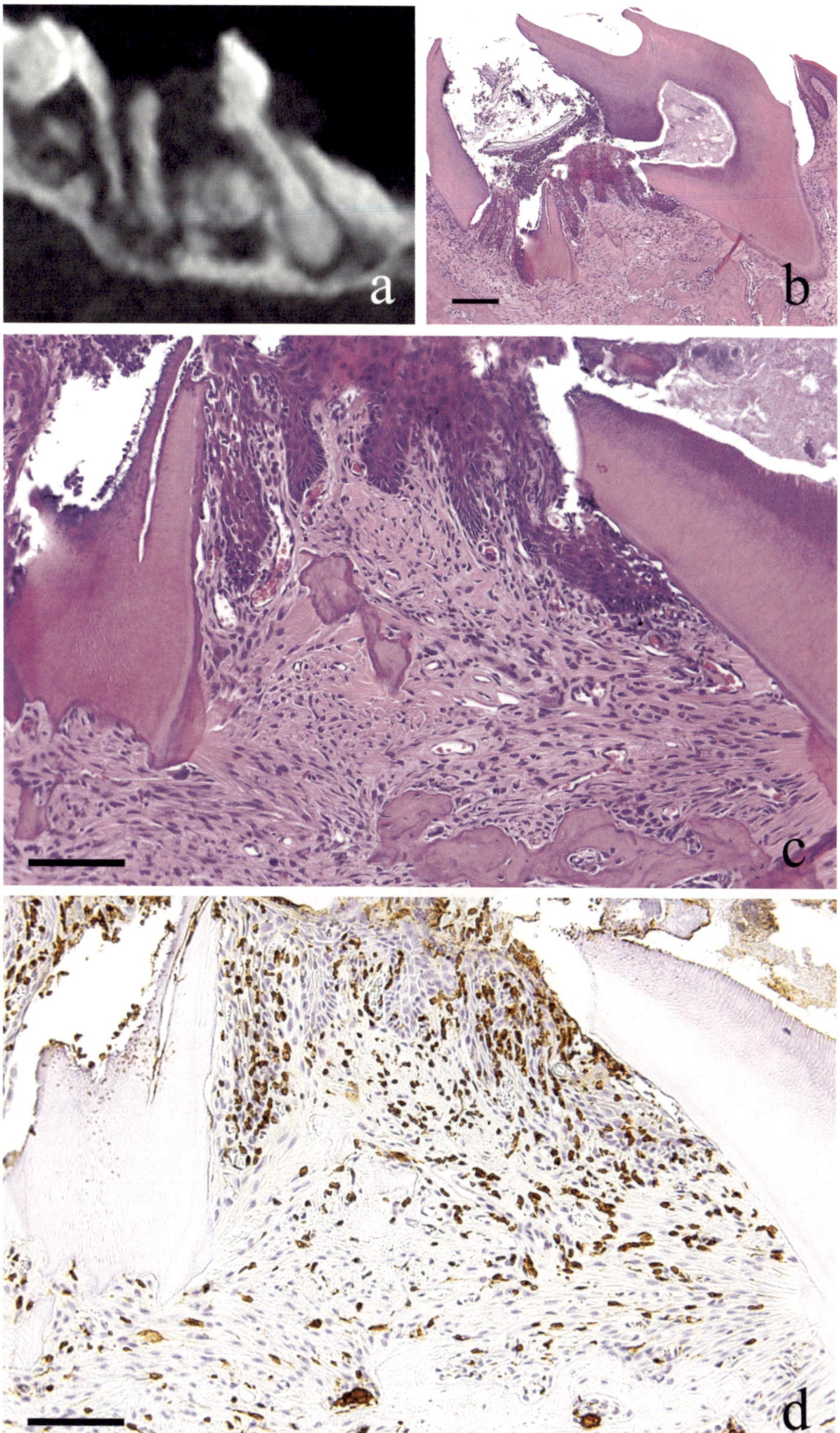

Figure 4.
6-month-specimen. A: m_CT image; b: Histopathological view of the same part of a, scale bar = 200 μm; c: Enlarged view of b, scale bar = 100 μm; d: IHC for GFP, scale bar = 100 μm.

and small oval cells decreased (**Figure 4**). The number of GFP-positive cells was reduced compared to that in the tissue at 3 months. However, many GFP-positive reactions appeared in the cells of mature granulation tissue.

A large number of GFP-positive cells appeared in periodontal polyps. Most of the positive cells were small oval cells. Over time, the number of GFP-positive fibroblasts increased. Therefore, these GFP-positive cells were derived from transplanted bone marrow cells. These GFP-positive cells were undifferentiated mesenchymal cells that migrated from the bone marrow to the pulp. From this, it was shown that the pulp has the potential to supply a large amount of BMDCs.

3. Cell differentiation of BMDCs recruited to the dental pulp

It is known that dental pulp tissue receives various stimuli even under physiological conditions. As a result, degenerative changes, such as atrophy are induced in the dental pulp cells. Moreover, activation of odontoblasts occurs because of stimulation, and new dentin is formed [28]. Histopathological investigations have been performed for a long time on the changes in dental pulp cells caused by stimulation [29]. Since external mechanical stress is applied to the pulp tissue even during orthodontic tooth movement, tissue changes in the pulp have been investigated experimentally [30–32]. Some studies have been performed using electron microscopy [33]. However, previous studies of dental pulp cell differentiation have not considered the presence of BMDCs in the pulp. Recently, many findings have been clarified regarding the factors that control cell differentiation regulation, and factors related to the differentiation of hard tissue cells, such as osteoblasts, have also been investigated. Sigehara et al. reported the gene expression status of osteocalcin, osteopontin, and HSPs [34]. Nakano et al. [35] investigated cell differentiation in the pulp caused by orthodontic mechanical stress using immunohistochemical techniques. The results of the study showed that the expression of Runx2 increased in the odontoblasts in the pulp, and the activity of odontoblasts may be increased. Runx2 is a transcriptional regulator belonging to the Runx family, including Runx1, Runx2, and Runx3 [30]. The Runx family is involved in cell differentiation and cell cycle progression [31] and is an essential transcriptional regulator of osteoblast differentiation and development [32]. Runx2 is a master regulator of odontoblast differentiation as well as osteoblasts [28]. No bone tissue was produced in the pulp. Therefore, the expression of Runx2 in the dental pulp strongly suggests odontoblast differentiation. Additionally, ALP expressed in the early stage of calcification associated with odontoblast differentiation is an index of odonoblastic activity [33]. In our previous studies, we induced the differentiation of dental pulp cells by adding injurious stimulation to the periodontium and pulp [10, 11]. Nabeyama et al. have shown that there is a weak positive reaction for Runx2 in the pulp tissue that has not been artificially stimulated [10]. This is similar to the results of the study conducted by Nakano et al. [35, 36], and it is presumed that it is a reaction to physiological stimuli, such as mastication and occlusion. Furthermore, Nabeyama et al. observed tissue changes in the pulp by stimulating the pulp with the immediate teeth separation method used for dental treatment for 30 min and observed the expression of Runx2 in odontoblasts, vascular endothelial cells of the pulp, and pulp-specific cells [10]. Additionally, its expression reached the maximum levels after 24 h, then gradually disappeared, and decreased to the same level as that of the control group at 1 week. It is considered that this is because BMDCs are recruited to the pulp and differentiated into pulp cells slightly after the local stimulation.

Regarding tooth separation in conservative dental treatment, the mechanical stress generated by the operation puts a stress load on the periodontal tissue, especially on the periodontal ligament [37]. However, at the same time, it is easy to understand that it also acts as an injury stimulus on the pulp tissue of the tooth. That is, compression of the periodontal ligament in the alveolar region causes strong injurious stimulation of the vessels and nerves. Because these vessels and nerves are connected to the pulp, the damaging stimulus propagates into the pulp. However, there has been little research on the type of damage that actually occurs in dental pulp cells, and within the scope of our literature, we mention the expression of HSPs in dental pulp tissue. Only a few papers have been published regarding this issue. Sens et al. immunohistochemically examined the expression of HSPs in the pulp of human third molars and examined odontoblasts, dentin cell projections, dental fibroblasts, pulp vascular endothelial cells, and some blood vessels. HSPs are expressed in membranous smooth muscle cells [38]. Additionally, Tate et al. and Suzuki et al. experimentally verified the expression of HSPs in odontoblasts of the pulp after laser cavity formation in dental conservative treatment [39, 40]. Furthermore, Matsuzaki et al. reported a study at the mRNA level that HSP27 increased in the pulp with aging [41]. There are also forecast papers that investigated the expression of HSP27 and Runx2 in the pulp under orthodontic mechanical stress loading [35, 36]. The results of these studies indicated that HSP27 expression is associated with the differentiation of dental pulp cells into odontoblasts. It is widely known that HSPs are expressed in response to injurious stimuli, and they work to maintain homeostasis of the injured tissue. HSPs are proteins acquired for survival in a harsh environment in which cells are placed. They are strongly induced by non-physiological stimuli and have anti-apoptotic functions as molecular chaperones [42]. In addition, it is known that most HSPs are expressed as a cell response to stress, suppress protein denaturation, and repair denatured proteins. In fact, HSPs are constitutively expressed even under non-stress conditions and are essential proteins for various cell activities, such as cell differentiation, proliferation, survival, and function maintenance, *in vitro* and *in vivo* [42]. HSPs, such as HSP70 and HSP90, are known to act as molecular chaperones that temporarily bind to immature proteins, mediate the folding and association of polypeptides, and assist in protein maturation [43]. It is speculated that low molecular weight HSPs also function as molecular chaperones in cells, but the details have not been clarified [44]. HSP27 was initially discovered as an inhibitor of actin polymerization [45]. Since then, it is known that HSP27 is present in high concentrations in cells, such as skeletal muscle cells and vascular smooth muscle cells, even in the non-stimulated state. Thus, it is considered that HSP27 plays a physiological role in the vascular system [46].

Saito et al. stimulated the pulp by the same experimental method as Nabeyama et al. and examined the expression of HSP27 [11]. The pulp showed a weak positive reaction for HSP27 from the immunohistochemical reaction of the control group. These results are similar to the experimental results by Nakano et al. [35], and it is inferred that this may be a reaction to the constant load of physiological mechanical stress, such as mastication and tongue pressure on the teeth. The HSP27-positive reaction observed in the pulp of the control group was weakly expressed in the pulp cells but was mainly expressed in the vascular endothelial cells. This indicates that HSP27 plays a physiological role in the vascular system [46]. Next, HSP27 was strongly expressed in the vascular endothelial cells of the dental pulp 30 min after the teeth separation treatment and was also observed in some odontoblasts. Additionally, this expression reached its maximum after 24 h, then gradually disappeared, and its expression decreased to the same level as that of the control group at 1 week. It is considered that this is because dental pulp cells are stimulated by the stress of teeth separation, and HSP27 is expressed as a vascular reaction to it and induction of odontoblast differentiation.

Since all cells derived from GFP transgenic mice express GFP, all bone marrow cells of GFP bone marrow transplanted mice also express GFP. BMDCs are recruited to various places and transformed into various cells. However, we can track BMDCs using GFP as a marker [26, 27]. We used an experimental system using GFP mice to perforate the pulp cavity of the maxillary left first molar. The growth of granulation tissue in the pulp was examined to clarify the origin of the cellular components involved in the formation of periodontal polyps. In other words, a large number of BMDCs were recruited to the pulp that has been stimulated by inflammation. BMDCs are thought to differentiate into various cells in the pulp. BMDCs appear not only in the pulp but also in the periodontal ligament. Cells with spindle-shape cells, blood vessels, and polynuclear giant cells that make up the periodontal ligament were positive for GFP. There were no GFP-positive cells among the epithelial cells, but it was found that the GFP-positive cells infiltrated the epithelial tissue. Therefore, GFP-positive cells are considered dendritic cells.

The cells in the capillaries of the periodontal polyp prepared by Osuka's experimental model can be identified by immunohistochemical examination of CD31 as a marker of vascular endothelial cells. The highest number of capillaries was observed at 3 months. Immunofluorescence double staining of GFP and S100A4 in tissues over 2 weeks to 6 months detected green fluorescence (**Figure 5-a**) showing GFP-positive cells and red fluorescence showing S100A4 positive fibroblast-like spindle-shaped cells. (**Figure 5-b**). The region with orange fluorescence included cells with both proteins (**Figure 5-c**). As a result of marking the nucleus with DAPI, orange fluorescence was observed around the nucleus that usually emits blue fluorescence (**Figure 5d**).

Immunofluorescent double staining for GFP and Runx2 detected both oval and spindle-shaped cells positive for GFP green fluorescence (**Figure 6-a**) and Runx2

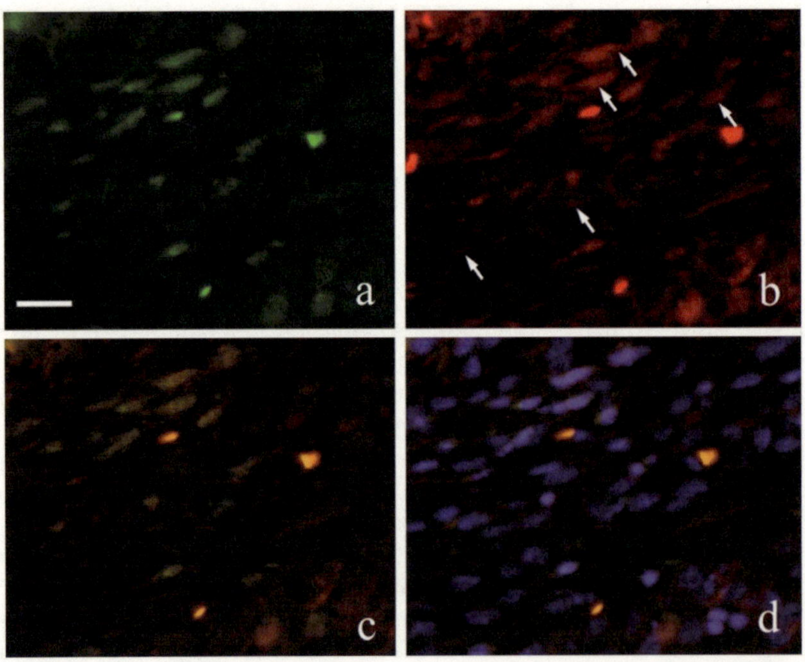

Figure 5.
FIHC images of periodontal polyp (a: GFP; b: S100A4; c: Merged image of GFP and S100A4; and d: Merged image of S100A4, GFP and DAPI; 2 week specimen; scale bar = 20 μm).

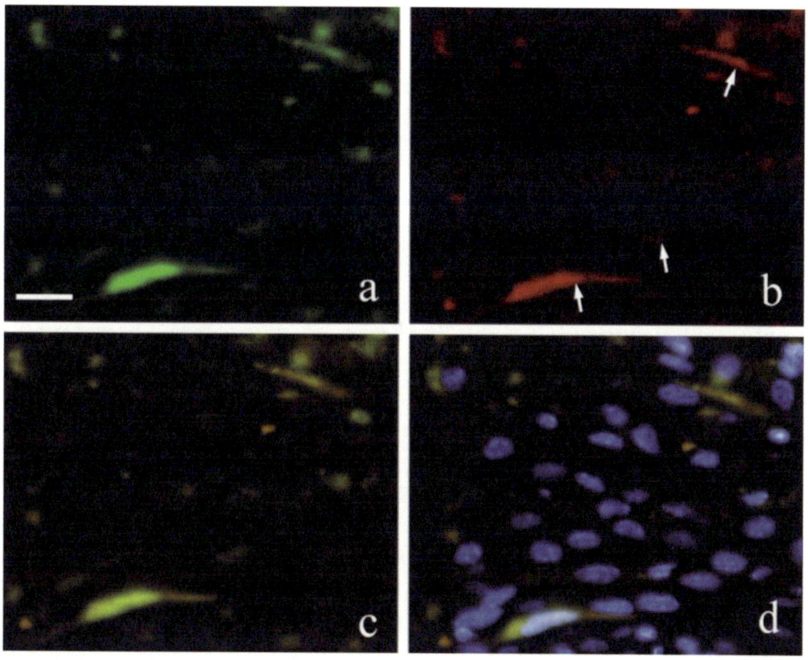

Figure 6.
FIHC images of periodontal polyp (a: GFP; b: Runx2; c: Merged image of GFP and Runx2; and d: Merged image of Runx2, GFP and DAPI; 2 week specimen; scale bar = 20 μm).

red fluorescence (**Figure 6-b**). In the superimposed image, cells showing orange fluorescence coexpressed two proteins (**Figure 6-c**). When the image was overlaid with DAPI, which showed blue fluorescence in the nucleus, orange fluorescence was seen in the cytoplasm (**Figure 6-d**). Runx2-positive and GFP-positive cells that showed orange fluorescence were observed at 2 weeks to 1 month of periodontal polyp formation and then decreased at 3 months. Even at 6 months, both Runx2- and GFP-positive cells appeared. However, there were many cells that were individually stained with GFP. Normally, no bone tissue is formed in the pulp. Runx2-positive cells in the pulp mean odontoblasts. This result indicates that the cells that proliferate in the pulp and differentiate into Runx2-positive odontoblasts are GFP-positive BMDCs.

4. Induction of differentiation of dental pulp stem cells into odontoblasts

Recently, the use of stem cells in molecular and cell biology has led to new therapeutic strategies for regenerating damaged oral tissue. It is well known that the pulp is rich in adult mesenchymal stem cells (MSCs), and the stem cells isolated from the pulp have high proliferative potential and may be able to differentiate into hard tissue-forming cells. Additionally, dental pulp stem cells play an important role in regenerative medicine for both oral and non-oral areas because of their high proliferation rate, pluripotency, and ease of collection [47]. Therefore, pulp stem cells are a promising source of MSCs used in a variety of clinical applications, such as bone formation, tooth tissue engineering, and nerve tissue regeneration [48]. We established a stable dental pulp cell line derived from GFP transgenic rats. It has the characteristics of dental pulp stem cells and exhibits stable odontoblast differentiation both *in vitro* and *in vivo*. To date, there are no reports of established cells showing stable osteoblastic and stem cell-like properties over time, both *in vitro* and *in vivo*. However, this dental pulp cell line forms dentin-like hard tissue *in vivo* but does not lead to the induction of polar odontoblasts. A scaffold is an integral part of tissue engineering. Various artificial biomaterials have been developed as scaffolds and are widely applied clinically. In recent years, some studies have focused on the geometry of biomaterials. This is because scaffold composition and optimal geometry are believed to be important for inducing cell proliferation and differentiation. Focusing on this, we have already succeeded in developing a new biomaterial, honeycomb tricalcium phosphate (TCP), which contains holes of various diameters. Previous studies have reported that the surface properties of TCP due to different sintering temperatures affect hard tissue inducibility and biocompatibility [49]. Furthermore, cartilage and bone formation can be controlled by changing the diameter of the through holes in the honeycomb TCP. In a skull defect rat model, active bone tissue formation was observed in honeycomb TCP containing a through hole with a diameter of 300 μm, suggesting its clinical applicability [50]. These findings indicate that this honeycomb TCP can potentially act as a bioactive carrier and reproduce the interaction between progenitor cells and the extracellular matrix microenvironment. Additionally, we successfully differentiated polar odontoblasts from dental pulp stem cells using honeycomb TCP.

Gronthos et al. reported the isolation and characterization of pulp stem cells from wisdom tooth pulp tissue of impacted teeth, and reported that pulp stem cells have higher cell proliferation and tissue regeneration capacity than bone marrow-derived mesenchymal stem cells [51]. Since then, many researchers have reported that dental pulp stem cells differentiate into a variety of cells, including nerve cells, adipocytes, chondrocytes, and bone [52, 53].

The TGC we created is a pulp-derived stem cell that can differentiate into functional odontoblast-like cells both *in vitro* and *in vivo*. *In vitro*, the bone-forming medium resulted in increased ALP activity of TGC and formation of calcium deposits (**Figure 7**).

Since transforming growth factor (TGF)-β is involved in dentin repair and dentin formation [54], we also investigated the effect of TGF-β on TGC.

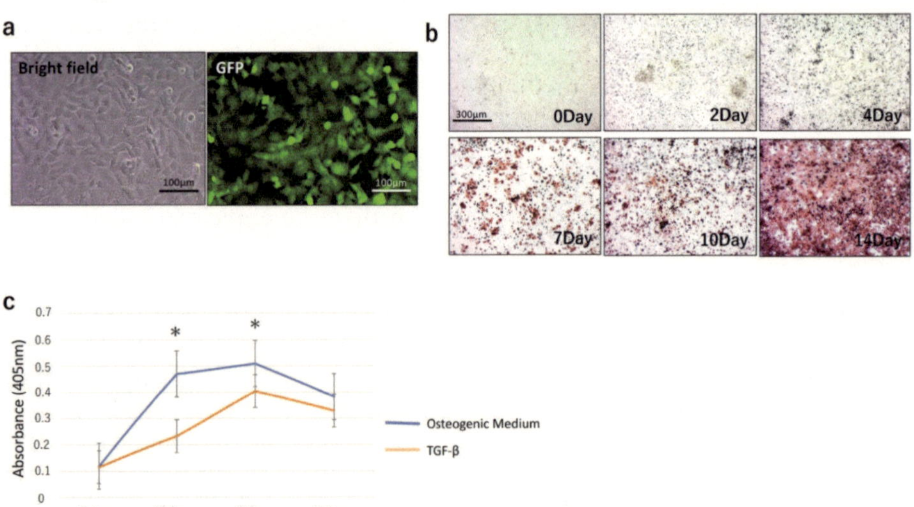

Figure 7.
(a) TGC showed a fibroblast-like shape (left), expression of green fluorescent protein (GFP) (right). (b) Alizarin red staining of TGC exposed to osteogenic medium from 0 to 14 days. (c) Alkaline phosphatase (ALP) activity of TGC cultivated with osteogenic medium or TGF-β. the ALP activity from osteogenic medium became significantly higher than that from TGF-β. $^{*}p < 0.05$.

Addition of TGF-β to TGC yielded results similar to those obtained with bone-forming medium. However, the increase in ALP activity by TGF-β was weaker than that of the bone-forming medium. One hypothesis that explains this weak stimulus is that TGC is already exposed to TGF-β because it can express the TGF family of proteins.

Regeneration using dental pulp cells and scaffolds has been reported. Ceramics, such as polylactic acid, poly (α-hydroxyl) acids, polylactic-co-glycolic acid, and TCP or hydroxyapatite have been used as scaffolds for dentin regeneration [55]. These artificial biomaterials have already been confirmed to be highly biocompatible and are used as scaffolds for odontoblast differentiation and bone induction. To date, there have been several reports of dentin-like hard tissue formation in experiments combining various scaffolds with dental pulp stem cells [56]. Among these artificial biomaterials, TCP has been reported to be highly biocompatible, and when transplanted into a living body, it is absorbed over time and self-assembled. However, previous studies using TCP and pulp cells to induce odontoblast differentiation have not led to the regeneration of polar dentin [6].

Many studies have used artificial biomaterials that are suitable for inducing differentiation into odontoblasts. However, no studies have effectively induced the differentiation into odontoblasts by changing the geometric structure of artificial biomaterials. We have shown by histological observation that changing the pore diameter of honeycomb TCP with multiple through-holes changes the type and amount of hard tissue formed in the pores. *In vivo* TGC transplantation experiments showed bone-like hard tissue formation at a pore diameter of 75 μm TCP and 500 μm TCP. However, for 300 μm TCP, hard tissue formation was observed to be added to the TCP surface, and the induced cells were dentin sialoprotein (DSP)-positive odontoblasts (**Figure 8**). In addition, these cells had a polar sequence and exhibited an odontoblast-like structure, which was present in the pulp cavity. Since the pore diameter of 300 μm resembles the width of the pulp cavity [57], it is considered that the 300 μm honeycomb TCP reproduces the dental pulp environment in the living body and differentiates polar odontoblasts to form dentin.

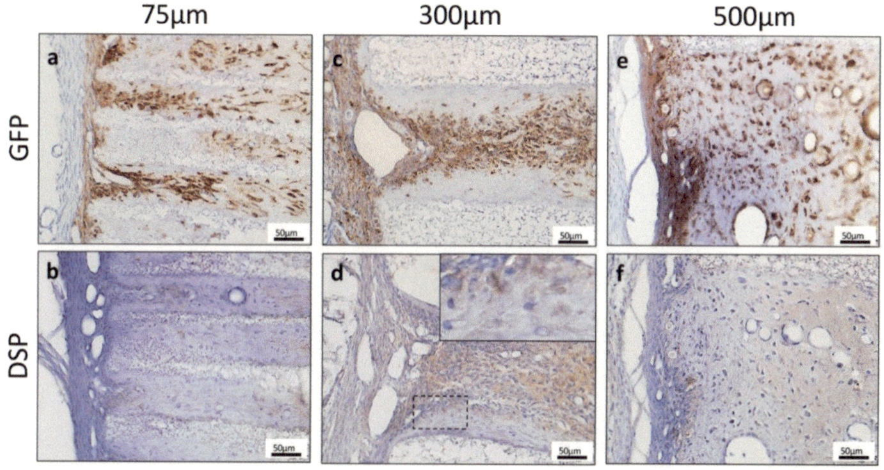

Figure 8.
The cells forming hard tissues in the TCP pores were GFP positive. Dentin Sialprotein (DSP) was not expressed in the cytoplasm of cells forming hard tissues in 75TCP and 500TCP. In contrast, in 300TCP, DSP was expressed in the cytoplasm of cells that were arranged with polarity on the TCP wall.

5. Conclusions

Maintaining tooth function is an important factor in ensuring health and quality of life. Unfortunately, illness, injury, or aging causes many people to lose their teeth and have a poor quality of life. As a result, it is necessary to develop an appropriate method for the restoration of tooth function. Tissue engineering provides an attractive perspective with the potential to regenerate fully functional organs to replace damaged or lost organs. This method required the integration of three key elements: progenitor or stem cells, extracellular matrix scaffold, and morphogens, which induce morphogenetic signals. Therefore, proper stem cell isolation and stable establishment are one of the points that must be achieved to perform regenerative therapy. Within the pulp, it is known that the pulp contains progenitor cells/stem cells, which proliferate and differentiate into various cells. Pulp stem cells can generate a new population of odontoblasts to repair damaged hard tissue. Induction of stem cell proliferation and differentiation is triggered by the release of morphogens from the pulp and periodontal tissue. Such releases occur in response to caries, therapeutic irritation, and injury. We established a cell line from the pulp of GFP transgenic rats, named it TGC, and used it for dentin regeneration. These rat pulp-derived cells were maintained in cultures for more than 80 passages without showing any changes in morphology or ability. Using this TGC and pore diameter 300 μm TCP as a scaffold, odontoblasts could be differentiated to develop polar dentin and create a structure similar to physiological dentin.

Acknowledgements

This work was supported by JSPS KAKENHI Grant Nos. JP19K19159, JP20K10178 and JP20K23079. And this research was supported by AMED under Grant No. JP20lm0203008.

Conflict of interest

The authors have declared that there is no conflict of interest.

Author details

Toshiyuki Kawakami[1], Kiyofumi Takabatake[2], Hotaka Kawai[2], Keisuke Nakano[2]*, Hidetsugu Tsujigiwa[3] and Hitoshi Nagatsuka[2]

1 Department of Hard Tissue Research, Matsumoto Dental University Graduate School of Oral Medicine, Shiojiri, Japan

2 Department of Oral Pathology, Graduate School of Medicine, Dentistry and Pharmaceutical Sciences, Okayama University, Okayama, Japan

3 Department of Life Science, Faculty of Science, Okayama University of Science, Okayama, Japan

*Address all correspondence to: keisuke1@okayama-u.ac.jp

References

[1] Popov BV, Serikov VB, Petrov NS, et al. Lung epithelial cells induce endodermal differentiation in mouse mesenchymal bone marrow stem cells by paracrine mechanism. Tissue Eng. 2007; 13: 2441-2450.

[2] Zou H, Otani A, Oishi A, et al. Bone marrow-derived cells are differentially involved in pathological and physiological retinal angiogenesis in mice. Biochem Biophys Res Commun 2010; 391: 1268-1273.

[3] Tsujigiwa H, Nishizaki K, Teshima T, et al. The engraftment of transplanted bone marrow-derived cells into the olfactory epithelium. Brain Res. 2005; 1052: 10-15.

[4] Bobis S, Jarocha D, Majka M. Mesenchymal stem cells: characteristics and clinical applications. Folia Histochem Cytobiol 2006; 44: 215-230.

[5] Zhang HK, Zhang N, Wu LH, et al. Therapeutic neovascularization with autologous bone marrow CD34+ cells transplantation in hindlimb ischemia. Zhonghua Wai Ke Za Zhi. 2005; 43: 1275-1278.

[6] Tsujigiwa H, Katase N, Sathi GA, et al. Transplanted bone marrow derived cells differentiated to tooth bone and connective tissues in mice. J Hard Tissue Biol. 2011; 20: 147-152.

[7] Matsuda H, Nakano K, Muraoka R, et al. BMPs and related factors appearing in the mouse periodontal tissues due to orthodontic mechanical stress. J Hard Tissue Biol. 2010; 19: 153-160.

[8] Watanabe T, Nakano K, Muraoka R, et al. Role of Msx2 as a promoting factor for Runx2 at the periodontal tension sides elicited by mechanical stress. Eur J Med Res. 2008; 13: 425-431.

[9] Watanabe T, Nakano K, Shimizu T, et al. Immunohistochemistry of the Periodontal Ligament Fibroblasts in Orthodontic Tension Sides. J Hard Tissue Biol. 2009; 18: 175-180.

[10] Nabeyama A, Nakano K, Saito S, Sato M, Okafuji N, Yamamoto A, et al. European Journal of Medical Research. 2011;**16**:507-513.

[11] Saito S, Nakano K, Nabeyama A, Sato M, Okafuji N, Yamamoto A, Kasahara E, Kawakami T. European Journal of Medical Research. 2011;**16**: 495-500.

[12] Watanabe T, Okafuji N, Nakano K, et al. Periodontal tissue reaction to mechanical stress in mice. Journal of Hard Tissue Biology. 2007; 16: 71-74.

[13] Tomida M, Tsujigiwa H, Nakano K, Muraoka R, Nakamura T, Okafuji N, et al. Promotion of transplanted bone marrow-derived cell migration into the periodontal tissues due to orthodontic mechanical stress. International Journal of Medical Science. 2013;**10**:1321-1326

[14] Kaneko K, Matsuda S, Muraoka R, Nakano K, Iwasaki T, Tomida M, et al. Histological evaluation of periodontal ligament in response to orthodontic mechanical stress in mice. International Journal of Medical Science. 2015;**12**: 689-694.

[15] Takabatake K, Tsujigiwa H, Nakano K, Inada Y, Qiusheng S, Kawai H, et al. Geometrical Structure of Honeycomb TCP to Control Dental Pulp-Derived Cell Differentiation. Materials. 2020;13(22):E5155. doi: 10.3390/ma13225155.

[16] Matsuda S, Yokoi Y, Moriyama K, Shoumura M, Osuga N, Nakano K and Kawakami T. Pathological examination of experimentally induced periodontal polyp in mice. J Hard Tissue Biol. 2015; 24: 397-400.

[17] Oka Y, Yoshikawa M, Takemura M, Yamamoto K and Toda T. Histological examination on periodontal tissue reaction of rat molar following perforation of the chamber floor. Jpn J Conserv Dent. 1991; 34: 1574-1579.

[18] Imaizumi I, Iwama A, Shibata N, Kumazawa M, Yamasaki M, Nakamura H and Kameyama Y. Experimental studies on lesion progression following perforation of the furcation area of rat molars. Aichi Gakuin J Dent Sci. 1996; 34: 717-723.

[19] Kudoh J. A study on the treatment of the furcation perforation using germfree rat. Jpn J Conserv Dent. 1989; 32: 201-213.

[20] Ishida T, Tachibana T, Sato K, Sawada M, Watanabe K, Endo M, Saito H, Takeda Y and Ishibashi M. Experimental study of endodontic treatment for furcation perforation. Jpn J Concerv Dent. 1985; 28: 1372-1382.

[21] Muraoka R, Tsujigiwa H, Nakano K, Katase N, Tamamura R, Tomida M, Okafuji N, Nagatsuka H and Kawakami T. Transplanted bone marrow-derived cell migration into periodontal tissues and cell differentiation. J Hard Tissue Biol. 2011; 20: 301-306.

[22] Osuga N, Matsuda S, Shoumura M, Moriyama K, Nakano K and Kawakami T. Establishment of experimental periapical inflammatory lesions in mice. J Hard Tissue Biol. 2013; 22: 517-520.

[23] Min S, Sato S, Saito M, Ebihara H, Arai Y and Ito K. Micro-computerized tomography analysis: dynamics of bone augmentation within a titanium cap in rabbit calvarium. Oral Surg Oral Med Oral Pathol Oral Radiol Endod. 2008; 106: 892-895.

[24] Arai Y, Yamada A, Ninomiya T, Kato T and Masuda Y. Micro-computed tomography newly developed for in vivo small animal imaging. Oral Radiol. 2005; 21: 14-18.

[25] Nakamura C, Hayashi T, Iso K and Nakamura F. A case of periondontal polyp, clinically resembled to pulp polyp. Matsumoto Shigaku (J Matsumoto Dent Univ Sci). 1979; 5: 89-93.

[26] Okabe M, Ikawa M, Kominami K, Nakanishi T and Nishimune Y. 'Green mice' as a source of ubiquitous green cells. FEBS Lett. 1997; 407: 313-319.

[27] Ikawa M, Yamada S, Nakanishi T and Okabe M. Green flourecsent protein (GFP) as a vital maker in mammals. Curr Top Dev Biol. 1999; 44: 1-20.

[28] Chen S, Gu TT, Sreenath T, Kulkarni AB, Karsenty G and MacDougall M. Spatial expression of Cbfa1/Runx2 isoforms in teeth and characterization of binding sites in the DSPP gene. Connect Tissue Res 2002; 43: 338-344

[29] Xia SH, Ben CR, Niu ZY, Kohchi T and Katayama I. Studies on the influence of composite resin filling material (Command Ultra fine) on the dental pulp. Meikai Daigaku Shigaku Zasshi 1990; 19: 349-355

[30] Durst KL and Hiebert SW. Role of Runx family members in transcriptional repression and gene silencing. Oncogene 2004; 23: 4220-4224

[31] Ito Y. Oncogenic potential of the RUNX gene family: Overview. Oncogene 2004; 23: 4198-4208

[32] Miyzaki T, Kanatani N, Rokutanda S, Yoshida C, Toyosawa S, Nakamura R, Takada S and Komori T. Inhibition of the terminal differentiation of odontoblasts and their transdifferentiation into osteoblasts in Runx2 transgenic mice. Arch Histol Cytol 2008; 71: 131-146

[33] Inoue T, Chen SH, Usuda J, Morohoshi Y and Shimono M. Osteogenic activity of cells from dental pulp, periodontal ligament, bone marrow and muscle in vitro:

an ultrastructural study and alkaline-phosphatase activity. Bull Tokyo Dent Coll 1992; 33: 7-12

[34] Shigehara S, Matsuzaka K and Inoue T. Morphohistological change and expression of HSP70, osteopontin and osteocalcin mRNAs in rat dental pulp cells with orthodontic tooth movement. Bull Tokyo Dent Coll 2006; 47: 117-124

[35] Nakano K, Muraoka R, Tomida M, Matsuura S, Okafuji N, Siar CH and Kawakami T. Possibility of odontoblasts activity up-regulation due to orthodontic mechanical stress in mice. J Hard Tissue Biol 2010; 19: 13-16

[36] Nakano K, Muraoka R, Tomida M, Matsuura S, Okafuji N, Siar CH and Kawakami T. Expression of HSP in dental root pulp cells due to experimental orthodontic mechanical stress. J Hard Tissue Biol 2009; 18: 127-130

[37] Muraoka R, Nakano K, Kurihara S, Yamada K and Kawakami T. Immuno-histochemical expression of heat shock proteins in the mouse periodontal tissues due to orthodontic mechanical stress. Eur J Med Res 15: 475-482, 2010.

[38] Sens DA, McGuirt JP, Khan W, Todd JH and Howell RM. Expression of heat shock protein27 in adult human third molar dental pulp. J Oral Pathol Med 25: 382-387, 1996.

[39] Tate Y, Yoshiba K, Yoshiba N, Iwaku M, Okiji T and Ohshima H. Odontoblast responses to GaAlAs laser irradiation in rat molars: an experimental study using heat-shock protein-25 immunohistochemistry. Eur J Oral Sci 114: 50-57, 2006.

[40] Suzuki T, Nomura S, Maeda T and Ohshima H. An immunocytochemical study of pulpal responses to cavity preparation by laser ablation in rat molars by using antibodies to heat shock protein(HSP)25 and classII MHC antigen. Cell Tissue Res 315: 311-319, 2004.

[41] Matsuzaka K, Muramatsu T, Katakura A, Ishihara K, Hashimoto S, Yoshinari M, Endo T, Tazaki M, Shintani M, Sato Y and Inoue T. Changes in the homeostatic mechanism of dental pulp with age: expression of the core-binding factor alpha-1, dentin sialoprotein, vascular endothelial growth factor, and heat shock protein27 messenger RNAs. J Endod 34: 818-821, 2008.

[42] Hratl FU. Molecular chaperone in cellular protein folding. Nature 381: 571-579, 1996.

[43] Gething MJ and Sambrook J: Protein folding in the cell. Nature 355: 33-44, 1992.

[44] Benndorf R, Hayess K, Ryazantsev S, Wieske M, Behlke J and Lutsch G. Phosphorylation and supermolecular organization of murine small heat shock protein HSP25 abolish its actin polymerization-inhibiting activity. J Biol Chem 269: 20780-20784, 1994.

[45] Miron T, Vancompernolle K, Vandekerckhove J, Wilchek M and Geiger B: A 25-kDa inhibitor of actin polymerization is a low molecular mass heat shock protein. J Cell Biol 114: 255-261, 1991.

[46] Inaguma Y, Goto S, Shinohara H, Hasegawa K, Ohshima K and Kato K. Physiological and pathological changes in levels of two small stress proteins, HSP27 and B-crystallin, in rat hind limb muscles. J Biochem 114: 378-384, 1993.

[47] Abe, F.; Takahashi, H.; Tanaka, A. Investigation on the action and effect of culture supernatant of human dental pulp stem cells using rats with medication-related osteonecrosis of the jaw. J. Hard Tissue Biol. 2019, 28, 349-358.

[48] Morsczeck, C.; Völlner, F.; Saugspier, M.; Brandl, C.; Reichert, T.E.; Driemel, O.; Schmalz, G. Comparison

of human dental follicle cells (DFCs) and stem cells from human exfoliated deciduous teeth (SHED) after neural differentiation in vitro. Clin. Oral Investig. 2010, 14, 433-440.

[49] Takabatake, K.; Yamachika, E.; Tsujigiwa, H.; Takeda, Y.; Kimura, M.; Takagi, S.; Nagatsuka, H. Effect of geometry of microstructure of honeycomb TCP scaffolds on bone regeneration. J. Biomed. Mater. Res. A. 2013, 102, 2952-2960.

[50] Watanabe, T.; Takabatake, K.; Tsujigiwa, H.; Watanabe, S.; Nakagiri, R.; Nakano, K.; Nagatsuka, H.; Kimata, Y. Effect of honeycomb β-TCP geometrical structure on bone tissue regeneration in skull defect. Materials 2020, 13, 7714.

[51] Gronthos, S.; Mankani, M.; Brahim, J.; Robey, P.G.; Shi, S. Postnatal human dental pulp stem cells (DPSCs) in vitro and vivo. Proc. Natl. Acad. Sci. USA 2000, 97, 13625-13630.

[52] Iohara, K.; Zheng, L.; Ito, M.; Tomokiyo, A.; Matsushita, K.; Nakashima, M. Side population cells isolated from porcine dental pulp tissue with self-renewal and multipotency for dentinogenesis, chondrogenesis, adipogenesis, and neurogenesis. Stem Cells 2006, 24, 2493-2503.

[53] Sato, N.; Isomura, M.; Kawai, R.; Yoshida, W.; Sugita, Y.; Kubo, K.; Funato, A.; Ueno, N.; Jinno, M.; Maeda, H. Osteogenic potential of rat dental pulp-derived cells on titanium surfaces. J Hard Tissue Biol. 2018, 27, 315-320.

[54] Yamakoshi, Y.; Kinoshita, S.; Izuhara, L.; Karakida, T.; Fukae, M.; Oida, S. DPP and DSP are necessary for maintaining TGF-β1 activity in dentin. J. Dent. Res. 2014, 93, 671-677.

[55] Duailibi, S.; Duailibi, M.T.; Zhang, W.; Asrican, R.; Vacanti, J.; Yelick, P.C. Bioengineered dental tissues grown in the rat jaw. J. Dent. Res. 2008, 87, 745-750.

[56] Chang, B.; Ahuja, N.; Ma, C.; Liu, X. Injectable scaffolds: Preparation and application in dental and craniofacial regeneration. Mater. Sci. Eng. R: Rep. 2017, 111, 1-26.

[57] Provenza, D.V. The blood vascular supply of the dental pulp with emphasis on capillary circulation. Circ. Res. 1958, 6, 213-218.

Chapter 6

Restoration of Endodontically Treated Teeth

Deepak M. Vikhe

Abstract

A tooth that has been properly treated endodontically should have a good prognosis. It can resume full function and if necessary serve satisfactory as an abutment for a fixed and removable partial denture. However special techniques are needed to restore such a tooth. Traditionally, a pulpless tooth received a dowel or post to "reinforce" it and a crown to "protect" it. Until the introduction of ZnPO4 cement in the last century. The major problem with their use was that of post retention. Currently, the clinician can use a variety of port and core systems for the different endodontic and restorative requirements. However, no single system provides the perfect restorative solution for every clinical circumstance, and each situation requires individual evaluation.

Keywords: abutment, dowel, endodontically, post, restorative

1. Introduction

Loss of vitality decreases the physical properties, translucency, and fracture resistance of the remaining tooth structure. A load applied on upper teeth makes them move towards labially i.e. up and outwards having no support from adjacent teeth treated endodontically will have no central core of dentine and so the stresses are mainly absorbed by margins. Unless there is bulk in this region simple restoration of the coronal form may be insufficient to reinforce the tooth. So to reinforce the crown, a post is placed in the root canal. By this, the potential point of fracture from the gingival margin can be shifted towards the root apex. Similarly loads on lower teeth cause down and inward movement which closes the arch and also gains support from adjacent teeth. So here reinforcement with the post is not as important compared to upper teeth. But still, as preparation of access cavity may leave little of dentine placement of post may be desirable. Endodontically treated teeth often require partial or complete coverage restorations according to the amount of remaining tooth structure. Endodontic treatment is usually the consequence of caries followed by pulpal infection or traumatic damage to a tooth. Therefore, these teeth also suffer from loss of structural integrity, necessitating restoration of the tooth for esthetic and functional rehabilitation. It was believed that the insertion of a post into an endodontically treated tooth reinforced and increased fracture resistance [1].

- **What is post? (Figure 1)**

It is that part of the prosthesis usually made of metal that is fitted into a prepared canal of a natural tooth

IntechOpen

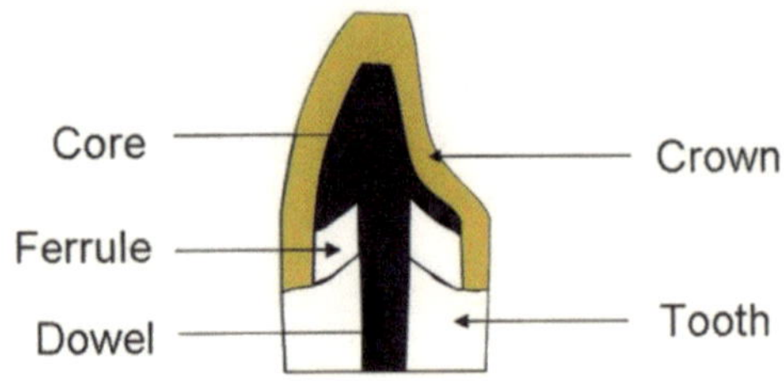

Figure 1.
Schematic illustration of an endodontically-treated tooth restored by the post-core system.

- Depending upon the design of the post the basic designs available are

  1. round ended
  2. tapered ended
  3. parallel ended

- Depending on surface texture it is divided into.

  1. smooth sided
  2. serrated
  3. threaded posts.

- Examples of some posts are

  flexi posts, endoposts, plastic impression posts, brasslers ER casting post, weissmans dentatus post, para post, v- lock active post etc.

- Parallel sided posts advantages

  Better retention, better distribution of forces.

- Disadvantages are.

  Fits only at the apical part of the canal,requires more dentine to be removed.

- Tapered posts advantages are.

  Better conforms to the canal, less removal of dentine.

- Disadvantages are.

  Less retentive than other posts, causes greater stress concentration and causes wedging affect.

- Here retention can be increased by controlled grooving.

- Of all the posts threaded posts are more retentive but these are well known to cause root fracture due to increase in forces at each coil of the threaded during insertion of the post.

According to Caputo and Standlee the self-threaded pins and friction lock pins should not be used in endodontically treated teeth [2].

According to Johnson and Sakamura, parallel sided posts resists tensile forces 4.5 times greater than tapered posts [3].

- What is parapost?

  parallel pins that are added to the prefabricated post, which provides resistance to rotation and some minimal additional retention.

According to colley parallel sided serrated posts of 5.5 mm long is more retentive than tapered post of 8 mm long [4].

- The ideal required length of the post is 2/3 the length of the root or the length of the clinical crown, whichever is longer and the diameter of the post is 1/3 of the diameter of the root [it is the maximum]

2. Recent advancements in posts

2.1 Fiber reinforced epoxy resin posts

Reinforced with black carbon fibers which are later coated with quartz fibers to mask the black color and to improve the easthetics. These posts possesses inherent flexibility that is similar to that of natural teeth [dentine], allowing the post to behave similar to the radicular dentine, which absorbs stresses and prevents root fracture. at the same time these posts causes failure of the cement seal at the margins of the artificial crown, especially when the ferrule is minimum [5].

2.2 Zirconia posts

These contain zirconium oxide, a medicine for orthopedic implants. These should be used along with composite cores. These have less tensile strength and may fracture when subjected to shear stresses [5].

2.3 Woven—fiber composite materials

These include cold—glass. Plasma treated poly ethylene woven fibers embedded in conventional resin composites. These are weaker than cast metal posts and cores. These have inferior strength combined with undesirable flexibility [5].

- **What is core? (Figure 1)**.

  It is the centre or base of the structure.

- core materials used for anterior teeth are:

  1. Plastic materials like amalgam or glass ionomer cement or composites.

  2. Resin or wax.

- core materials used for posterior teeth are.

  1. Cast gold core.

2. Resin core or composite core with metal post.

3. Resin or composite core with a cast pins.

In vitro studies states that, when load is applied on a tooth, root fracture is less in teeth restored with resin core, compared with amalgam and cast gold cores [6].

Trauma and decay are often associated with an extensive loss of tooth structure, requiring a restoration for esthetic and functional rehabilitation of the tooth. Often caries leads to loss of tooth structure and vitality of the pulp. Endodontic treatment is necessary in such cases. Adequate anchorage for restoration cannot be achieved if a significant amount of coronal section of the tooth is lost i.e. when only one wall or no wall is remaining. To increase the retention of the restoration post and core treatment is required.

Endodontic treatment influences the strain values and fracture resistance of the remaining tooth [7]. Most of the endodontic treatment failures are influenced by masticatory load. In general, failure rates tend to increase concomitantly as occlusal load increases. Failure loads have been shown to increase as parallelism approaches the load angle between the long axes of the teeth i.e. under lateral loading, failure tends to occur more readily [8]. Teeth which are nearer to transverse horizontal axis are subjected to increased amount of load as compared to anterior teeth. The fracture resistance of the tooth is also directly proportional to remaining bulk of dentin. Post space preparation can increase the amount of dentin removed thus affecting the load bearing capacity of the tooth. To prevent the major tragedy of vertical root fracture (VRF) cases, researchers have been focusing on materials used for post fabrication, designs of the post, luting agents, and the ferrule effect.

Various types of post and core systems have been introduced in dentistry. Endodontic post and core may be cast using material such as gold and nickel-chromium (Ni-Cr), or they may be prefabricated, such as titanium, stainless steel posts and fiber posts. For many years, the custom made posts have been the choice of restoration for endodontically treated teeth. However custom-made posts are technique-sensitive. The elution of the metal ions from these posts can cause metal allergy [9]. Another disadvantage of cast post being higher modulus of elasticity than dentin, which increases the risk of catastrophic failure [10]. Due to these disadvantages, these posts are progressively being replaced by titanium post. Use of a straight titanium posts requires excessive post space preparation in the curved canals [11]. This disadvantage of straight titanium post can be overcome by bendable titanium posts due to its flexible nature. Bendable titanium post can be used for various purposes, for instance, it can be included in preparation of the core when the axis of the crown of the tooth being restored has to be altered to place two or more posts, if necessary, or they can be placed in curved root canals since they can be contoured to follow the canal anatomy, thus bending internally, creating a mechanical lock for the resin core and increasing the retention surface.

Evidence remains controversial regarding the most efficient form of post for restoring endodontically treated teeth. The reduced load bearing capacity of the endodontically treated teeth being the one of the major concerns; fracture resistance provided by different posts needs to be compared.

3. Review of literature

Standlee J, Caputo A, Collard E (1972) [12], compared three post systems in regard to their design, methods of insertion, their length and their abilities to transmit forces to their supporting structures. According to the photoelastic stress analysis, post design affects stress distribution. Stresses tended to concentrate under the post shoulder, especially if sharp angles were present. Also ascertained was the fact that the post length should approximate the length of the anatomic crown.

Guzy G, Nicholls J (1979) [13], compared the breaking loads of endodontically treated teeth, with and without cemented posts, to determine if the post reinforces the root against fracture. Study was performed using maxillary central incisors and maxillary and mandibular canines. Load was applied at an angle of 130 degrees to the long axis of tooth with a speed of 5 cm/min. It was concluded that teeth without posts fractured through the middle or coronal one third of the root whereas teeth with posts fractured through the body of the post and there was no statistical significant reinforcement with cementation of posts.

Davy D, Dilley G, Krejci R (1981) [14], compared a series of designs for endodontic dowel posts, using maxillary central incisor. The tooth was examined under two load conditions, lateral load and compressive load. Both loads were treated as being concentrated along the incisal edges. They concluded the effect of taper was found to be slight if the local tapered-post diameter was comparable to the cylindrical post diameter in the high-stress region. The tapered-post design experienced slightly higher tensile and slightly lower shear stresses than the cylindrical post. Using the peak stresses in the dentin and at the dentin-post interface as a criterion, the cylindrical post with the largest diameter was the best design.

Eshelman E, Sayegh F (1983) [15], compared three post systems for fracture resistance. He concluded that between three post systems, ParaPost (stainless steel), custom made gold dowels and custom made composite dowels, the materials used for fabrication were not necessarily significant, but the angle of the load influenced the amount of force required to cause fracture and its location.

Reinhardt R, Krejci R, Stannard J (1983) [16], studied the effect of alveolar bone loss on the magnitude and distribution of stress in dentin of post-reinforced teeth. Dentin stresses from simulated functional loads to post-reinforced tooth models with four levels of periodontal support were calculated using finite element analysis. As bone levels diminished, stresses increased dramatically and were found to concentrate in the small amount of dentin remaining near the post apex.

Sorensen JA, Martinoff JT (1984) [17], evaluated 1273 endodontically treated teeth and compared the clinical success rate of six coronal-radicular stabilization methods, recorded the failure of dowel systems and the effect on endodontically treated teeth, and determined the effect of dowel length on the clinical success rate. Authors concluded the cast parallel-sided serrated dowel and core and the parallel-sided serrated dowel with an amalgam or composite resin core recorded the highest success rate. The tapered cast dowel and core displayed a higher failure rate than teeth treated without intracoronal reinforcement.

Kersten H, Fransman R, Velzen T (1986) [18], studied the effect of shape of the root canal in the success of the root canal treatment, apart from the efficiency of different root canal filling techniques especially in oval shaped canals. It was shown that close canal adaptation with minimal tooth structure removal provides a conservative and long lasting treatment for the restoration of endodontically treated teeth.

Plasmans PJJM, Visseren GH, Vrijhoef MA, Iyser AKF (1986) [19], evaluated the failure resistance of some restoration methods utilizing amalgam under an oblique load. The results suggested that intracoronal reinforcement with a prefabricated dowel did not significantly increase the in vitro resistance. Hence, the authors concluded that this in vitro study supports the approach of not removing too much remaining tooth structure to adapt the tooth for a cast dowel and core. Preservation of sound dentin and adapting the amalgam core to the teeth leaves more tooth structure and makes easy rebuilding possible with a restoration which is strong enough to resist forces of about 1,000 N.

Leary J, Aquilino S (1987) [20], evaluated the effect of various post lengths on the strength or rigidity of the root within the elastic limit of dentin. Extracted maxillary centrals, maxillary and mandibular canines were the specimens selected for study. For the study the minimum root length acceptable was 12 mm measured from the cemento-enamel junction on the facial surface. This length allowed three incremental increases in post length of 3 mm, still leaving a 3 mm minimum for the apical seal. Load was applied 10 mm from the CEJ at 90 degrees to the long axis of the test specimen. They concluded that as internal tooth structure is removed from the tooth the tooth becomes weaker, that teeth with posts do show more reinforcement than teeth without post with the same manipulation characteristics, and that some load transfer appears to exist with cemented posts.

Hunter A, Feiglin B, Williams J (1989) [21], examined the effect of root canal preparation, post preparation, and posts on the relative stresses in the cervical and apical regions of tooth models representing an intact maxillary central incisor. The authors concluded that removal of internal tooth structure during root canal therapy is accompanied by a proportional increase in stresses at the cervical area, particularly on the tension side. Post length appeared more important than post diameter in determining relative stresses at the cervical region. However, short wide posts led to elevated stress concentrations in this region. Post placement beyond two thirds of the root depth did not further decrease cervical stresses but usually increased stresses in the apical region.

Greenfeld R, Roydhouse R, Marshall F, Schoner B (1989) [22], compared a new parallel-tapering, threaded, split-shank post with a well-accepted parallel serrated post under applied compressive-shear loads. The posts were placed in paired, contralateral human teeth to attempt to minimize variation in the tooth model. Both initial and ultimate failure modes were observed, and the clinical significance was reported. The Flexi-post system compared favorably with the Para-Post system under the conditions of this research.

Burns DA, Krause WR, Douglas HB, Burns DR (1990) [23], compared the stress distribution during insertion and function of three prefabricated endodontic posts with different designs using the criteria of post length and diameter. It was reported that larger diameter posts at increased depths distributed stress more efficiently than the smaller, shorter posts when loaded obliquely.

Hatzikyriakos A, Reisis G, Tsingos N (1992) [24], conducted a longitudinal clinical study of patients treated with three traditional techniques (1) screw post and light-curing composite resins, (2) cemented post with parallel sides and light-curing composite resins, and (3) a cast and core technique. All post and core fabrications demonstrated remarkable success in the 3-year period regardless of the technique. The posts and cores with the techniques described performed for patients with existing prosthodontics, were satisfactory. The statistical analysis revealed that only the factor "type of abutment" (RPDs and FPDs) had some effect on the failure of the restorations.

Sedgley C, Messer H (1992) [25], compared the biomechanical properties of endodontically treated teeth. It was concluded that Vital dentin was 3.5% harder than dentin from contralateral endodontically treated teeth ($p = 0.002$). The similarity between the biomechanical properties of endodontically treated teeth and their contralateral vital pairs indicated that teeth do not become more brittle following endodontic treatment.

Assif D, Bitenski A, Pilo R, Oren E (1993) [26], examined the effect of post design on the fracture resistance of endodontically treated premolars restored with cast crowns The experimental model used cast posts and cores to test the effect of post design in a post-core system with identical rigidity. Samples were loaded on an Instron testing machine until failure revealed that post design did not influence the fracture resistance of endodontically treated premolars restored with complete cast crowns. In their study they concluded that endodontically treated teeth having a dowel-core system of identical rigidity and restoration with a complete cast crown having a 2 mm margin on healthy tooth structure. The selection of a dowel should be based on a system that preserves the most tooth structure and possesses suitable retention of the core for restoration of the tooth. If the anatomic crown is sufficiently preserved and core retention can be achieved from within the natural crown, or if completion of the coronal surface is unnecessary, a dowel is not required.

Mentink A, Creugers N, Meeuwissen R, Leempoel P, Kayser A (1993) [27], conducted a clinical trial to assess the clinical performance of several post and core systems. During the period 1974–1986, 112 post and core build-ups were inserted in 74 patients. The build-ups consisted of a metal prefabricated post in combination with a composite core. After an average follow-up period of 7.9 years, they concluded that the Dentatus post in combination with composite tends to yield a high failure rate. The results of the Unimetric and Radix posts in combination with composite appear to be acceptable.

Goodacre C, Spolink K (1994) [28], reviewed the management options of endodontically treated teeth and concluded that crowns should generally be used on endodontically treated posterior teeth but are not necessary on relatively sound anterior teeth. The primary purpose of post is to retain a core that can be used to retain the definitive prosthesis. Loosening of the post and tooth fractures were the two most common failures reported. Considering the post design threaded posts are the most retentive followed by cemented parallel sided posts, cemented tapered post is least retentive posts. Threaded post forms are the most likely to cause root fracture and split, and threaded flexible posts do not reduce stress concentration during function. Cemented posts produce the least root stress.

Torbjorner A, Karlsson S, Odont D, Odman P (1995) [29], evaluated the dental records of 638 patients treated with 788 posts and cores to analyze failure rate and failure characteristics for two post designs. Frequency of the technical failures, loss of retention, root fracture, and post fracture were recorded 4 to 5 years after post cementation. Two types of posts were compared: custom-cast tapered posts and parallel-sided serrated posts. The cumulative failure rate was 15% for 456 tapered posts and 8% for 332 Para-Post posts. Loss of retention was the most frequent reason for failure for both types of posts, whereas root fractures had the most serious consequences, and all resulted in extraction. A significantly higher success rate was recorded for parallel-sided serrated posts, compared with custom-cast posts, regarding the total failure rate and the severity of the failure.

Purton D, Love R (1996) [30], compared the properties in two different 1-mm diameter root canal posts — smooth carbon fiber posts (Endopost) and serrated stainless steel posts (Parapost). Ten posts of each type were tested for rigidity in a three point bend test. Ten posts of each type were cemented with resin cement into the roots of endodontically treated, extracted teeth. The tensile force required to remove the posts was recorded. The Paraposts proved to be significantly more rigid under load and significantly more strongly retained in the tooth roots. The Parapost appears to be a mechanically superior post for the restoration of root-filled teeth with narrow diameter root canals.

Mendoza D, Eakle W, Kahl E, Robert H (1997) [31], evaluated the ability of resin-bonded posts to reinforce teeth that are structurally weak in the cervical area against fracture. Forty canine roots were endodontically treated and randomly distributed into four groups of 10. Parallel-sided preformed posts were cemented into the roots of these teeth after their crowns were removed. The cervical third of the canals were flared to simulate teeth weakened in this area as a result of caries or endodontic therapy. Three resin cements and a zinc-phosphate cement, which was used as the control, were used to secure the posts into the roots. Cemented posts were loaded with a gradually increasing force at a 60-degree angle to the long axis of the root until the root fractured. Authors concluded that the roots in which the posts were cemented with Panavia were significantly more resistant to fracture than those where zinc phosphate was used.

Asmussen E, Peutzfeldt A (1999) [32], investigated the direction of shrinkage of a light-curing resin composite in relation to the attachment and the thickness of the material. The resin composite was applied in cylindrical brass molds in such a manner that a flash, serving as attachment, was produced at one side of the specimens, while the material was flush with the mold at the other side. The specimens were now irradiated from either the flash or the flush side, and the convexity or the concavity of the specimens was measured. At a material thickness of 3 mm, the shrinkage was towards the light source, irrespective of the position of the flash. At 4 and 5 mm thickness of the molds, the direction of shrinkage could be directed towards or away from the light source, depending on the position of the flash. The number of light quanta emitted from the light source and passing through the material was compared with the number of molecules of camphorquinone present in a resin composite of 3, 4, or 5 mm thickness. It was concluded that under the conditions of the present study, the direction of shrinkage was the result of an interplay between the direction of the light, the attachment of the material, and the thickness of the material.

Hazaimeh N, Gutteridge D (2001) [33], investigated the effect of a ferrule preparation on the fracture resistance of crowned central incisors incorporating a prefabricated post (Parapost) cemented with Panavia-Ex and with a composite core. The test group consisted of 10 post crowned natural central incisor teeth with a 2-mm wide ferrule preparation, whilst the control group of 10 teeth had no ferrule. The specimens were mounted on a Lloyd universal testing machine and a compressive load was applied at an angle of 135 degrees to the palatal surface of the crown until failure occurred. He concluded that when composite cement and core materials are utilized with a Parapost prefabricated system in vitro the additional use of a ferrule preparation has no benefit in terms of resistance to fracture.

Cormier C, Burns D, Moon P(2001) [34], evaluated 6 post systems over 4 simulated clinical stages of tooth restoration to (1) determine quantitatively the fracture resistance strength at each stage when a static loading force is applied to cause failure; (2) determine the failure mode for each post system at each simulated clinical stage 12 and (3) determine the feasibility of removing failed post systems. Ten post systems made with various materials and designs were tested at the following 4 stages of simulated clinical treatment: stage #1: posts only, loaded using a 3-point loading model to failure, to determine transverse strengths and failure modes for each post system; stage #2: posts alone, bonded into teeth; stage #3: posts bonded into teeth with core build up; stage #4: post and core build up and full veneer restoration. For stages #2 through #4, the coronal portion of 60 mandibular premolars was amputated at the cemento-enamel junction, the canals were treated endodontically, and the specimens were mounted in acrylic blocks. A testing force was applied to the posts at 90° to the long axis of the tooth, 4 mm from the cemento-enamel junction. The fiber posts evaluated provided an advantage over a conventional post that showed a higher number of irretrievable posts and unrestorable root fractures. At the stage of final restoration insertion, there was no difference in force to failure for all but the FibreKor material, which continued to be weaker than all other tested materials. The fiber posts were readily retrievable after failure, whereas the remaining post systems tested were non retrievable.

Raygot C, Chai J, Jameson L (2001) [35], evaluated the fracture resistance and mode of fracture of endodontically treated incisors restored with cast post-and-core, prefabricated stainless steel post, or carbon fiber–reinforced composite post systems. Ten endodontically treated teeth restored with each technique were subjected to a compressive load delivered at a 130-degree angle to the long axis until the first sign of failure was noted. The fracture load and the mode of fracture were recorded. They concluded that the use of carbon fiber–reinforced composite posts did not change the fracture resistance or the failure mode of endodontically treated central incisors compared to the use of metallic posts.

Akkayan B, Dent M, Gulmez T (2002) [36], compared the effect of 1 titanium and 3 esthetic post system on fracture resistance and fracture patterns of crowned endodontically treated teeth. A total of 40 recently extracted human maxillary canines with their crowns removed were endodontically treated. Four groups of 10 specimens were formed. Teeth were restored with titanium, quartz fiber, glass fiber, and zirconia posts and numbered as groups 1, 2, 3, and 4, respectively. All posts were cemented with Single Bond dental adhesive system and dual-polymerizing RelyX ARC adhesive resin cement. All teeth were restored with composite cores, and metal crowns were fabricated and cemented with glass ionomer cement. Each specimen was embedded in acrylic resin and then secured in a universal load-testing machine. A compressive load was applied at a 130-degree angle to the long axis of the tooth until fracture, at a crosshead speed of 1 mm/min. He concluded that significantly higher failure loads were recorded for root canal treated teeth restored with quartz fiber posts. Fractures that would allow repeated repair were observed in teeth restored with quartz fiber and glass fiber posts.

Pontius O, Hutter J (2002) [37], evaluated the survival rate and fracture resistance of maxillary central incisors restored with different post and core systems. The post and core systems investigated were a prefabricated high precious metal post with cast core (group A), zirconia post with a prefabricated bonded ceramic core (group B), and a resin-ceramic interpenetrating phase composite post (experimental) with a prefabricated bonded ceramic core (group C). The all-ceramic copings were cemented using Panavia 21 TC. In the group without corono radicular reinforcement, the access cavity was closed with a light-cured composite in combination with a dentine-bonding agent (group D). Each specimen was intermittently loaded and thermocycled before final stress tests. With the help of results they concluded that the samples restored with a cast post and core demonstrated more vertical root fractures and the preservation of both internal and external tooth structure is of utmost importance when restoring endodontically treated teeth.

Nergiz I, Schmage P, Platzer U, Ozcan M (2002) [38]; investigated the effect of length and diameter on the retentive strength of sandblasted tapered prefabricated titanium posts. The results of the study were that retention was affected strongly with the increase in the length (approximately 100%) than with the increase in the diameter (approximately 60%).

Kishen A, Kumar GV, Chen N (2004) [39], evaluated biomechanical perspective of fracture predilection in post-core restored teeth using computational, experimental and fractographic analysis. These experiments aided in correlating the stress–strain response in structural dentine with cracks and catastrophic fractures in post-core restored teeth. They observed that the inner dentine displayed distinctly high strains, while the outer dentine demonstrated high stresses during tensile loading. Hence they concluded that energy fed into the material as it is extended will be spread throughout the inner dentine, and there is less possibility of local increase in stress at outer dentine, which can lead to the failure of dentine structure.

During post endodontic restoration with increase in loss of inner dentin the fracture resistance factor contributed by inner dentine is compromised, which in turn disposes the tooth to catastrophic fracture.

Tan PL et al (2005) [40], investigated the resistance to static loading of endodontically treated teeth with uniform and nonuniform ferrule configurations. Fifty extracted intact maxillary human central incisors were randomly assigned to 1 of 5 groups: CRN, no root canal treatment (RCT), restored with a crown; RCT/CRN, no dowel/core, restored with a crown; 2 FRL, 2-mm ferrule, cast dowel/core and crown 0.5/2 FRL, nonuniform ferrule (2 mm buccal and lingual, 0.5 mm proximal), cast dowel/core and crown; and 0 FRL, no ferrule, cast dowel/core and crown. The teeth were prepared to standardized specifications and stored for 72 hours in 100% humidity prior to testing. Testing was conducted with a universal testing machine with the application of a static load, and the load (N) at failure was recorded. With the help of their results they demonstrated that central incisors restored with cast dowel/core and crowns with a 2-mm uniform ferrule were more fracture resistant compared to central incisors with nonuniform (0.5 to 2 mm) ferrule heights. Both the 2-mm ferrule and nonuniform ferrule groups were more fracture resistant than the group that lacked a ferrule.

Ng CC, Dumbrigue HB, Al-Bayat MI, Griggs JA, Wakefield CW (2006) [41], investigated the fracture resistance of restored endodontically treated teeth when residual axial tooth structure was limited to one half the circumference of the crown preparation. Fifty extracted maxillary anterior teeth were sectioned 18 mm from their apices, endodontically treated, and divided into 5 groups of 10 teeth each. Four groups were prepared with full shoulder crown preparations having axial wall heights of 2 mm around the preparation circumferences. In 3 of the groups with axial tooth structure, one half of the axial tooth structure was removed, palatally, labially, or proximally, and groups were identified according to the site of retained coronal tooth structure. For the fifth group, all axial tooth structure was removed to the level of the preparation shoulder. Thus, in 1 group the axial walls were circumferential, 360 degrees around the preparations (Complete group), in 3 groups the axial walls were continuous for 180 degrees (Palatal, Labial, and Proximal groups), and the last group had no retained coronal tooth structure incisal to the finish line (Level group). All 50 prepared teeth were then restored with quartz fiber posts (Bisco), composite resin (Bisco) cores, and metal crowns. A universal testing machine compressively loaded the tooth specimens from the palatal at a crosshead speed of 0.5 cm/min at an angle of 135 degrees to the long axis of teeth until failure occurred. Authors observed that for restored endodontically treated teeth that do not have complete circumferential tooth structure between the core and preparation finish line, the location of the remaining coronal tooth structure may affect their fracture resistance.

Dietschi D, Ardu S, Gerber A, Krejci I (2006) [42], evaluated the influence of post material physical properties on the adaptation of adhesive post and core restorations after cyclic mechanical loading. Composite posts and cores were made on endodontically treated deciduous bovine teeth using 3 anisotropic posts (made of carbon, quartz, or quartz-and-carbon fibers) and 3 isotropic posts (zirconium, stainless steel, titanium). Specimens were submitted to 3 successive loading phases – 250,000 cycles at 50 N, 250,000 at 75 N, and 500,000 at 100 N – at a rate of 1.5 Hz. Restoration adaptation was evaluated under SEM, before and during loading (margins) and after test completion (margins and internal interfaces). With the help of results they concluded that regardless of their rigidity, metal and ceramic isotropic posts proved less effective than fiber posts at stabilizing the post and core structure in the absence of the ferrule effect, due to the development of more interfacial defects with either composite or dentin.

Salvi GE, Siegrist Guldener BE, Amstad T, Joss A, Lang NP (2007) [43], assessed the survival rates and complications of root-filled teeth restored with or without post-and-core systems over a mean observation period of 4 years. A total of 325 single- and multirooted teeth in 183 subjects treated in a private practice were root filled and restored with either a cast post-and-core or with a prefabricated titanium post and composite core. Root-filled teeth without post-retained restorations served as controls The restored teeth served as abutments for single unit metal-ceramic or composite crowns or fixed bridges. Teeth supporting cantilever bridges, overdentures or telescopic crowns were excluded. In their observation they concluded that the, provided that high-quality root canal treatment and restorative protocols are implemented, high survival and low complication rates of single- and multirooted root-filled teeth used as abutments for fixed restorations can be expected after a mean observation period of ± 4 years.

Maccari PC, Cosme DC, Oshima HM, Burnett LH Jr, Shinkai RS (2007) [44]; evaluated the fracture strength of teeth with flared canals and restored with two fiber-reinforced resin systems and one custom cast base metal (Ni-Cr) post and core system. The results suggested that teeth restored with cast posts had fracture strength twice that of teeth restored with resin posts. Fiber-reinforced resin posts failed at a compressive force comparable to clinical conditions, but all failures were repairable. While with the cast posts involved with root fractures.

Hinckfuss S, Wilson P (2008) [45], evaluated the fracture resistance of bovine teeth restored with one-piece cast core/crowns and no ferrule, compared to teeth restored with amalgam cores and full coverage crowns, with and without a dentine ferrule. In this study thirty bovine incisors were selected and modified to ensure all teeth had axial dentine walls of similar size. The teeth were then randomly allocated to one of the three groups: control group restored with amalgam core and cast crown without ferrule; ferrule group restored with amalgam core and cast crown with a 2-mm dentine ferrule; one-piece group restored with one-piece cast core/crown without ferrule. Each tooth was loaded to the point of fracture. It was observed that the maximum load resistance was significantly enhanced by a 2-mm ferrule compared with teeth with no ferrule and teeth restored with one-piece cast core/crowns. Teeth restored with one-piece cast core/crowns were significantly more resistant to loading than teeth restored with amalgam cores and crowns without a ferrule.

Kivanc B, Gorgul G (2008) [46], investigated the fracture strength of three post systems cemented with a dual cure composite resin luting cement by using different adhesive systems. Sixty three extracted anterior teeth with single roots were endodontically prepared and filled. Teeth were randomly assigned to one of three post systems placed into the prepared canals: Group I - titanium posts, Group II - glass fiber posts and Group III zirconia posts. Each group was again randomly divided into three subgroups according to the bonding materials used [Single Bond ($n = 7$), Clearfil SE Bond ($n = 7$), and Prompt L Pop ($n = 7$)]. A dual cured resin cement (Rely X ARC) was used for bonding the posts into the root canals. Standard cores were made by a composite resin (Clearfil Photocore) using core build-ups. The samples were tested in the compression test machine for 1 mm/min and fracture resistance of the teeth were recorded. This study concluded that endodontically treated anterior teeth restored with glass fiber posts exhibited higher failure loads than teeth restored with zirconia and titanium posts. Self-etching adhesives are better alternatives to etch-and rinse adhesive systems for luting post systems.

Alikhasi M, Dorriz H (2009) [47], compared the fracture resistance of endodontically treated teeth restored with different post and core systems in combination with complete metal crowns in teeth with no coronal structure. Fifty extracted mandibular premolars were divided into five groups. The coronal portion of each tooth was removed at the cemento-enamel junction (CEJ) in all groups except Group 1. In this group the teeth were sectioned 1 mm above the CEJ to create a ferrule. After root canal preparations, cast posts were placed in the first four groups. Prefabricated glass fiber posts and composite cores were placed in the fifth group. An opaque porcelain layer was applied to the metal post surfaces in the third group and an alloy primer was applied to the posts in the fourth group before using Panavia F2 resin cement. No bonding agent or surface treatments were used for the first and sec.ond groups. It was concluded that either a ferrule preparation or bonding with the use of an opaque porcelain layer can increase the fracture resistance of teeth with little remaining tooth structure that are restored with cast crowns following endodontic therapy.

Ma P, Nicholls J, Junge T, Phillips K (2009) [48], correlated different ferrule lengths with the number of fatigue cycles needed for failure of the crown cement for an all-ceramic crown cemented with a resin cement. Fifteen maxillary central incisors were divided into 3 groups (n = 5), with ferrules of 0.0 mm, 0.5 mm and 1.0 mm respectively. Each tooth was restored with a 0.050-inch glass-filled composite post) and a composite resin core. The posts were cemented with resin cement, and the composite resin cores were bonded to dentin using a dentine bonding agent. Each specimen was prepared with a 7-mm total preparation height, a 1.5-mm lingual axial wall, and a 1.0-mm shoulder around the tooth. The crowns for all specimens were pressed with a pressable ceramic material and cemented with resin cement. Load of 6-kg cyclic test was applied to each specimen at 135 degrees to the long axis of the tooth. After looking at the result they concluded that specimens with a 0.0-mm ferrule survived few fatigue cycles despite the fact that both the post and crown were bonded with resin cement. Teeth with a 0.5-mm ferrule showed a significant increase in the number of fatigue cycles over the 0.0-mm group, whereas teeth with the 1.0-mm ferrule exhibited a significantly higher fatigue cycle count over the 0.0-mm but not the 0.5-mm group.

Signore A, Benedicenti S, Kaitsas V, Barone M, Angiero F, Ravera G (2009) [49], compared the long-term survival of endodontically treated, maxillary anterior teeth restored with either tapered or parallel-sided glass-fiber posts and full-ceramic crown coverage. Authors stated that the choice of appropriate definitive restoration of endodontically treated maxillary anterior teeth should be guided by the amount of remaining hard tissues as well as functional and esthetic considerations. However, in cases of inadequate remaining coronal tooth structure, post-retained cores are often required to support complete crown restorations. The preparation of a post space significantly weakens endodontically treated teeth. A post did not significantly strengthen endodontically treated teeth.

Silva NR, Raposo L, Versluis A, Julio A, Neto F, Soares C (2010) [50], evaluated the effect of post, core, crown type, and ferrule presence on the deformation, fracture resistance, and fracture mode of endodontically treated bovine incisors. One hundred and eighty bovine incisors were selected and divided into 12 treatment groups (n = 15). The treatment variations were: with or without ferrule, restored with cast post and core, glass fiber post with composite resin core, or glass fiber post with fiber-reinforced core, and metal- or alumina-reinforced ceramic crown (n = 15). The restored incisors were loaded at a 135-degree angle, and the deformation was measured using strain gauges placed on the buccal and proximal root surfaces. Specimens were subsequently loaded to the point of fracture. It was concluded that core type did not affect the deformation and fracture resistance of endodontically treated incisors restored with alumina-reinforced ceramic crowns. The presence of a ferrule improved the mechanical behavior of teeth restored with metal crowns, irrespective of core type.

Jang JH et al (2012) [51], examined the stress distribution in endodontically treated maxillary central incisors restored with various lengths of either titanium or fiber reinforced composite (FRC) post-and-core systems, using two-dimensional finite element analysis models. Eight models of the maxillary central incisor were formed, surrounded by cortical bone, cancellous bone, and the periodontal ligament. Two different post-and-core systems, titanium and FRC posts (D.T Light Post), were modeled. In each restorative system, four models were designed by changing the post lengths cemented to the root at 10 mm, 9 mm, 8 mm, and 7 mm. A 100-N load was applied at a 45 angle to the long axis of each model. In the end they observed that the possibility of fracture of the FRC post is relatively low, compared to the titanium post, even for a short post. The same criteria for installation of a metal post should not be applied to an FRC post.

Hegde J, Ramakrishna, Bashetty K, Srirekha, Lekha, Champa (2012) [52], evaluated the fracture strength and mode of failure of endodontically treated teeth with flared canals restored with two fiber reinforced systems (glass fiber and quartz fiber) and one base metal cast post and core system. Forty five anterior teeth were decoronated at cemento-enamel junction and were endodontically treated. Post space was prepared and randomly divided into three groups according to the post system. Specimens were loaded at 45° in a universal testing machine at a cross head speed of 0.5 mm/min until failure. The mode of failure was classified as repairable or non-repairable. They concluded that the results of this study showed that fracture strength and mode of failure in anterior teeth with flared canal varied according to the type of post used to support a crown.

Juloski J, Radovic I, Goracci C, Vulicevic JR, Ferrari M (2012) [53], summarized the results of research conducted on different issues related to the ferrule effect. They said that presence of a 1.5- to 2-mm ferrule has a positive effect on fracture resistance of endodontically treated teeth. If the clinical situation does not permit a circumferential ferrule, an incomplete ferrule is considered a better option than a complete lack of ferrule. Including a ferrule in preparation design could lead to more favorable fracture patterns. Providing an adequate ferrule lowers the impact of the post and core system, luting agents, and the final restoration on tooth performance. In teeth with no coronal structure, in order to provide a ferrule, orthodontic extrusion should be considered rather than surgical crown lengthening. If neither of the alternative methods for providing a ferrule can be performed, available evidence suggests that a poor clinical outcome is very likely.

Santos-Filho P, Verıssimo C, Soares PV, Saltarello RC, Soares CJ, Martins LR (2014) [54], evaluated the influence of post system, length, and ferrule on biomechanical behavior of endodontically treated anterior teeth. The investigation was conducted by using laboratory tests and 3-dimensional finite element analysis. Eighty bovine incisors were selected and divided into 8 treatment groups ($n = 10$) with absence of ferrule and 2.0 mm of ferrule, restored with glass fiber post or cast post and core, and 12.0 and 7.0 mm of post length. The specimens were loaded at 135 angle, and the strain was measured by using strain gauge method. Specimens were subsequently loaded until fracture. Three-dimensional models of a maxillary central incisor were generated with the same treatment variations used in laboratory tests. Each model was subjected to 100 N oblique loads. They concluded that the post length influenced only the cast post strain and stress distribution. The ferrule groups always showed more satisfactory stress distribution and fracture resistance.

Maroulakos G, Nagy W, Kontogiorgos E (2015) [55], investigated the fracture resistance and mode of failure of severely compromised teeth restored with 3 different adhesively bonded post and core systems. Thirty extracted endodontically treated maxillary anterior teeth were randomly divided into 3 groups, CPC, gold cast post and core; TPC, titanium prefabricated post/composite resin core; and FPC, quartz fiber reinforced post/composite resin core. All posts were adhesively cemented. All cores resembled a central incisor preparation with no remaining tooth structure above the finish line. Cast gold crowns were fabricated and cemented adhesively. The specimens were aged with thermocycling and cyclic loading. Two specimens per group were randomly selected for micro-computed tomographic imaging before and after aging. Failure was induced with a universal testing machine. The mode of failure was characterized by the interface separation. They observed that the severely compromised endodontically treated teeth restored with bonded gold cast post and cores showed significantly higher fracture resistance.

Upadhyayal V, Bhargava A, Parkash H, Chittaranjan B, Kumar V (2016) [56], evaluated the effect of design and material of post with or without ferrule on stress distribution using finite element analysis. A total of 12 three-dimensional (3D) axisymmetric models of post retained central incisors were made, six with ferrule design and six without it. Three of these six models had tapered posts, and three had parallel posts. The materials tested were titanium post with a composite resin core, nickel chromium cast post and core, and fiber reinforced composite (FRC) post with a composite resin core. The load of 100 N at an angle of 45° was applied 2 mm cervical to the incisal edge on the palatal surface. In their study they concluded that a rigid material with high modulus of elasticity for the post and core system creates the most uniform stress distribution pattern. Ferrule provides uniform distribution of stresses and decreases the cervical stresses.

Kim AR, Lim HP, Yang HS, Park SW (2017) [57], evaluated the fracture resistance with regard to ferrule lengths and post reinforcement on endodontically treated mandibular premolars incorporating a prefabricated post and resin core. One hundred extracted mandibular premolars were randomly divided into 5 groups (n = 20): intact teeth (NR); endodontically treated teeth (ETT) without post (NP); ETT restored with a prefabricated post with ferrule lengths of either 0 mm (F0), 1 mm (F1), or 2 mm (F2). Prepared teeth were restored with metal crowns. A thermal cycling test was performed for 1,000 cycles. Loading was applied at an angle of 135 degrees to the axis of the tooth using a universal testing machine with a crosshead speed of 2.54 mm/min. In their study they observed fracture resistance of ETT depends on the length of the ferrule, as shown by the significantly increased fracture resistance in the 2 mm ferrule group (F2) compared to the groups with shorter ferrule lengths (F0, F1) and without post (NP).

Marchionatti A, Wandscher V, Rippe M, Kaizer O, Valandro L (2017) [58], compared the clinical performance and failure modes of teeth restored with intra-radicular retainers. Evaluated retainers were fiber (prefabricated and customized) and metal (prefabricated and cast) posts, and follow-up ranged from 6 months to 10 years. Most studies showed good clinical behavior for evaluated intra-radicular retainers. In their review they concluded that the metal and fiber posts present similar clinical behavior at short to medium term follow-up. Remaining dental structure and ferrule increase the survival of restored pulpless teeth.

Onofre R, Fergusson D, Cenci MS, Moher D, Cenci P (2017) [59], assessed the influence of the number of remaining coronal walls, the use or disuse of posts, and their type on the clinical performance of these restorations. Randomized controlled trials and controlled clinical trials for ETT restored with a combination of post/crown or no post/crown were searched for in MEDLINE, Embase, and the Cochrane Library. In their review they concluded that the restoration of ETT should focus on the maintenance of the coronal structure. Until more studies with longer follow-up periods are available, posts with a high elastic modulus appear to present with better performance when restoring ETT with no ferrule.

Naumann M, Sterzenbach G, Dietrich T, Bitter K, Frankenberger R, Lausnitz MS (2017) [60], evaluated the dentin-like glass fiber posts (GFPs) compared with rather rigid titanium posts (TPs) for post-endodontic restoration of severely damaged endodontically treated teeth with 2 or fewer remaining cavity walls. Ninety-one subjects in need of post-endodontic restorations were randomly assigned to receive either a tapered GFP (n = 45) or TP (n = 46). Posts were adhesively luted by using self-adhesive resin cement, followed by composite core build-up and preparation of 2-mm ferrule design. Primary endpoint was loss of restoration for any reason. Hence they concluded that when using self-adhesively luted prefabricated posts, resin composite core build-up, and 2-mm ferrule to reconstruct severely damaged endodontically treated teeth, tooth survival is not influenced by post rigidity. Survival decreased rapidly after 8 years of observation in both groups.

Lazari P, Carvalho M, Altair A, Curry D, Magne P (2018) [61], investigated the restoration of extensively damaged endodontically treated incisors without a ferrule using glass–ceramic crowns bonded to various composite resin foundation restorations and 2 types of posts. Sixty decoronated endodontically treated bovine incisors without a ferrule were divided into 4 groups and restored with four different post-and-core foundation restorations. NfPfB = no-ferrule (Nf) with glass-fiber post (Pf) and bulk-fill resin foundation restoration (B); NfPfP = no-ferrule (Nf) with glass-fiber post (Pf) and dual-polymerized composite resin core foundation restoration (P); NfPt = no-ferrule. They concluded that the survival of extensively damaged endodontically treated incisors without a ferrule was slightly improved by the use of a fiber post with a bulk-fill composite resin core foundation restoration. However, none of the post-and-core techniques was able to compensate for the absence of a ferrule. The presence of the posts always adversely affected the failure mode.

Meng Q, Ma Q, Wang T, Chen Y (2018) [62], evaluated the effect of ferrule design on the fracture resistance of endodontically treated mandibular first premolars after simulated crown lengthening and orthodontic forced eruption methods restored with a fiber post-and-core system. Forty extracted and endodontically treated mandibular first premolars were decoronated to create lingual to-buccal oblique residual root models, with a 2.0 mm height of the lingual dentine wall coronal to the cemento-enamel junction, and the height of buccal surface at the cemento-enamel junction. The roots were divided randomly into five equal groups. With the help of results they concluded that increased apically complete ferrule preparation resulted in decreased fracture resistance of endodontically treated mandibular first premolars, regardless of whether surgical crown lengthening or orthodontic forced eruption methods were used.

Zarow M et al (2018) [63], reviewed the status of root filled teeth to analyze the most important factors in decision-making and discuss the current restorative concepts and classified both the evidence and clinical practice in a way that seeks to be clear, understandable and helpful for clinicians. They concluded that the decision-making process in the restoration of root filled teeth is complex and should consider the following factors: amount and quality of tooth structure, tooth position in the arch and anatomy and function. Fiber posts are recommended in anterior teeth and premolars with compromised tooth structure (<50%) and/or with high tooth length over bone crest. A ferrule is highly beneficial for the prognosis of root filled teeth. If a ferrule cannot be provided and the patient still prefers to save the tooth, a gold cast could be a possible option.

Fadag A et al (2018) [64], evaluated the fracture resistance of endodontically treated maxillary central incisors with different post systems. Fifty-six extracted intact maxillary permanent central incisors were used, treated endodontically (except for the control group), and distributed into the following seven test groups (n = 8) depending on the post type: UHT (control group: root-filled teeth without endodontic post), ZRP (prefabricated zirconia post), GFP (prefabricated glass fiber post), CFP (prefabricated carbon fiber post), CPC (custom-made cast post and core), TIP (prefabricated titanium post), and MIP (prefabricated mixed post). The specimens were loaded in a universal testing machine until fracture occurrence. In their, they observed endodontically treated teeth restored with zirconia post, glass fiber post, titanium post, or mixed post were more resistant to fracture loads compared with those that were not restored (control group) or restored with either carbon fiber post or cast post and core.

Pinto CL et al (2019) [65], evaluated the influence of different post systems on the biomechanical behavior of teeth with a severe loss of remaining coronal structure. Fifty standardized bovine teeth (n = 10 per group) were restored with: cast post-and-core (CPC), prefabricated metallic post (PFM), parallel glass-fiber post (P-FP), conical glass-fiber post (C-FP), or composite core (no post, CC). The survival rate during thermomechanical challenges (TC), the fracture strength (FS), and failure patterns (FP) were evaluated. Hence they concluded that the type of intracanal post had a relevant influence on the biomechanical behavior of teeth with little remaining coronal structure.

Bakirtzoglou E, Kamalakidis S, Pissiotis A, Michalakis K (2019) [66], evaluated the retention and resistance form of complete coverage restorations supported by two different cast post and core designs. Forty extracted maxillary central incisors were randomly divided into four groups of 10 specimens each. All specimens were endodontically treated and a uniform post space of 9 mm was created. All prepared teeth had a 360 degree chamfer ferrule of 2 mm in axial height measured 0.5 mm coronally from the cemento-enamel junction (CEJ) and an axial wall thickness of 1.5 mm. Both cast post and core designs offer equal retention.

Veeraganta S et al (2020) [67], evaluated the influence of post material and post diameter on the fracture resistance of endodontically treated mandibular premolars. In addition, the influence of tooth substance loss was evaluated by comparing 1 with 2 residual dentinal walls. Sixty-four extracted mandibular first premolars were endodontically treated and divided into 8 test groups based on the number of residual walls (1 or 2), post material (glass fiber or titanium) and post diameter (International Standards Organization [ISO] 70 or ISO 90). After luting the posts, the specimens received a composite resin core and a crown preparation with a 2-mm ferrule. Cast Co-Cr crowns were cemented with glass ionomer cement. After 1200000 mastication cycles with a load of 49 N and simultaneous thermocycling (5–55°C), specimens were loaded at 30 degrees to the longitudinal axis of the tooth until fracture. In their study they observed that fracture loads ranged from 954 ± 35 N (1 residual wall glass fiber ISO 70) to 1286 ± 202 N (1 residual wall glass fiber ISO 90). Titanium posts showed a statistically significant higher fracture resistance than glass fiber posts. A statistically significant increase in fracture resistance was also observed with increasing post diameter. However, no significant difference was found with respect to the number of residual walls. Hence they concluded that teeth restored with titanium posts exhibited higher fracture resistance than teeth restored with glass fiber posts, especially when smaller diameter posts were used.

One of the most frequent procedures of restorative dentistry is the restoration of mutilated and endodontically treated teeth. It is also difficult to repair these teeth since significant quantities of the coronal tooth structure is lost as a result of decay, prior restorative treatment, endodontic access and fractures. Restoration of an endodontically treated tooth needs a good understanding of its physical as well as biomechanical properties, along with sound knowledge of its anatomy as well as endodontic, periodontal, restorative and occlusal principles. Even though the availability of various restorative materials for endodontically treated teeth has increased over few years, the principle of restoring it remains the same [68]. When a significant coronal section has been lost, resulting in the presence of one wall or no wall remaining, then adequate anchorage for the restoration cannot be achieved [69].

With the aid of a post, anchorage can be gained in such conditions. A post is described as the restoration segment inserted into the root canal to help maintain a core component. It can be made of metal or non-metallic compounds. The main objective of the post is to provide retention for the core and the coronal restoration [29, 70]. Sorensen in 1984 stated that the reason for placing a post in the root canal is to retain a crown and not to reinforce the tooth. Posts should not be positioned arbitrarily because post space preparation introduces a degree of risk to a restorative operation by disrupting the seal of the root canal filling, which can lead to microleakage. The risk of perforation increases due to the removal of sound tooth structure. Tooth fracture can also occur because of weakening of roots due to removal of sound tooth structure.

It is preferred that physical properties of the tooth i.e. the dentin should match with the physical properties of post system. An ideal post should distribute the functional stresses along the root surface in such a manner that minimum stresses are developed. Esthetics of the post should be compatible with the surrounding tissue. An ideal post should have easy retrievability, good retention and should be compatible with core material. They should also be available at a reasonable cost and should be easy to use. The indications for a post have been modified over the years based on the advantages of the adhesive restoration principles, which may obviate the need for the posts [71]. The remaining amount of tooth structure determines the stability for the restoration. In addition, the tooth's prognosis is influenced by different factors such as occlusal contacts, its location in dental arch and ferrules [71].

1.5 to 2 mm height of ferrule is the minimum requirement to obtain sufficient fracture resistance. 20 The ferrule with the help of core and dentin reduces the stress on the entire restoration. However, researchers have indicated that it is possible to overcome the lack of fracture protection that may occur in the absence of ferrules using adhesive agents [70, 71].

A further benefit of flexible posts is that dentine elimination is reduced by following the morphology of the channels in curved channels, while direct positioning in the post increases dentine elimination as the length (surface area) increases. Another explanation for this is that the curvature region starts after the 7 mm mark. This is where the thickness of the dentine decreases and there is a very high chance of strip perforation [72].

3.1 Considerations [anterior teeth]

Its not always necessary to have a complete coverage except when a plastic restoration has limited prognosis. Teeth which are badly destructed due to caries, which can be used for RPD or FPD.

Posterior teeth are subjected to greater stresses because of their position i.e. closer to the insertion of the muscles of mastication. This combined with their morphologic characteristics makes them more susceptible to fracture.

Complete coverage is recommended on teeth with a high risk of fracture especially maxillary premolars as they have long, thin and curved roots which gives best protection against fracture but at the same time considerable tooth reduction must be done and in these cases a post and core foundation is needed for better retention of the prosthesis.

- Its commonly believed that endodontically treated teeth are weak than normal teeth which may be due to low moisture content.[not proved experimentally]. so attempts have been made to increase strength by adding posts.

Studies reveal that no significant reinforcement results with the post, because teeth when loaded, stresses are more at the facial and lingual aspects of the root and post being at centre is minimally stressed and does not help prevent fracture. However some contradicts this assumption.

Disadvantages of placement of the post:

It requires an additional operative procedure. Additional tooth structure must be removed. if post fails it is difficult to restore the tooth later for a complete crown. Post can prevent future endodontic treatment.

when a complete coverage is not necessary, post is contraindicated in that tooth. when there is extensive loss of tooth structure which can be used for a FPD or RPD a complete coverage is mandatory.

3.2 Preparation aspects

All most all the principles of normal tooth preparation applies to the endodontically treated teeth. Ideally coronal half of the post hole will have been left open at the time of obturation. if not care must be taken not to deviate from the canal while opening. Guidance can be achieved by softening the guttapurcha with an heated instrument. A reamer can then be inserted to remove the guttapurcha and the direction of the canal is identified. Use of magnifying lens and fiber optic light is helpful in this process. After opening to the required length it is reamed to the appropriate size to accept a post. The minimum length required for a post hole is either the size of that tooth crown or two-thirds the length of the root whichever is longer.

3.3 Conservation aspects

- Root canal- as the thickness of the remaining is the prime variable in fracture resistance of the root, care should be taken only to remove mimimal tooth structure from the canal. Over enlargement can perforate or weaken the root which may split while cementing the post.

- Studies reveal that post of 1.8 mm diameter fracture more easily than those with 1.3 mm and also internal stresses are less with thinner posts. It is recommended to enlarge the root only the amount required because most of the roots are narrow mesio distally and also have proximal concavities where the remaining dentine is thin which can favor perforation by the post or acts as a fracture point.

Enlargement seldom needs to exceed once or twice additional file sizes beyond that used for endodontic treatment. so it is wise to check the treatment record of endodontic therapy for proper and limited enargement of the canal.

3.4 Crown aspect

In most of the endodontically treated teeth the coronal part has been lost from caries, previous restoration or during access cavity opening so most tooth structure should be conserved as it helps in reducing the stress concentration at the gingival margins.

Indeed if more than 2 mm of coronal tooth is left the post design probably plays little role in the fracture resistance of the restored tooth. 1 mm of the vertical height of the crown provides FERRULE EFFECT.

FERRULE EFFECT: It is defined as a metal ring or cap put around the end of tool, cane etc. to give added strength. This effect is used in the dowes preparation in the form of a circumferential contrabevel which reinforces the coronal aspect of the dowel preparation. it also aids in affecting a positive occlusal seat and acts as antirotational device [73].

FERRULE EFFECT: If the artificial crown extends apical to the margin of the core and encircles sound tooth structure for 360 degrees, the crown serves as a reinforcing ring or ferrule to help protect the root from vertical fracture.

SECONDARY FERRULE: A contrabevel has been advocated when preparing a tooth for a cast post and core to produce a cast core with a collar of metal that encircles the tooth and serves as a secondary ferrule, independent of the ferrule provided by the cast crown [5].

3.5 Retention aspects

3.5.1 Anterior teeth

Retention is mainly two types.

1. Active retention.: It is due to threads or the serrations or any irregularities present on the post surface.

2. Passive retention: It is due to the sealer or the cement used for the luting of the post.

Retention of the post is affected by preparation geometry, post length, post diameter, surface texture and luting agent.

Preparation geometry: Taper should be restricted to 6 degrees or nearly parallel walls should be attained. Under cuts should be removed

Studies reveal that threaded posts are most retentive of all provided the post fits the canal properly.

1. **Length**: Increase in length increases the retention and post that is too long may damage the apical seal or may perforate the apical third of the root that is curved. in general normal crown length is 10.5 mm and root length is 13 mm.so leaving a 4 mm of guttapurcha at the apex for better seal is impossible and a compromised situation may requires a serrated post which is more retentive at shorter lengths. Increase in the length of the post, shifts the point of fracture from gingival part to apical part of the root, so that the horizontal force required to get fracture is more when compared to shorter post.

2. **Diameter**: One group says increase in diameter increases the retention while other do not confirm this. But increase in diameter in an attempt to increase the retention may weaken the remaining root.- caution..the commonly used diameter ranges from 0.8 mm to 2 mm and different types used are boston, dentatus, flexi, kerr, parapost, v lock passive post etc.

3. **Surface texture**: Roughned post is more retentive than a smooth one.

4. **Luting agent**: This has little affect in retention aspects. But recent advancements like adhesive resin shows an increase in retention of the post which are dislodged due to lack of retention.new generation lutings like adhesive resins and tuble-seal promises the role of this, in retention.

3.5.2 Posterior teeth

- Usual cause of loss of vitality of the posterior teeth is extensive caries, micro leakage beneath a large restoration. Therefore much of the central core of dentine is missing and the remaining enamel is undermined and weakened. so simple restoration of crown of the tooth with G I C OR COMPOSITE cannot impart sufficient strength to with stand laterally directed occlusal load. so it is desirable to rebuild with amalgam to support the posts before placing crown.

- Ditches and grooves will help in retention but as there is little dentine left it is not possible to place them.

- Relatively long posts with a circular cross section provide good retention and support in anterior teeth but should be avoided in posterior teeth which often have curved roots i.e. elliptical or ribbon shaped canals. so for these teeth retention is better provided by relatively short posts in the divergent canals.

- If more than 4 mm of coronal tooth structure is remaining use of the root canal for retention is not necessary.

- If a cast core is used it can be made in sections that have different paths of withdrawal.

4. Resistance aspects

One of the function of the post and core is to improve resistance to laterally directed forces by distributing them over as large as an area as possible.

According to studies• Stresses are more at shoulder and apex region.

- Stresses can be decreased by increasing the post length.

- Parallel sided posts distributes stresses more evenly than tapered posts[which has wedging effect]

- Sharp angles should be avoided.

5. Rotational resistance

Rotation of the post can be prevented by axial walls.where more coronal tooth structure is present. When most of dentine is destroyed a small groove placed in the canal can serve as an anti rotational element. it should be placed in the bulkiest part of root [usually lingual side]. auxillary pins also acts as anti rotational elements. Alternatively rotation of the threaded post can be prevented by preparing a small cavity, half in the post and half in the root then condensing amalgam in to it after cementation of the post.

6. Procedure

It involves 3 stages:

1. Removal of root canal material to appropriate depth

2. Enlargement of canal

3. Preparation of the coronal tooth structure

A post cannot be placed if the canal is filled with a full length silver point and these should be retreated with gutta purcha.

7. Methods to remove Gutta Purcha

- With a warm endodontic instrument and rotary instrument[some times with a chemical agent chloroform].

However warm method is preferred as it will not disturb the apical seal.

before removing the G.P. calculate the length of the post to be placed.

Make sure the post length equal to height of the anatomic crown or 2\3 the length of the root whichever is longer.

- Do not disturb the apical 4 to 5 mm of the G P. if this is not done the prognosis of the tooth is compromised.

If working length of the tooth is known the length of the post can be easily determined.

Then apply rubber dam to prevent aspiration. Select an condenser large enough to hold heat well, mark it at app length W.L minimum 5 mm and place in canal to soften the G P.

- If GP is old and lost its thermoplasticity use rotary instrument. Make sure that instrument does not engage the dentine.

- It was stated that gates glidden drill conforms to the original canal more consistently than the para post drill.

- Choose the rotary slightly narrow than the canals.

- Rotary should follow the centre of the gutta purcha preserving the dentine.

- Rotary shoukd not be used immediately after obturation as it disturbs the apical seal.

After removing, shape the canal as needed. The purpose is to remove the undercuts and prepare the canal to receive the posts.

posts should not be no more than 1\3 the diameter of the root dimension.

8. Enlargement

Prior to enlargement of the canal, decision must be made regarding the type of post used.

Parallel sided prefabricated posts are recommended for conservatively prepared root canals with circular cross section.

Flared canals can best be managed with custom made post.

9. For pre fabricated post

- Parallel sided posts are more retentive and distributes stresses better than tapered, but they do not conform to the shape of the canal. in this situation it may not be possible to enlarge the canal sufficiently for the post, then a tapered custom made post is preferred.

- Tapered post better conform to the canal than parallel post but it is less retentive and will cause greater stress concentration although retention may be improved by controlled grooving.

10. For custom made posts

These are used in canals that have a noncircular cross section or extreme taper.

Little preparation is sufficient for custom made post. i.e. removal of undercuts and additional shaping.

CAUTION: Mandibular molars distal wall of mesial root is particularly susceptible. in maxillary molars the curvature of the mesio buccal root makes mesial or distal perforation more likely.

11. Preparation of coronal tooth structure

After post space is prepared then extracoronal restoration is done.

Anterior teeth requiring post and core can be best restored with metal ceramic crown

Prepare the remaining crown as it was an undamaged tooth.

Sufficient reduction in the facial surface gives good easthetics.

Remove the undercuts and undermined enamel

The prepared crown must be perpendicular to the post so that it can act as a positive stop and prevent over seating of tooth.

Rotation of the post can be prevented by preparing a flat surfaces parallel to the post and when little tooth structure remains an antirotational groove should be placed in the canal.

Complete the preparation by giving smooth finish lines.

12. Post fabrication

12.1 Pre fabricated posts

- The only advantage is simplicity of the technique.

- Post is selected to match the canal and minimum adjustments are made to seat it.

- Coronal part may not exactly fit and this is adjusted by adding material to the core while it is fabricated.

Available materials are pt- au- pd. \ p-g-p,cr-co, s.s, ni- cr-ti and non oxidizing noble alloys.

- Studies reveal that corrosion of these base metal leads to root fracture and this is attributed to the electrolytic action of the dissimilar metals used to the post and core which causes a v olume change that split the root.

Prefabricated posts have high modulous of elasticity, elongated grain structure which contributes to the physical properties as compared to cast posts and also more rigid.

13. Custom made posts

These can be cast either by direct pattern or by indirect pattern.
In single canals ————direct pattern is used.
In multiple canals———indirect pattern is used.

14. Direct pattern

Lubricate the canal—select a dowel, it should extend full deapth of the canal. Apply resin [bead brush tech,]
Here resin can be applied in two types.

1. Applying at the orifice of the canal only

2. Resin is rolled and placed in canal

Now moisten the dowel with monomer and insert in the canal. Donot allow the resin to set fully and now loosen the dowel and reseat it. repeat this u ntill the resin sets. Remove the dowel. Trim any excess or undercuts on it…. the completed post pattern should not bind the canal.

15. Indirect pattern

Here a wire reinforcement should be done to prevent distortion and to get an accurate impression of the root canal.
An orthodontic wire cut in J shape is selected. it should be loosely fit in canal and must extend to full depth of the canal. Coat it with an adhesive. Lubricate the canal to facilitate removal of the wire.
Fill the canal with impression material using lentulo spiral. Seat the wire in the canal. Syringe more material around the wire and tooth and place the tray. Now remove the tray along with the post pattern. Evaluate it and pour the cast.
Using this cast take a plastic post or toothpick which extends full deapth, and apply sticy wax to it and seat it in the canal.like this wax pattern is fabricated. Which should completely adapt to post space.

16. Core fabrication

Replace the missing coronal tooth structure, restoring its original anatomy. It can be shaped either in resin or wax which is added to the post before the assembly is casr in metal. This prevents failure at the post-core interface.
It can be cast on to the prefabricated post system or make the core with a plastic material like amalgam or G I C or composites.

Advantages with plastic materials.

1. Undercuts need not be removed. so tooth structure can be conserved.

2. Less visits to the patient.

3. Less lab procedure.

4. Good adaptation to the tooth structure.

Disadvantages:

1. No long term success due to corrosion.

2. Temperature fluctuations leads to micro leakage.

3. Difficulty may be encountered with rubber dam or matrix application.[with grossly decayed teeth].

17. Procedure with amalgam

- Rubber dam is applied. Remove the G P cone from the pulp chamber. if crown structure is less than 4 mm remove the G P from the root canal up to 2–4 mm.

- Remove the unfermined enamel and carious dentin.

- When cusps are missing, pins are not usually required because adequate retention can be gained by extending the amalgam into the root canal.

- When pulp chamber is thin, protect the chamber from condensing pressures while inserting the base. When lack of tooth structure makes the application of matrix difficult then apply orthodontic or copper band. Condense the materials into the canals with endodontic plugger.

- Fill the pulp chamber and carve the amalgam to desired shape and make an impression.

- Alternatively the amalgam can be built up to anatomic contour and later prepared for a compedte crown.under these circumstance care must be taken to avoid forces that would fracture the tooth or newly placed restoration.

18. Cast metal advantages

Can be cast directly onto a prefabricated post.
An indirect procedure can be applied making restoration of posterior teeth easier.
High noble alloys can be used.

19. Direct procedure for the single rooted teeth

- Take a pre fabricated post[metal or acrylic]

- By bead technique apply resin to the post, light cure resin can also be used

- Slightly overbuild the core and let it polymerize.shape the core with burs. Use water spray to prevent overheating of resin. if any defects correct it with wax.

- Remove the pattern sprue it and invest it.

20. For multirooted teeth

Both direct and indirect techniques can be used

- Limited access makes the indirect tech easier.

- Single core with auxiliary post can be used or multisection core can be used. Multisection is preffered in indirect approach.

- Core is cast directly on to the post of one canal., while the other canals already have prefabricated posts that passes through the hole in the core.

20.1 Direct approach

Fit the prefabricated posts in the canals. One of the posts is roughened and others are smoothened. All the posts should extend beyond the preparation. Now build up the core with resin by bead tech. Shape the core and finish it.

Now grip the smoothened posts. With forceps and remove the post, invest and cast The core with the single rough post. After this the holes for the auxiliary posts can be refined with the appropriate twist drill. Verify it and cement the core and auxiliary posts to place.

20.2 Indirect approach

Wax the custom made posts, build part of the core around the first post. Remove the undercuts adjacent to other post holes and cast the first section. Now wax the other section and cast them.

Use of dove tails to interlock the sections makes the procedure more complicated and is probably of limited benefit.

21. Provisional restorations

TO prevent drifting of opposing or adfacant teeth an endodontically treated teeth requires a proper provisional restoration immediately following completion of endodontic treatment

These provide good proximal contacts to prevent tooth migration leading to unwanted root proximity

22. Investing and casting

The prepared prosthesis should fit some what loosely in the canal.tight fit may cause root fracture.

Casting should be slightly undersized which can be accomplished by restricting expansion of the invest ment [by omitting the ring liner or casting at a lower mold temperature.]

A sound casting technique is essential because any undetected porosity could lead to a weakened casting that might fail in function.

23. TRY — IN

Care should be exercised such that casting defects should not interfere with seating of the post, lest root fracture results.

Post and core should be inserted with gentle pressure. no adjustments should be made immediately after cementation because vibration from the bur could fracture the setting cement and cause premature failure.

24. Cementation

It is important that the luting agent should fill all the dead space within the root canal system. a rotary paste filler or cement tube is used to fill the canal.post and core is inserted gently to reduce hydrostatic pressure which could cause root fracture.

It is recommended that a groove placed along the side of the post to allow excess cement to escape, if a parallel sided post is being used.

25. Cements and disadvantages

- Zinc phosphate: Solubility in oral fluids.
- Polycarboxylate: Undergoes plastic deformation
- Glass ionomer cement: Do not reach its maximum strength for many days. Therefore Any recontouring of the core may disturb the set of the cement and weaken the immature cement fibers.
- Resin modified GIC: exhibits delayed expansion of the cement.

26. Removal of existing posts

Occasionally a failed post and core must be removed, then if sufficient post length is exposed coronally, it can be retrieved with thin beaked forceps.

Vibrating the post with a ultrasonic scaler will weaken the cement and facilitates easy removal. Here a thin scaler tip is recommended or alternatively a post puller is used. [post puller cannot be used for fractured post.]

Fractured posts should be drilled out but care should be taken not to deviate from the canal. This is best limited to short fractured posts

27. Masserann 1966 handling

He used a hallow end cutting tubes o r trephines to prepare a thin trench around the post. Post retrieved can be facilitated by using an adhesive to attach a hallow tube extractor or by using a threaded extractor.

Newer Concepts:

Zarow, M proposed new classification was to help the clinician to select the most appropriate treatment plan for restoring root filled teeth when choosing between a composite core alone, a composite core reinforced by fiber post, a gold cast post or implant treatment. **The following is the classification:-** [74]

1. Class 0 (no post – composite core build-up).

2. Class 1 (fiber post).

3. Class 2 (pre-restorative procedures are needed: orthodontic extrusion or crown lengthening).

4. Class 3 (gold cast post).

5. Class 4 (extraction).

The three categories given by Motasum Abu-Awwad in 2019 are [75].

1. Minimally destructed teeth, which could be managed simply through intracoronal composite resin restorations.

2. Moderately destructed teeth, which could be managed through adhesive overlays

3. Severely destructed teeth, which could be managed through fiber post–core–crown combination, or through endocrowns [9].

28. Summary

- Restoration of endodontically treated teeth can be done successfully if the available procedures are performed well.

- Where most of the crown is preserved an anterior teeth can be safely restored with a plastic filling material.

- To prevent fracture of posterior teeth, cast restoration with cuspal coverage is recommended.

- Anterior teeth can best built up with a cast metal post and core or a metal core cast on to a prefabricated wire.

- Amalgam can be used on posterior teeth, although if much coronal tooth structure is missing a casting may be preferred.

29. Conclusion

The rational for the post placement is two folds that is,

1. To retain the restoration, and.

2. To protect the remaining tooth structure.

The success rate will be high if the rationales for the results are understood, appreciated and propagated accordingly. A technique with more advantages and fewer disadvantages in the given restoration should be chosen. It is important to preserve as much tooth structure as possible, particularly in the root canal. The post should be adequate length for good stress distribution but not as long as to jeopardize the apical seal. In the final analysis the quality of the root canal thereby combined with the quality of its final restoration determines the clinical success of pulpless tooth with post and core.

Acknowledgements

I am thankful to Rural Dental College,Pravara institute of medical sciences,Loni. Dr.Mukund Singh, Dr.Milind Jagdale, Dr.Agey Pathak.

Conflict of interest

None.

Author details

Deepak M. Vikhe
Department of Prosthodontics, Crown and Bridge, Rural Dental College and Hospital, Pravara Institute of Medical Science (DU), Pravara Medical Trust, Loni, Maharashtra, India

*Address all correspondence to: drdeepak_mvikhe@yahoo.com

References

[1] Suna Toksavul, Muhittin Toman, Mehmet Sankanat, Ibrahim Nergiz and Petra Schmage , Effect of Noble Metal Alloy Post and Core Material on the Fracture Resistance of Endodontically Treated Teeth , European Journal Of Prosthodontics & Restorative Dentistry. March 2010,Vol 18, Issue 1.

[2] Standlee J.P.Caputo A.A.Hanson E.C. Retention of endodontic dowels: Effects of cement, dowel length, diameter, and design.J Prosthet Dent. 1978; 39: 401

[3] Sorensen J.A.Martinoff J.T.Intracoronal reinforcement and coronal coverage: a study of endodontically treated teeth.J Prosthet Dent. 1984; 51: 780-784

[4] Colley IT Hampson EL Lehman ML , Retention of post crown: An assessment of the relative efficiency of posts of different shapes and sizes.Br Dent J. 1968; 124: 63-69

[5] Goodacre CJ. Designing tooth preparations for optimal success. Dent Clin North Am. 2004;48(2):v-385.

[6] Chan, R. W., & Bryant, R. W. (1982). Post-core foundations for endodontically treated posterior teeth. The Journal of Prosthetic Dentistry, 48(4), 401–406. doi: 10.1016/0022-3913(82)90074-9

[7] Valdivia ADCM, Correia AD, Raposo LHA, Simamoto-Junior PC, Novais VR, Soares CJ. The effect of fiber post presence and restorative technique on the biomechanical behavior of endodontically treated maxillary incisors: An in vitro study. J Prosthet Dent 2012 Sep;108(3):147-157.

[8] Rosenstiel SF, Land MF, Fujimoto J. Contemporary Fixed Prosthodontics. 3rd edition. Year Book Medical Pub; 2001. p.868.

[9] Santos-Filho PCF, Veríssimo C, Soares PV, Saltarelo RC, Soares CJ, Martins LRM. Influence of ferrule, post system, and length on biomechanical behavior of Endodontically treated anterior teeth. J Endod. 2014 Jan; 40(1): 119-123.

[10] Schwartz R, Robbins J. Restoration of Endodontically treated teeth: A literature review. J Endod 2004 May;30 (5):289-301.

[11] Baba ZN, Goodacre CJ. Contemporary restoration of endodontically treated teeth. Ingle's endodontics 7th edition. PMPH USA, 2019.

[12] Standlee JP, Caputo AA, Collard EW, Pollack MH. Analysis of stress distribution by endodontic posts. Oral Surg Oral Med Oral Pathol. 1972;33 (6):952-960.

[13] Guzy GE, Nicholls JI. In vitro comparison of intact endodntically treated teeth with and without endo-post reinforcement. J Prosthet Dent 1979 Jul;42(1):39-44.

[14] Davy DT, Dilley GL, Krejci RF. Determination of stress patterns in root-filled teeth incorporating various dowel designs. J Dent Res. 1981 Jul;60(7):1301–1310.

[15] Eshelman EG Jr, Sayegh FS. Dowel materials and root fracture. J Prosthet Dent. 1983 Sep;50(3):342–344.

[16] Reinhardt RA, Krejci RF, Pao YC, Stannard JG. Dentin stresses in post-reconstructed teeth with diminishing bone support. J Dent Res. 1983 Sep;62 (9):1002-1008.

[17] Sorensen JA, Martinoff JT. Clinically significant factors in dowel design. J Prosthet Dent. 1984 Jul;52(1):28-35.

[18] Kersten HW, Fransman R, Thoden Velzen SK. Thermomechanical

compaction of gutta-percha. II. A comparison with lateral condensation in curved root canals. May 1986;19(3): 134-140.

[19] PJJM, P JJ, Visseren LGH, Vrijhoef MMA, Käyser AF. In vitro comparison of dowel and core techniques for endodontically treated molars. J Endod;1989; 12(9):382-387.

[20] Leary JM, Aquilino SA, Svare CW. An evaluation of post length within the elastic limits of dentin. J Prosthet Dent. 1987 Mar;57(3):277–281.

[21] Hunter AJ, Feiglin B, Williams JF. Effects of post placement on endodontically treated teeth. J Prosthet Dent. 1989 Aug;62(2):166–172.

[22] Greenfeld RS, Roydhouse RH, James Marshall F, Schoner B. A comparison of two post systems under applied compressive-shear loads. J Prosthet Dent.1989;61(1): 17-24.

[23] Burns DA, Krause WR, Douglas HB, Burns DR. Stress distribution surrounding endodontic posts. J Prosthet Dent.1990 Oct;64(4):412-418.

[24] Hatzikyriakos AH, Reisis GI, Tsingos N. A 3-year postoperative clinical evaluation of posts and cores beneath existing crowns. J Prosthet Dent. 1992 Apr;67(4):454–458.

[25] Sedgley CM, Messer HH. Are endodontically treated teeth more brittle? J of Endod. 1992 Jul;18(7): 332-335.

[26] Assif D, Bitenski A, Pilo R, Oren E. Effect of post design on resistance to fracture of endodontically treated teeth with complete crowns. J Prosthet Dent. 1993 Jan;69(1):36-40.

[27] Mentink AGB, Creugers NHJ, Meeuwissen R, Leempoel PJB, Kayser AF. Clinical performance of different post and core systems - results of a pilot study. J Oral Rehabil. 1993 Nov;20(6):577-584.

[28] Goodacre CJ, Spolnik KJ. The prosthodontic Management of Endodontically Treated Teeth: A literature review. Part I. success and failure data, treatment concepts. J Prosthodont. 1994 Dec;3(4):243-250.

[29] Torbjorner A, Karlsson S, Dr O, Odman PA. Survival rate and failure characteristics for two post designs. J Prosthet Dent. 1995 May;73(5):439-444.

[30] Purton DG, Love RM. Rigidity and retention of carbon fibre versus stainless steel root canal posts. Int Endod J.1996 Jul;29(4):262-265.

[31] Mendoza DB, Stephan Eakle W, Kahl EA, Ho R. Root reinforcement with a resin-bonded preformed post. J Prosthet Dent. 1997 Jul;78(1):10-14.

[32] Asmussen E, Peutzfeldt A. Direction of shrinkage of light-curing resin composites Acta Odontologica Scandinavica. Jan 2000.57(6):310-315.

[33] Al-Hazaimeh N, Gutteridge DL. An in vitro study into the effect of the ferrule preparation on the fracture resistance of crowned teeth incorporating prefabricated post and composite core restorations. Int Endod J. 2001 Jan;34(1):40-46.

[34] Cormier CJ, Burns DR, Moon P. In vitro comparison of the fracture resistance and failure mode of fiber, ceramic, and conventional post systems at various stages of restoration. J Prosthodont. 2001 Mar;10(1):26–36.

[35] Christophe G, Chai J, Jameson L. Fracture Resistance and Primary Failure Mode of Endodontically Treated Teeth Int J Prosthodont 2001;14:141–145.

[36] Akkayan B, Gülmez T. Resistance to fracture of endodontically treated teeth restored with different post systems.J Prosthet Dent.2002; 87(4):431-7.

[37] Pontius O, Hutter J. Survival rate and fracture strength of incisors restored with different post and Core systems and Endodontically treated incisors without Coronoradicular reinforcement. J of Endod.2002;28(10): 710-715.

[38] Nergiz I, Schmage P, Platzer U, Ozcan M. Bond strengths of five tapered root posts regarding the post surface. J. Oral Rehabil.2020 ;29(4):330-335.

[39] Kishen A, Kumar GV, Chen N-N. Stress-strain response in human dentine: Rethinking fracture predilection in postcore restored teeth. Dent Traumatol. 2004 Apr;20(2):90–100.

[40] Tan PLB, Aquilino SA, Gratton DG, Stanford CM, Tan SC, Johnson WT, et al. In vitro fracture resistance of endodontically treated central incisors with varying ferrule heights and configurations. J Prosthet Dent. 2005 Apr;93(4):331–336.

[41] Ng CCH, Dumbrigue HB, Al-Bayat MI, Griggs JA, Wakefield CW. Influence of remaining coronal tooth structure location on the fracture resistance of restored endodontically treated anterior teeth. J Prosthet Dent. 2006 Apr;95(4): 290–296.

[42] Dietschi D, Ardu S, Rossier-Gerber A, Krejci I. Adaptation of adhesive post and cores to dentin after in vitro occlusal loading: Evaluation of post material influence. J Adhes Dent. 2006 Dec;8(6):409–419.

[43] Salvi GE, Siegrist Guldener BE, Amstad T, Joss A, Lang NP. Clinical evaluation of root filled teeth restored with or without post-and-core systems in a specialist practice setting. Int Endod J. 2007 Mar;40(3):209–215.

[44] Maccari PC, Cosme DC, Oshima HM, Burnett LH, Shinkai RS. Fracture strength of Endodontically treated teeth with flared root canals and restored with different post systems. J Esthet Restor Dent.2007;19(1):30-36.

[45] Hinckfuss S, Wilson PR. Effect of core material and restoration design on strength of endodontically treated bovine teeth: A laboratory study. J Prosthodont. 2008 Aug;17(6):456–461.

[46] Gorgul G, Kivanç BH. Fracture resistance of teeth restored with different post systems using new-generation adhesives. J Contemp Dent Pract. 2008 Nov 1;9(7):33-40.

[47] Alikhasi M, Dorriz H, Mirfazaelian A, Hooshmand T. Effect of ferrule and bonding on the compressive fracture resistance of post and Core restorations. J Contemp Dent Pract. Feb 2009;10(1):1-8.

[48] Ma PS, Nicholls JI, Junge T, Phillips KM. Load fatigue of teeth with different ferrule lengths, restored with fiber posts, composite resin cores, and all-ceramic crowns. J Prosthet Dent. 2009 Oct;102(4):229-234

[49] Signore A, Benedicenti S, Kaitsas V, Barone M, Angiero F, Ravera G. Long-term survival of endodontically treated, maxillary anterior teeth restored with either tapered or parallel-sided glass-fiber posts and full-ceramic crown coverage. J Dent. 2009 Feb;37(2): 115-121.

[50] Da Silva NR, Raposo LHA, Versluis A, Fernandes-Neto AJ, Soares CJ. The effect of post, core, crown type, and ferrule presence on the biomechanical behavior of endodontically treated bovine anterior teeth. J Prosthet Dent. 2010 Nov;104(5): 306-317.

[51] Jang J-H, Park S-J, Min K-S, Lee B-N, Chang H-S, Oh W-M. Stress behavior of cemented fiber-reinforced composite and titanium posts in the upper central incisor according to the post length: Two-dimensional finite element

analysis. Journal of Dental Sciences. 2012 Dec;7(4):384–389.

[52] Hegde J, Bashetty K, Ramakrishna, Srirekha, Lekha, Champa. An in vitro evaluation of fracture strength of endodontically treated teeth with simulated flared root canals restored with different post and core systems. J Conserv Dent 2012 ;15 (3): 223-227.

[53] Juloski J, Radovic I, Goracci C, Vulicevic ZR, Ferrari M. Ferrule effect: a literature review. J Endod. 2012 Jan;38 (1):11–19.

[54] Santos-Filho PCF, Verissimo C, Soares PV, Saltarelo RC, Soares CJ, Marcondes Martins LR. Influence of ferrule, post system, and length on biomechanical behavior of endodontically treated anterior teeth. J Endod. 2014 Jan;40(1):119–123.

[55] Maroulakos G, Nagy WW, Kontogiorgos ED. Fracture resistance of compromised endodontically treated teeth restored with bonded post and cores: An in vitro study. J Prosthet Dent. 2015 Sep;114(3):390-397.

[56] Upadhyaya V, Bhargava A, Parkash H, Chittaranjan B, Kumar V. A finite element study of teeth restored with post and core: Effect of design, material, and ferrule. Dental research journal. May 2016;13(3):233.

[57] Kim A-R, Lim H-P, Yang H-S, Park S-W. Effect of ferrule on the fracture resistance of mandibular premolars with prefabricated posts and cores. J Adv Prosthodont. 2017;9(5):328.

[58] Marchionatti AME, Wandscher VF, Rippe MP, Kaizer OB, Valandro LF. Clinical performance and failure modes of pulpless teeth restored with posts: a systematic review. Braz Oral Res. 2017. Jul 3;31-64.

[59] Sarkis-Onofre R, Fergusson D, Cenci MS, Moher D, Pereira-Cenci T. Performance of post-retained single crowns: A systematic review of related risk factors. J Endod. 2017;43:175–183.

[60] Naumann M, Sterzenbach G, Dietrich T, Bitter K, Frankenberger R, Von Stein-Lausnitz M. Dentin-like versus rigid endodontic post: 11-year randomized controlled pilot trial on No-wall to 2-wall defects. J Endod. 2017 Nov;43(11):1770–1775.

[61] Lazari PC, de Carvalho MA, Del Bel Cury AA, Magne P. Survival of extensively damaged endodontically treated incisors restored with different types of posts-and-core foundation restoration material. J Prosthet Dent. 2018 May;119(5):769-776.

[62] Meng Q, Ma Q, Wang T, Chen Y. An in vitro study evaluating the effect of ferrule design on the fracture resistance of endodontically treated mandibular premolars after simulated crown lengthening or forced eruption methods. BMC Oral Health. 2018 May 10; 18(1):83.

[63] Zarow M, Ramírez-Sebastià A, Paolone G, de Ribot Porta J, Mora J. A new classification system for the restoration of root filled teeth. Int Endod J. 2018 Mar;51(3):318-334.

[64] Fadag A et al. Fracture resistance of Endodontically treated anterior teeth restored with different post systems: An In vitro study. Eur Endod J. 2018;3(3): 174-178.

[65] Pinto CL, Bhering CLB, de Oliveira GR, Maroli A, Reginato VF, Caldas RA. The influence of post system design and material on the biomechanical behavior of teeth with little remaining coronal structure. J Prosthodont. 2019 Jan;28(1):350–356.

[66] Bakirtzoglou E, Kamalakidis SN, Pissiotis AL, Michalakis K. In vitro assessment of retention and resistance failure loads of complete coverage

restorations made for anterior maxillary teeth restored with two different cast post and core designs Journal of Clinical and Experimental Dentistry.2019 Mar; 11(3):e225-e230.

[67] Veeraganta SK, Samran A, Wille S, Kern M. Influence of post material, post diameter, and substance loss on the fracture resistance of endodontically treated teeth: A laboratory study. J Prosthet Dent ; 2020 Aug 2:S0022-3913 (20)30362-0.

[68] Cheung W. A review of the management of endodontically treated teeth. Post, core and the final restoration. J Am Dent Assoc. 2005 May; 136(5):611–619.

[69] Peroz I, Blankenstein F, Lange KP, Naumann M. Restoring endodontically treated teeth with posts and cores—A review. Quintessence Int 2005;36:737–746.

[70] Ree M, Schwartz RS. The Endo-restorative Interface: Current concepts. Dent Clin North Am. 2010;54(2):345–374.

[71] Valea MC, Pena VA. Titanium posts and bonded amalgam core longevity A 22- year clinical survival retrospective study. J Am Dent Assoc. 2017 Feb;148 (2):75-80.

[72] Abou-Rass M, Jaan MJ, Jobe D and Tsutsui F. Preparation of space for posting: Effect on thickness of canal walls and incidence of perforation in molars. J Am Dent Assoc,1982 Jun;104 (6):834-837.

[73] Delgado MM. The ferrule effect: An important aspect of rehabilitation involving using fiber posts. Rev ADM. 2014;71(3):120-123.

[74] Zarow, M, Ramírez-Sebastià, A, Gaetano, P, de Ribot Porta, J, Mora, J, Espona, J, Durán-Sindreu, F, Roig, M. A new classification system for the restoration of root filled teeth. International Endodontic Journal, 51, 318– 334, 2018.

[75] Abu-Awwad M. A modern guide in the management of endodontically treated posterior teeth. Eur J Gen Dent [serial online] 2019 [cited 2020 Aug 19]; 8:63-70.

Chapter 7

The Application of Zirconia in Tooth Defects

Feng Luo, Hongyan Luo, Ruyi Li, Changxing Qu, Guang Hong and Qianbing Wan

Abstract

Dental caries is among the most prevalent chronic diseases of childhood, affecting larger part of children and adults. Non-treated enamel caries can lead to destruction and then spreads into the underlying softer and sensitive dentine layer. Dental restorative materials are applied to treat and reconstruct damaged teeth clinically and recover their functions. Currently, there are various dental restorative materials available, and many appropriate materials are used to restore dental carious teeth. The applicability of biomimetic principles can elicit innovations in restorative dentistry for tooth conservation and preservation. There are three types of materials commonly used in dental restorations: resin, alloys, and ceramic. During the past decade, zirconia-based ceramics have been successfully introduced into the clinic due to acceptable biocompatibility, lower price compared with gold restorations, and better appearance than traditional metal-ceramic restorations. Recently, zirconia restoration is an acceptable treatment option in restorative dentistry and a developing trend in esthetic dentistry.

Keywords: dental caries, dental restorative materials, biomimetic principles, resin, zirconia

1. Introduction

Human teeth have a complex structure with an inner core of highly vascular, soft, and delicate pulp surrounded by the highly mineralized enamel and dentin tissues (**Figure 1**) [1]. The structure of teeth can be altered by diet, age, or diseases such as caries and sclerosis. Currently, dental caries is among the most prevalent chronic diseases of childhood, affecting 60–90% of school-aged children and the larger part of adults [2]. Non-treated enamel caries can lead to destruction and then spreads into the underlying softer and sensitive dentine layer. Dental caries could attack the cement of the root and cause gum recession and periodontitis [3]. Dental enamel is composed of long and parallel mineralized crystals containing 90–92% hydroxyapatite, 1–2% organic matrix proteins, and 4–12% water [4]. In addition, the thickness of enamel is different in different anatomical parts of different teeth. For instance, the enamel thickness at the cementum-enamel junction (CEJ) is thinner than the occlusal/incisal surface. Further, the average enamel thickness of incisal edge, premolar cusp, and molar cusp are 2 mm, 2.3–2.5 mm, and 2.5–3 mm, respectively [5]. Dentin is composed of inorganic (50% by volume) and organic material (30% by volume; 90% of which is type 1 collagen and 10%

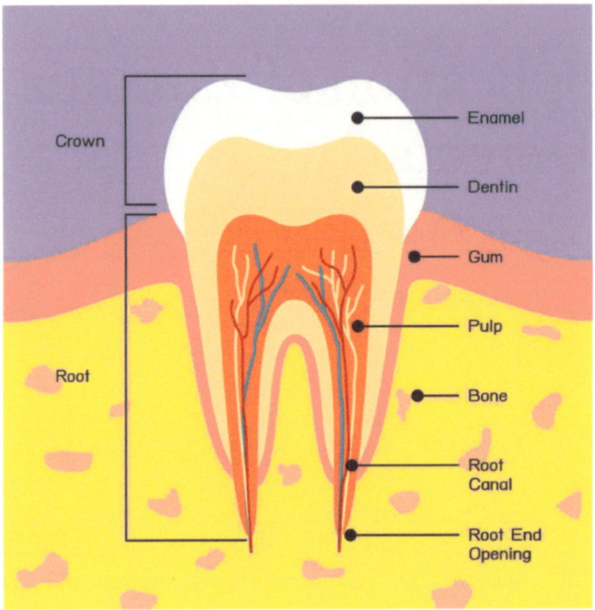

Figure 1.
Structure of human tooth. Human teeth have a complex structure with an inner core of highly vascular, soft, and delicate pulp surrounded by the highly mineralized enamel and dentin tissues.

non-collagenous proteins) [6]. Dentin covers most of the tooth structure, and it is externally covered by enamel and cementum.

Unfortunately, dental caries is non-avoidable disease. The tooth's hard tissue, included the enamel and dentin, is typically damaged by dental caries. The shape and function of the teeth are also impaired. In spite of much effort in oral health promotion and preventive methods, dental restorations are still needed. Natural teeth are always considered to be a reference while employing biomimetic approaches to restore diseased or fractured dental tissues [7]. The main goal of restorative dentistry is to create a restoration that can mineralize initial enamel and dentinal lesions in native form. Besides, restorative dentistry aims to develop material that can mimic natural teeth' structural, functional, and biological properties.

Dental restorative materials are applied to treat and reconstruct damaged teeth clinically and recover their functions [8]. Currently, there are various dental restorative materials available, and many appropriate materials are used to restore dental carious teeth. At a macrostructural level, various biomimetic restorative materials can be applied to achieve the teeth' biomechanical, structural, and aesthetic integrity. For this purpose, materials scientists take natural teeth as a reference during the development of dental restorative materials. The widespread application of bionic principles in the field of dentistry can also promote the innovation of restorative dentistry, especially in the field of protection and preservation of teeth. For example, when restoring damaged parts of teeth, dentists should pay more attention to factors, such as color tone, internal coronal anatomy, mechanics, and tooth position in the dental arch [9]. There are three types of materials commonly used in dental restorations: resin, alloys, and ceramic [10]. In dental clinical, resin dental composites and glass-ionomer cements are commonly used to restore features depending on the extent of damage and aesthetic requirement. While alloy and ceramic materials are mainly used for fixed restorations (e.g., fixed dentures), removable restorations mainly use nano-resins and alloys. Recently, the most prevalent clinical materials in oral restorations are ceramics and nano-resins.

2. Dental restorative materials

2.1 Resin

Most dental ceramics and hybrid resin composites have the potential to mimic the enamel and dentin, respectively. However, it has been suggested that moderate damage to teeth could be restored with resin composites. For the resin composites restorations, minimal preparation of teeth is required, reducing the likelihood of pulpal involvement and tooth fracture [11].

The filling resin composite can strengthen the remaining tooth structure in some cases. For example, cemented porcelain restorations are recommended for severely damaged, worn, or broken teeth in dental clinics. Besides, alumina and nano-hydroxyapatite are also widely used in dentistry [12]. Alumina is recommended because it has good fracture resistance, abrasion resistance, and high compressive strength. In addition, nano-hydroxyapatite is an essential part of teeth and bones. Therefore, it should achieve biomimetic properties in the restoration. Glass ionomer cement has a bactericidal effect because it releases fluoride and can stimulate hardened dentin [13]. In addition, these cements have properties comparable to dentin, thus realizing the concept of bionics. Glass-ionomer cements are used as restorative materials in deep class I or II cavities in pedodontics and restoration of class V cavities [14]. Glass-ionomer cements are not generally recommended in load-bearing posterior dentition due to low tensile strength. Therefore, in the context of mismatched elastic modulus between enamel and the direct restorative materials, more stresses may be transferred to teeth, leading to either tooth damage or failure of the restoration.

Nowadays, many clinicians take direct resin composite posterior restoration as their first choice in treating carious lesions or other tooth defects, including restoration of large cavities [15]. However, partial indirect restorations (inlay, onlay, and overlay) for excessive posterior tooth defects have started to replace direct resin composite restorations since the development of modern chairside computer-aided design/computer-aided manufacturing (CAD/CAM) systems [16].

One of the most important advancements in chairside CAD/CAM systems is the production of resin composite blocks [17, 18]. Paradigm MZ100, as an industrial polymerized version of direct resin composite (Z100), is the first product in this field [19]. Paradigm MZ100 contains bisphenol A-glycidyl methacrylate (Bis-GMA), triethylene glycol dimethacrylate, and 85% (by weight) zirconia-silica filler. Therefore, its degree of polymerization and mechanical properties are better than Z100 [20]. Later, a new resin composite block containing urethane dimethacrylate instead of Bis-GMA was produced under high temperature and pressure. This kind of resin was developed with the ambition of increasing the degree of polymerization [21, 22]. Recently, the flexibility and convenience of CAD/CAM resin composite are similar to resin composites, combined with durability, and surface finish characteristics are identical to ceramics. In addition, compared with glass ceramics, the resin composite block has minor wear on the relative teeth and can maintain its gloss for a longer time. Their non-fusion and composite-like properties make them easier to grind, polish, and adapt. Due to the less brittleness, the resin composite block has better edge characteristics. Furthermore, these materials produced less blunting on the drills during milling. They can also be repaired using resin composites with cutback or adding techniques. Besides, physical (color stability, water sorption, and water solubility) and mechanical (fracture-resistant, wear, compressive strength, hardness, and elastic modulus) properties of resin composite blocks were found better than that of conventional resin composite because of their higher degree of polymerization [23, 24].

Tunac et al. evaluate the 2 year clinical performance of computer-aided design/computer-aided manufacturing (CAD/CAM) resin composite inlay restorations in comparison with direct resin composite restorations. According to FDI standards, the results show that the 2 year clinical performance of CAD/CAM resin composite inlay restorations is similar to that of direct resin composite restorations. After 2 years of clinical trials, CAD/CAM resin composite inlays have shown exemplary performance in class II cavities and meet clinical needs [25].

Despite the above advantages, due to the high degree of polymerization, discoloration, tarnishing, and fracture of the resin composite block overtime after the repair, the adhesion failure of the cement interface is a problem that may need to be considered for its long-term clinical performance [26]. However, data on CAD/CAM resin composite partial crowns (inlays, onlays, and overlying) restorations are limited. Therefore, more clinical trials are needed to draw further conclusions about its clinical behavior.

2.2 Alloy

Porcelain fused to metal (PFM) restoration comprises a metal coping that supports overlying ceramic (**Figure 2**) [27]. PFM restorations have a long clinical track record. However, the PFM fixed partial denture (FPD) failure rates were 4% after 5 years, 12% after 10 years, and 32% after 15 years [28].

To date, PFM restorations remain the most widely and successfully used option for FPDs because their failure rates are often low (8–10% within 10 years) [29]. It was reported that clinical survival rates of FPDs are between 72% and 87% after 10 years, between 69% and 74% after 15 years, and 53% after 30 years [30, 31]. However, as is well-known, the metals used in PFM restorations can cause allergic or toxic reactions within soft or hard tissue [32]. Besides, PFM is known to cause graying of the gingival margin because of metal show-through [33].

Compatibility between the ceramic and the metal alloy is of paramount importance. PFM ceramic veneers consist of an opaque ceramic (e.g., a titanium oxide glass) that is required to mask the color of the underlying metal and provides the bond with the metal alloy [34, 35].

Opaque ceramics are combined with metal alloys through an oxide layer formed on the metal surface. This process is called degassing [36]. The degassing process can also remove contaminants on the surface of the alloy—coating dentin/body ceramics on opaque ceramics. Dentin ceramics can mimic natural dentin. Then apply the incisal ceramic to the dentin/body ceramic on the incisal third. The restoration can also be polished by using low-melting glazed ceramics or self-glazing.

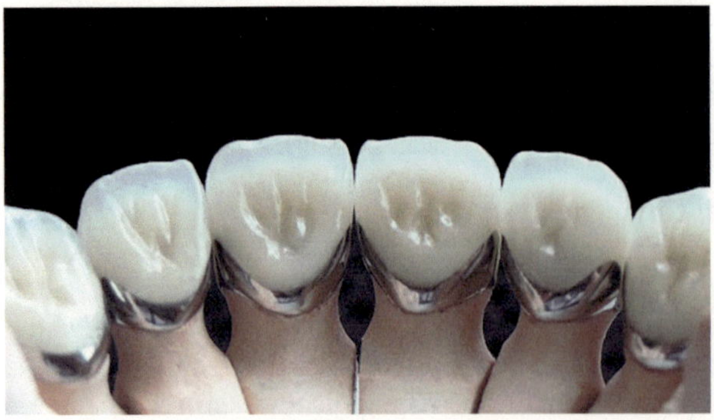

Figure 2.
Porcelain fused to metal (PFM). Porcelain fused to metal (PFM) restoration comprises a metal coping that supports overlying ceramic.

One of PFM restoration's main disadvantages is its inability to transmit light, thus having a negative effect on the aesthetic outcome of the restoration because it may appear dark in color [37]. This drawback is noticeable at the restoration's cervical area, where it is sometimes difficult to get enough room. Therefore, a sufficient tooth structure should be removed to accommodate the ceramic material, mask the underlying metal without overly modifying the restoration. In addition, the metal braces should stop 1 mm from the buccal finish line, and ceramic edges (shoulder ceramics) are recommended. Another disadvantage of a PFM restoration is allergic reactions in some patients to metal elements such as nickel in the metal alloy [32].

2.3 Ceramic

All-ceramic restorations refer to ceramic restorations made entirely of ceramic materials [38]. There are two kinds of all-ceramic restorations. One is monolithic (single layer), which composes of a single ceramic material. The other is a two-layer all-ceramic restoration which consists of a ceramic core material covered with a ceramic veneer [39, 40]. In the bi-layered, all-ceramic restoration, the ceramic core supports the restoration and gives it strength, while the veneer provides the restoration with its final shape, shade, and aesthetic [41]. Nevertheless, the veneer-core bond strength is considered one of the weakest links of the bi-layered all-ceramic restorations because they are prone to delamination and fracture [39]. Nowadays, with the increasing interest in aesthetics, a bi-layered all-ceramic restoration is widely applied in dentistry. However, the main disadvantages associated with this repair include delamination and fracture of the veneer [42]. In addition, it is sometimes difficult to achieve excellent occlusal contact with the structure of the opposing tooth. Finally, to achieve a lasting repair, the compatibility of the core and veneer materials is crucial [43].

When aesthetics is the priority, dental ceramics are the material of choice because they can successfully mimic the tooth substance's character (**Figure 3**) [44]. Ceramics can successfully simulate the visual characteristics of the tooth substance. Ceramics are biocompatible and inert material and have a high degree of intra-oral stability. Therefore, they can be safely used in the oral cavity. For example, the use of all-ceramic restorations has increased in recent years [45]. However, there are many ceramic materials and systems on the market that can be used in dentistry. The increased use of ceramics for restorative procedures and the need to improve clinical performance has led to the development and introduction of several new ceramic restorative materials and techniques [46].

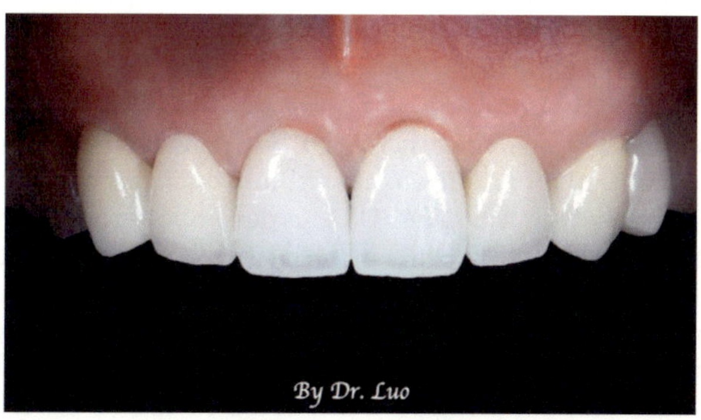

Figure 3.
Ceramics. Ceramics can successfully simulate the visual characteristics of the tooth substance. Ceramics are biocompatible and inert material and have a high degree of intra-oral stability.

The all-ceramic restorations can be used as a bi-layered restoration, in which the more aesthetic ceramic veneer is the core or framework. They can also be used as full-contour (monolithic) restorations, which can be stained when required [47].

In the past decade, countless types of all-ceramic crown systems have been introduced unprecedentedly. Many of these systems have been criticized for their failure in restorations. It was reported that the survival rate of all-ceramic restorations ranges from 88–100% after 2–5 years of use and can still reach 97% after 5–15 years of use [48]. Although all-ceramic restorations have been greatly improved, zirconia is still the best all-ceramic restoration currently available. Since the end of the 1990s, due to many clinical and basic scientific research, this form of partially stabilized zirconia has been popularized for application in dentistry due to its excellent strength and excellent fracture resistance [49]. Currently, two main types of all-ceramic FDP systems have been proposed. The first of these systems involves the use of a single material to make full-contour crowns. For instance, a single crown in anterior teeth and premolars is made by reinforced glass materials successfully [50]. Further, a full-contour crown in the molar region is prepared with polycrystalline zirconia with improved translucency [51]. For the second system, porcelain and other glass materials are fused into a frame made of high-strength ceramics [52]. Dense sintered polycrystalline zirconia-based materials are expected to be used in FDP frameworks [53].

Yttrium partially stabilized tetragonal zirconia polycrystalline (Y-TZP), due to its superior mechanical properties and excellent fracture resistance, has drawn lots of attention in clinical applications. For instance, the fracture toughness of Y-TZP ranges from 5 to 10 MPa $m^{1/2}$, and bending strength varies from 900 to 1400 MPa [54]. Y-TZP-based systems are a recent addition to the high-strength, all-ceramic systems used for crowns and fixed partial dentures.

Zirconia is a white crystalline oxide of zirconium with high mechanical strength, toughness, and corrosion resistance. Besides, zirconia has excellent biocompatibility, which can significantly reduce dental plaque [55]. However, zirconia is degradable at low temperatures, and this is a gradual, spontaneous phenomenon. Recently, the introduction of stabilized zirconia is supposed to overcome this drawback and promote the application of zirconia in dental restorations [56].

Marchack et al. proposed a custom-designed powerful grinding ceramic core technology for all-ceramic crowns [57]. This technique can eliminate the porcelain covering of the zirconia inner crown and frame to reduce the incidence of chipping or cracking of the porcelain veneer. The fracture of veneering ceramic is the most common complication for zirconia restorations. Thus, some suggestions for optimizing the manufacturing process of zirconia-based FPDs have been issued, including changes to the firing protocol. It was recommended because it can reduce the chipping rate. In addition, zirconia-ceramic FDP shows more clinical problems like prolonged fracture of the veneer ceramic [58]. Therefore, dentists should pay more attention to zirconia-ceramic FDP generated by CAD/CAM system before all treatment procedures [29]. On the other hand, with the development of ceramics on zirconia, people invented the framework of lithium disilicate glass-ceramics.

Cercon ht (Dentsply Intl., York, PA, USA) is developed from a clinically proven Cercon-based yttria-stabilized zirconia material formulation. It represents a new generation of zirconia with excellent transparency and can be used for esthetic restorations without build-up porcelain [29]. In order to better reproduce the color of natural teeth, some zirconia-based materials have been developed as translucent [59]. Among them, zirconia is widely applied as crown and FDP without veneer or pressed ceramics. Zirconia has a high flexural strength of more than 1200 MPa and has excellent veneer properties [60]. In the dental clinic, zirconia has proven to be a durable and reliable frame material that can inhibit crack propagation and prevent catastrophic failure. However, there are clinical studies show that zirconia has an abrasive effect on the dentition, leading to excessive wear of the tooth structure [61]. The in vivo studies indicated that polished zirconia has higher wear resistance and lower resistance to wear than porcelain [62]. Currently, the new zirconia materials make the surface of the antagonist smooth, just like natural tooth enamel [63]. Although more and more research is focused on zirconia, there is still much to be understood about the production of zirconia and the production of zirconia inner crowns and frames. Dentists and researchers need further studies with larger sample sizes and extended follow-up periods to investigate the possible influencing factors of technical failures.

Ceria-stabilized tetragonal zirconia polycrystalline (Ce-TZP) is a newly developed ceramic material, which has not yet been used in the dental field. Its fracture toughness is 19 MPa $m^{1/2}$, which is significantly better than Y-TZP. However, Ce-TZP has lower bending strength and hardness than Y-TZP [64]. Then, Ce-TZP/alumina nanocomposite (Ce-TZP/A) was developed to improve the property of Ce-TZP [65]. Ce-TZP/A contains nano-sized Al_2O_3 particles and Ce-TZP particles dispersed in Ce-TZP grains and grain boundaries [66]. This uniform dispersion of alumina in the Ce-TZP matrix plays a positive role in grain growth. However, it also negatively affects flexural strength, hardness, and hydrothermal stability of tetragonal zirconia. As reported, Ce-TZP/A is currently the toughest zirconia material available, and its fracture toughness reaches 19 MPa $m^{1/2}$, and the flexural strength is high as 1400 MPa [65]. More importantly, Ce-TZP/A is entirely resistant to low-temperature aging degradation (LTAD), a critical drawback of Y-TZP [67]. The tremendous improvement of these characteristics is expected to extend the clinical application of dental ceramics to all-ceramic restorations and other areas, such as implant abutments, implants, removable denture bases, and components.

3. Conclusions

In conclusion, various dental restorative materials are available, and many appropriate materials are used to restore dental carious teeth. Among them, zirconia-based ceramics have been successfully introduced into the clinic due to acceptable biocompatibility, lower price compared with gold restorations and better appearance than traditional metal-ceramic restorations. In summary, zirconia restoration is an acceptable treatment option in restorative dentistry and a developing trend in esthetic dentistry.

Acknowledgements

This study was supported by the CSA Clinical Research Foundation for Young Scholars-All Ceramic Material Research Project (CSA-P2019-01).

Conflict of interest

The authors declare no conflict of interest.

Author details

Feng Luo[1*], Hongyan Luo[2], Ruyi Li[1], Changxing Qu[1], Guang Hong[3,4] and Qianbing Wan[1]

1 State Key Laboratory of Oral Diseases, National Clinical Research Center for Oral Diseases, West China School of Stomatology, Sichuan University, Chengdu, China

2 Department of Psychological Counseling, People's Hospital of Lianhua County, Jiangxi Province, China

3 Liaison Center for Innovative Dentistry, Graduate School of Dentistry, Tohoku University, Sendai, Japan

4 Faculty of Dental Medicine, Department of Prosthetic Dentistry, Airlangga University, Surabaya, Indonesia

*Address all correspondence to: luofeng0122@scu.edu.cn

References

[1] Liu CH, Jeyaprakash N, Yang CH. Material characterization and defect detection of additively manufactured ceramic teeth using non-destructive techniques. Ceramics International. 2020

[2] Yadav K, Prakash S. Dental caries: A microbiological approach. Journal of Clinical Infectious Diseases & Practice. 2017;**2**(1):1-15

[3] Coll PP, Lindsay A, Meng J, et al. The prevention of infections in older adults: Oral health. Journal of the American Geriatrics Society. 2020;**68**(2):411-416

[4] Ruan Q, Zhang Y, Yang X, et al. An amelogenin–chitosan matrix promotes assembly of an enamel-like layer with a dense interface. Acta Biomaterialia. 2013;**9**(7):7289-7297

[5] Xue J, Zavgorodniy AV, Kennedy BJ, et al. X-ray microdiffraction, TEM characterization and texture analysis of human dentin and enamel. Journal of Microscopy. 2013;**251**(2):144-153

[6] Lee EY, Kim ES, Kim KW. Scanning electron microscopy and energy dispersive X-ray spectroscopy studies on processed tooth graft material by vacuum-ultrasonic acceleration. Maxillofacial Plastic and Reconstructive Surgery. 2014;**36**(3):103

[7] Lei C, Jiyao L, HKXH, et al. Demineralization and remineralization. In: Dental Caries. Berlin, Heidelberg: Springer; 2016. pp. 71-83

[8] Khan AS, Syed MR. A review of bioceramics-based dental restorative materials. Dental Materials Journal. 2019;**38**(2):163-176

[9] Santheep PC, Kumar R, Simon EP, et al. Biomimetics in conservative dentistry and endodontics. Dental Bites. 2017:32

[10] Priyadarsini S, Mukherjee S, Bag J, et al. Application of nanoparticles in dentistry: Current trends. In: Nanoparticles in Medicine. Singapore: Springer; 2020. pp. 55-98

[11] Sabbagh J, McConnell RJ, McConnell MC. Posterior composites: Update on cavities and filling techniques. Journal of Dentistry. 2017;**57**:86-90

[12] Mazumder S, Nayak AK, Ara TJ, et al. Hydroxyapatite composites for dentistry. Applications of Nanocomposite Materials in Dentistry. 2019:123-143

[13] Sidhu SK, Nicholson JW. A review of glass-ionomer cements for clinical dentistry. Journal of Functional Biomaterials. 2016;7(3):16

[14] Heck K, Frasheri I, Diegritz C, et al. Six-year results of a randomized controlled clinical trial of two glass ionomer cements in class II cavities. Journal of Dentistry. 2020;**97**:103333

[15] Lempel E, Lovász BV, Bihari E, et al. Long-term clinical evaluation of direct resin composite restorations in vital vs. endodontically treated posterior teeth—Retrospective study up to 13 years. Dental Materials. 2019;**35**(9):1308-1318

[16] Amesti-Garaizabal A, Agustín-Panadero R, Verdejo-Solá B, et al. Fracture resistance of partial indirect restorations made with CAD/CAM technology. A systematic review and meta-analysis. Journal of Clinical Medicine. 2019;**8**(11):1932

[17] Alamoush RA, Satterthwaite JD, Silikas N, et al. Viscoelastic stability of pre-cured resin-composite CAD/CAM structures. Dental Materials. 2019;**35**(8):1166-1172

[18] Choi BJ, Yoon S, Im YW, et al. Uniaxial/biaxial flexure strengths and elastic properties of resin-composite block materials for CAD/CAM. Dental Materials. 2019;**35**(2):389-401

[19] Tsujimoto A, Barkmeier WW, Takamizawa T, et al. Influence of thermal cycling on flexural properties and simulated wear of computer-aided design/computer-aided manufacturing resin composites. Operative Dentistry. 2017;**42**(1):101-110

[20] Tekce N, Pala K, Demirci M, et al. Influence of different composite materials and cavity preparation designs on the fracture resistance of mesio-occluso-distal inlay restoration. Dental Materials Journal. 2016;**35**(3):523-531

[21] Phan AC, Tang M, Nguyen JF, et al. High-temperature high-pressure polymerized urethane dimethacrylate—Mechanical properties and monomer release. Dental Materials. 2014;**30**(3):350-356

[22] Béhin P, Stoclet G, Ruse ND, et al. Dynamic mechanical analysis of high pressure polymerized urethane dimethacrylate. Dental Materials. 2014;**30**(7):728-734

[23] Sulaiman TA. Materials in digital dentistry—A review. Journal of Esthetic and Restorative Dentistry. 2020;**32**(2):171-181

[24] Moldovan M, Balazsi R, Soanca A, et al. Evaluation of the degree of conversion, residual monomers and mechanical properties of some light-cured dental resin composites. Materials. 2019;**12**(13):2109

[25] Tunac AT, Celik EU, Yasa B. Two-year performance of CAD/CAM fabricated resin composite inlay restorations: A randomized controlled clinical trial. Journal of Esthetic and Restorative Dentistry. 2019;**31**(6): 627-638

[26] Stanislawczuk R, Pereira F, Muñoz MA, et al. Effects of chlorhexidine-containing adhesives on the durability of resin–dentine interfaces. Journal of Dentistry. 2014;**42**(1):39-47

[27] Abrisham SM, Tafti AF, Kheirkhah S, et al. Shear bond strength of porcelain to a base-metal compared to zirconia core. Journal of Dental Biomaterials. 2017;**4**(1):367

[28] Zarone F, Russo S, Sorrentino R. From porcelain-fused-to-metal to zirconia: Clinical and experimental considerations. Dental Materials. 2011;**27**(1):83-96

[29] Pradeep C, Gupta S, Sisodia S. Zirconia in dentistry: An overview. Guident. 2020;**13**(10)

[30] Ahmed KE, Li KY, Murray CA. Longevity of fiber-reinforced composite fixed partial dentures (FRC FPD)—Systematic review. Journal of Dentistry. 2017;**61**:1-11

[31] von Stein-Lausnitz M, Nickenig HJ, Wolfart S, et al. Survival rates and complication behaviour of tooth implant–supported, fixed dental prostheses: A systematic review and meta-analysis. Journal of Dentistry. 2019;**88**:103167

[32] Levi L, Barak S, Katz J. Allergic reactions associated with metal alloys in porcelain-fused-to-metal fixed prosthodontic devices—A systematic review. Quintessence International-Journal of Practical Dentistry-English Edition. 2012:871

[33] Monaco C, Caldari M, Scotti R. Clinical evaluation of 1132 zirconia-based single crowns: A retrospective cohort study from the AIOP clinical research group. International Journal of Prosthodontics. 2013;**26**(5)

[34] Alikhasi M, Monzavi A, Ebrahimi H, et al. Debonding time and

dental pulp temperature with the Er, Cr: YSGG laser for debonding feldespathic and lithium disilicate veneers. Journal of Lasers in Medical Sciences. 2019;**10**(3):211

[35] Zhang Y, Kelly JR. Dental ceramics for restoration and metal veneering. Dental Clinics. 2017;**61**(4):797-819

[36] Yoo SY, Kim SK, Heo SJ, et al. Effects of bonding agents on metal-ceramic bond strength of Co-Cr alloys fabricated by selective laser melting. Materials. 2020;**13**(19):4322

[37] Trushkowsky RD. Esthetic and functional consideration in restoring endodontically treated teeth. Dental Clinics. 2011;**55**(2):403-410

[38] Warreth A, Elkareimi Y. All-ceramic restorations: A review of literature. Saudi Dental Journal. 2020

[39] Li SL, Zhang Q, Wu FF, et al. Research progress on all ceramic zirconia core/veneer interface: A review. Science of Advanced Materials. 2020;**12**(1):5-14

[40] Toyama DY, Alves LMM, Ramos GF, et al. Bioinspired silica-infiltrated zirconia bilayers: Strength and interfacial bonding. Journal of the Mechanical Behavior of Biomedical Materials. 2019;**89**:143-149

[41] Xie Z, Wang X, Chen J, et al. The effects of core material and cooling rate on fabrication defects in the veneer of bi-layered all-ceramic systems. Ceramics International. 2019;**45**(13):15876-15882

[42] Aboushelib MN, De Jager N, Kleverlaan CJ, et al. Microtensile bond strength of different components of core veneered all-ceramic restorations. Dental Materials. 2005;**21**(10):984-991

[43] Kang W, Park JK, Kim SR, et al. Effects of core and veneer thicknesses on the color of CAD-CAM lithium disilicate ceramics. The Journal of Prosthetic Dentistry. 2018;**119**(3):461-466

[44] Shahmiri R, Standard OC, Hart JN, et al. Optical properties of zirconia ceramics for esthetic dental restorations: A systematic review. The Journal of Prosthetic Dentistry. 2018;**119**(1):36-46

[45] Tezulas E, Yildiz C, Kucuk C, et al. Current status of zirconia-based all-ceramic restorations fabricated by the digital veneering technique: A comprehensive review. International Journal of Computerized Dentistry. 2019;**22**(3):217-230

[46] Al Hamad KQ, Obaidat II, Baba NZ. The effect of ceramic type and background color on shade reproducibility of all-ceramic restorations. Journal of Prosthodontics. 2020;**29**(6):511-517

[47] Altamimi AM, Tripodakis AP, Eliades G, et al. Comparison of fracture resistance and fracture characterization of bilayered zirconia/fluorapatite and monolithic lithium disilicate all ceramic crowns. International Journal of Esthetic Dentistry. 2014;**9**(1):98-110

[48] Moscovitch M. Consecutive case series of monolithic and minimally veneered zirconia restorations on teeth and implants: Up to 68 months. International Journal of Periodontics & Restorative Dentistry. 2015;**35**(3)

[49] Sulaiman TA, Abdulmajeed AA, Shahramian K, et al. Effect of different treatments on the flexural strength of fully versus partially stabilized monolithic zirconia. The Journal of Prosthetic Dentistry. 2017;**118**(2):216-220

[50] Beuer F, Stimmelmayr M, Gueth JF, et al. In vitro performance of full-contour zirconia single crowns. Dental Materials. 2012;**28**(4):449-456

[51] Rosentritt M, Preis V, Behr M, et al. Fatigue and wear behaviour of zirconia materials. Journal of the Mechanical Behavior of Biomedical Materials. 2020;**110**:103970

[52] Takeichi T, Katsoulis J, Blatz MB. Clinical outcome of single porcelain-fused-to-zirconium dioxide crowns: A systematic review. The Journal of Prosthetic Dentistry. 2013;**110**(6): 455-461

[53] Zarone F, Di Mauro MI, Spagnuolo G, et al. Fourteen-year evaluation of posterior zirconia-based three-unit fixed dental prostheses: A Prospective clinical study of all ceramic prosthesis. Journal of Dentistry. 2020;**101**:103419

[54] Ab-Ghani Z. Non-aqueous sol-gel derived calcia partially stabilized zirconia: Synthesis and characterizations. Malaysian Journal of Microscopy. 2020;**16**(1)

[55] Yu T, Zhang Z, Liu Q, et al. Extrusion-based additive manufacturing of yttria-partially-stabilized zirconia ceramics. Ceramics International. 2020;**46**(4):5020-5027

[56] Camposilvan E, Leone R, Gremillard L, et al. Aging resistance, mechanical properties and translucency of different yttria-stabilized zirconia ceramics for monolithic dental crown applications. Dental Materials. 2018;**34**(6):879-890

[57] Marchack BW, Sato S, Marchack CB, et al. Complete and partial contour zirconia designs for crowns and fixed dental prostheses: A clinical report. The Journal of Prosthetic Dentistry. 2011;**106**(3):145-152

[58] Vigolo P, Mutinelli S. Evaluation of zirconium-oxide-based ceramic single-unit posterior fixed dental prostheses (FDPs) generated with two CAD/CAM systems compared to porcelain-fused-to-metal single-unit posterior FDPs: A 5-year clinical prospective study. Journal of Prosthodontics: Implant, Esthetic and Reconstructive Dentistry. 2012;**21**(4): 265-269

[59] Capa N, Tuncel I, Tak O, et al. The effect of luting cement and titanium base on the final color of zirconium oxide core material. Journal of Prosthodontics. 2017;**26**(2):136-140

[60] Tabatabaian F. Color in zirconia-based restorations and related factors: A literature review. Journal of Prosthodontics. 2018;**27**(2):201-211

[61] Huang Z, Huang J, Li C, et al. The application of 3D printed self-glazed zirconia for full-mouth rehabilitation in a patient with severely worn dentition: A case report. Advances in Applied Ceramics. 2020;**119**(5-6):305-311

[62] Zhang F, Spies BC, Vleugels J, et al. High-translucent yttria-stabilized zirconia ceramics are wear-resistant and antagonist-friendly. Dental Materials. 2019;**35**(12):1776-1790

[63] Shi A, Wu Z, Huang J, et al. Wear performance of self-glazed zirconia crowns with different amount of occlusal adjustment after 6 months of clinical use. Advances in Applied Ceramics. 2018;**117**(8):445-451

[64] Abi CBE. Toughening mechanisms in dental composites. Toughening Mechanisms in Composite Materials. 2015:321-337

[65] Hagiwara Y, Nakajima K. Application of Ce-TZP/Al_2O_3 nanocomposite to the framework of an implant-fixed complete dental prosthesis and a complete denture. Journal of Prosthodontic Research. 2016;**60**(4):337-343

[66] Omori S, Komada W, Yoshida K, et al. Effect of thickness of

zirconia-ceramic crown frameworks on strength and fracture pattern. Dental Materials Journal. 2013;**32**(1):189-194

[67] Hussein AI, Ab-Ghani Z, Che Mat AN, et al. Synthesis and Characterization of Spherical Calcium Carbonate Nanoparticles Derived from Cockle Shells. Applied Sciences. 2020;**10**(20):7170

Section 3

Dental Trauma

Chapter 8

Short and Long Term Oral Hygiene Maintenance Protocols for Traumatic Dental Injuries

Girish Suragimath and Ashwinirani SR

Abstract

Traumatic dental injuries (TDIs) occur when a person undergoes trauma due to variety of reasons. Traumatic injuries are part of the growing up years and can have ever lasting wounds with scarring on the affected individuals. Treatment and rehabilitation of the teeth with traumatic injuries are essential for long term survival of the teeth. Immediate care, appropriate diagnosis and treatment with comprehensive follow-up are essential for a favorable prognosis of the affected teeth. A coordinated effort from different specialties including general dentist, oral radiologist, pediatric dentist, periodontist, oral surgeon, orthodontist and endodontist is essential for success of the treatment. Team efforts involving these different specialists will help the patient to receive successful long term outcome. Proper oral hygiene maintenance during and after traumatic dental injury, is required to stop the deterioration of the tooth and periodontal structures. The caregiver in children and the adult with traumatic dental injuries should be educated and guided about the proper oral hygiene techniques especially in the areas with dental injury. Dentist must be aware of the treatments rendered to the teeth with trauma and should have up-to-date knowledge of the oral hygiene measures to be inculcated in the subjects with dental trauma. This chapter highlights the oral hygiene measures to be followed by the subjects with TDIs and also includes measures to be followed by the dentist in such a scenario.

Keywords: dental trauma, interdental cleaning aids, mouth wash, oral hygiene, toothbrush, traumatic dental injuries

1. Introduction

Trauma to the hard and soft tissues occurs when a subject undergoes injuries due to motor vehicle accidents, physical fights; self-infested wounds, assaults, bicycle accidents or while playing sports. Other reasons of traumatic injury can be domestic abuse in adults and child abuse in children. Anterior teeth in both primary and permanent dentition are most commonly affected by dental trauma. Primary and permanent anterior teeth are not only important for esthetics but also essential for phonetics, mastication, integrity of supporting tissues, psychological and mental wellbeing [1]. Traumatic injuries are part of the growing up years and can have ever lasting wounds with scarring on the affected individuals. Dental trauma refers to injury to the oral and perioral structures i.e. teeth (enamel, dentin, pulp and cementum), gums, periodontal ligament, alveolar bone and also involves nearby soft tissues around the teeth such as the lips, tongue, etc. Traumatic dental injuries (TDI's) are part of body injury and occur frequently in children and young adults accounting to 5% of all the bodily injuries [2]. School going children up to 25% experience dental trauma and 33% of adult's less than 19 years of age have permanent dentition trauma [3]. Incisor teeth both in maxilla and mandible are the most commonly affected teeth with highest incidence in maxillary central incisors. A prospective study in 2017 found that among patients with maxillofacial fractures, 41.8% of them had concomitant dental injuries of two or more teeth [4]. Immediate care, appropriate diagnosis and treatment with comprehensive follow-up are essential for a favorable prognosis of the affected teeth.

Dental treatment of TDI's is usually delayed and not given as much attention as general medical treatment. Immediate dental consultation and treatment could improve long-term prognosis of the injured teeth [5]. Timing of the dental care rendered to patient who have undergone trauma is critical in management and saving of the teeth. Dentist must have the essential knowledge regarding the management of patients with trauma especially during the emergency phase of treatment. Appropriate management of patients with dental trauma requires coordinated efforts of different specialties including general dentists, oral radiologist, pediatric dentist, periodontist, oral surgeon and endodontist. Team efforts involving these different specialists will help the patient to receive successful long term outcome.

When a subject undergoes a traumatic incident, he or she is mentally disturbed and may tend to get disoriented with time and space. The person with dental trauma will experience difficulty in maintaining daily oral hygiene and this leads to dental plaque accumulation. The neglect of oral hygiene during and after dental trauma will lead to gingivitis which if untreated may lead to periodontitis and tooth loss. Studies have also shown that Oral Health-Related Quality of Life (OHRQoL) is affected by TDI's and it negatively impacts on the OHRQoL of children and their families [6]. It is imperative that oral hygiene standards are maintained during and post dental trauma for the long term survival of teeth with dental trauma. Twice daily brushing with soft bristled manual brush or electric toothbrush with toothpaste, interdental cleaning with dental floss or interdental brush and use of mouth rinse every day is apt to keep the teeth and mouth clean. Dentist must educate about oral hygiene maintenance and special instructions to be followed during TDI's to patients.

2. Epidemiology

The prevalence of injury and TDI's has been observed in children and young adults of every country of the world. Different authors have reported different incidences and prevalence's of TDI's from many countries. A 12-year review of the literature reports that 25% of all school children experience dental trauma and 33% of adults have experienced trauma to the permanent dentition, with the majority of injuries occurring before age nineteen [7].

A study on prevalence of TDI's conducted in India reported 59.2% of males and 40.8% of female's experienced dental injury and they concluded that males experienced more TDI's due to the outdoor activities [8]. Study conducted on Saudi Arabian children mention a incidence of TDI's is 1–3% and prevalence of 20–30%, similar results were also observed in studies conducted in Europe [9, 10]. The prevalence of missing anterior teeth as a result of dental trauma is reported as 12 per 1000 children in one cross-sectional epidemiological study [11]. A 2017 prospective study found that among patients with maxillofacial fractures, 41.8% of them had concomitant dental injuries to two or more teeth [4]. The trauma prevalence in one study showed 10.13% children suffered TDI's and only 3.37% of the children had undergone treatment for those injuries [12]. Studies have concluded that anterior teeth with increased incisal over jet and inadequate lip coverage were significant predictors for the occurrence of TDI's [13]. Children and adolescents in the poor socio economical conditions had greater incidence of TDI's and they had not received proper treatment for those TDI's.

3. Management of traumatic dental injuries

Timing of the dental care rendered to patient who have undergone trauma is critical in management and saving of the teeth. Dentist should be aware of management and treatment of patients with trauma especially during the emergency phase (**Table 1**). A coordinated efforts of different specialty including general dentists, pediatric dentist, periodontist, oral surgeon and endodontist is essential. Team efforts involving these different specialists will help the patient receive successful long term prognosis [15]. Avulsion of permanent teeth is one of the most serious dental injuries, prompt and correct emergency management is essential for attaining the best outcome after this injury [16].

Description	Primary dentition	Permanent dentition
Concussion/subluxation	Observe, soft foods for 1 week, dental radiograph to rule out root fracture	Observe, soft foods for 1 week, dental radiograph to rule out root fracture
Luxation	Reposition tooth or extract, do not splint	Dental radiograph, reposition tooth, splint for 4 week
Extrusion	Reposition tooth or extract, do not splint	Dental radiograph, reposition tooth, splint for 2 week
Intrusion	Dental radiograph, observe and allow to re erupt, extract if alveolar plate is compromised	Dental radiograph, observe and allow to re erupt, surgical or orthodontic repositioning, root canal treatment
Uncomplicated crown fracture	Restore tooth, smooth sharp edges, dental radiograph to rule out root fracture	Restore tooth, smooth sharp edges, radiograph to rule out root fracture
Complicated crown fracture	Dental radiograph, pulp treatment, restore or extract tooth, observe for infection	Dental radiograph, pulp treatment, restore tooth, observe for infection, may require root canal treatment
Root fracture	Dental radiograph, extract if root fracture is in middle or cervical third of root	Dental radiograph, splint, may require root canal treatment; if in cervical third, may need to extract
Avulsion	Do not replant, dental radiograph to rule out intrusion if tooth is not located	Do not handle the root, replant within30 min or place in recommended transport medium (balanced salt solution, cold milk); dental radiograph, replant and splint as soon as possible; systemic antibiotics, soft diet, chlorhexidine, close follow-up

Table 1.
Dental treatment plan for traumatic injuries in the primary and permanent dentition [14].

Dentist must assess the periodontal ligament (PDL) cells of the avulsed tooth, before commencing treatment: [16].

- The PDL cells are most likely viable. The tooth has been replanted immediately or within a very short time (about 15 minutes) at the place of accident.
- The PDL cells may be viable but compromised. The tooth has been kept in a storage medium (e.g., milk, HBSS (Save-a-Tooth or similar product), saliva, or saline, and the total extra-oral dry time has been <60 minutes).
- The PDL cells are likely to be non-viable. The total extra-oral dry time has been more than 60 minutes, regardless of the tooth having been stored in a medium or not.

The treatment of TDIs patients involves five phases [2, 17–22].

- Emergency phase
- Follow up phase
- Restorative phase
- Rehabilitation phase
- Maintenance phase

3.1 Emergency phase

When a patient with trauma arrives at the dental clinic, certain necessary actions have to be taken to start the treatment. Proper history of the etiology of the injury preferably in a structured checklist will be beneficial. The dentist can follow these steps for treating patients with dental trauma.

a. The dentist must thoroughly evaluate the injury to the dental and adjacent tissues. Careful extra oral and intraoral clinical examination and radiographic investigation is essential to arrive at the diagnosis of exact damage caused by the trauma.

b. Patient's general health and history of systemic diseases must be collected to plan the treatment accordingly.

c. History of previous dental injuries and the treatment received by the patient for the current injury should be ascertained before starting the treatment protocol.

d. Symptoms of central nervous system injury like vomiting, nausea, confusion, blurred vision, bleeding or fluid from ear or nose, difficulty in speech, loss of consciousness, amnesia should be assessed. The patient has to be referred to a neurologist for consultation of Central Nervous System (CNS) symptoms.

e. Areas of pain should be re-examined properly and source, etiology and pain relief measures and medications should be prescribed accordingly.

f. Radiographic assessment including Orthopantomogram (OPG), Intraoral periapical radiographs (IOPA) and occlusal radiographs will aid in proper judgment about the injury and its extent. Cone beam computed tomography (CBCT) can be availed in case of serious injuries such as crown/root, root and alveolar fractures, as well as luxation injuries.

g. Thorough decontamination and disinfection of intraoral and extra oral wounds should be carried out, to rid of all the contaminants.

h. Areas of bleeding should be detected and pressure pack, cautery or suturing of the artery can be used to stop the bleeding.

i. Injection of Tetanus vaccine, also known as tetanus toxoid (TT) can be given to prevent spasms in the muscles.

j. If there is fracture of maxilla or mandible, reduction of the fracture segments should be carried out and they can be stabilized with help of arch bar wiring or plates.

k. Sutures can be placed in open wounds and dressing can be used over the extra oral wounds.

3.2 Immediate follow-up phase

During the subsequent visits after three days, dentist should evaluate healing of the primary lesions and occlusion of teeth should be checked for any discrepancies. Sensitivity tests should be carried out on all teeth with trauma and the opposing teeth. Cold testing is recommended over electric pulp testing in young patients. The pulp test has to be carried out during the follow-up visits as the teeth with trauma are nonresponsive for several weeks. Dentist should help achieve complete healing of soft and hard tissue structures. Healing complications are more common in teeth with vertical fracture of teeth, trauma in supporting tissues and avulsion. Complications usually occur in the first three months and necrotic pulp was the most common complication [23].

3.3 Restorative phase

The Restorative phase should include restoration of fractured and decayed teeth. Fractured teeth have to be carefully examined, for type and extent of the fracture and the need for endodontic and periodontal treatments. A multidisciplinary approach will improve the prognosis of the teeth. Non-surgical periodontal therapy (NSPT) including scaling, root planing, patient education and local drug delivery should be carried out, to keep the tissues in healthy state. Dentist must observe the gums for any inflammation and periodontal examination for periodontitis and check for ulcers or irritation due to prosthetic appliances.

3.4 Rehabilitation phase

Rehabilitation phase includes occlusal corrections with orthodontic tooth movement. Psychological counseling among children will help children to overcome and forget traumatic events of TDI's. Patient should be educated and motivated to maintain healthy teeth, gums and periodontium for long term rehabilitation.

3.5 Maintenance phase

Maintenance phase or oral hygiene phase should be carried out during all the phases of treatment of TDI's. Regular oral hygiene maintenance with either manual or powered toothbrush should be started in immediate follow-up phase and maintained throughout life. Brushing twice daily once early morning and once before going to bed is best advised. The interdental areas between the teeth should be kept clean with appropriate interdental cleaning aids. Mouthwashes should be routinely used to maintain the overall health of oral structures like teeth, gums, periodontium, oral mucosa and tongue.

Regular visit to the dentist for periodic checkup and examination should be followed by the patients who experienced TDI's. Dentists must keep the patients with TDI's on maintenance therapy for regular interaction and follow-ups.

4. Oral hygiene aids

> *"Correct and routine tooth brushing will soon iron out, so to speak, all the irregularities in, and restore normal colour and contour to, the gingivae ... thus, since the toothbrush may also readily aid in the resolution of these incipient symptoms, its potentiality in their prevention is evident."*
>
> *- Hirschfeld [4].*

Hirschfeld advocated tooth brushing to keep teeth and gums clean free from dental caries or periodontal diseases [24]. Cleaning of teeth and oral hygiene maintenance are carried out using toothbrushes and interdental cleaning aids. Commercially available varieties of dental products can be used to keep the mouth clean. Toothbrush with toothpaste is the most commonly employed teeth cleaning oral hygiene aid. American Dental Associations (ADA) advocates brushing of teeth twice daily, use of interdental cleaning aids regularly and oral rinse with mouthwashes every day to keep good oral health. Tooth brushing and interdental cleaning remain the mainstays of prevention of periodontal diseases. The primary approach requires individually tailored instruction for implementation of a systematic oral hygiene regimen [25].

Toothbrushes come in different designs and function.

- Manual tooth brush
- Powered toothbrush
- Sonic, Ultrasonic and Ionic toothbrushes

4.1 Manual toothbrush

Manual tooth brush with toothpaste is commonly used all over the world to clean the teeth. Manual toothbrushes come in different sizes and design and basically classified according to the diameter of the bristles as soft, medium and hard.

Different brushing techniques are used to clean the teeth by different individuals. Tooth brushes can be used with horizontal scrub, vertical scrub, vibratory, sweeping, rotatory motion or combination of them. Various researchers have recommended different brushing techniques like Bass, Charter's, Stillman, Fone, Leonard, Hirchfeld's, Smith-Bell and many more. Modified Bass technique also called sulcus cleansing method is advised for healthy patients with no gingival disease. Fone's technique or circular method of brushing is advised for children as it is easy to learn. Modified Stillman's method is recommended in patients with gingival recession for gingival massage. Charter's method is most useful in patients with fixed prosthesis or orthodontic appliances and post periodontal surgery.

4.2 Powered/electric toothbrush

Powered toothbrush are also called electric toothbrush, they make rapid automatic bristle movements, either to and fro or rotatory-oscillation to clean the teeth. Electric brushes can be classified according to their type of action as side to side vibration, Counter oscillation, Rotation or Circular. Compared to manual toothbrushes; electric-powered ionic ones were significantly efficient in removing plaque in the premolar and molar areas [26, 27]. Powered toothbrush manufacturers do not recommend a specific brushing method, the Swiss Dental Society, in 2001 developed an instruction manual for use of electric tooth brushes. Instructions for brushes with a sweeping and/or oscillating rotary motion are as follows:

- The brushes are positioned on the tooth surfaces in a 45-or 90-degree angle to the incisal plane.
- Only when positioned should the brush be switched to "on."
- The mouth should be almost closed.
- The brush should be moved slowly over and around each tooth for 3 to 5 seconds, making sure that the bristles clean the crevices between the teeth.
- The brush head can be lifted distally and mesially into the interproximal areas to reach the interdental area; the brush always remains on a single tooth.
- After a period of approximately 5 seconds, the brush is moved to the next tooth surface and repositioned [27].

4.3 Sonic, ultrasonic and ionic toothbrushes

Sonic tooth brushes bristles vibrate at lower frequency and ultrasonic, indicates a brush action where the bristles vibrate at ultrasonic frequencies (> 20 kHz). An ionic brush releases an electrical charge to the tooth surface which disrupts the attachment of dental plaque [28].

4.4 Interdental cleaning aids

Interdental cleaning aids are usually dental floss, toothpick or small interdental brush and Uni-tufted brushes. The use of interdental cleaning aid depends upon the spacing between the teeth and gingival tissue in the interdental spaces. Interdental cleaning of teeth is best achieved by using interdental brushes and these brushes should therefore be the first choice in patients with open interdental spaces [29].

Several interdental cleaning aids are available for cleaning of interdental areas. The use interdental cleaning device and method can vary depending upon the type of interdental embrasure (**Table 2**).

Dental floss: Dental floss is most useful in cleaning the interdental areas where the contacts between the teeth are tight and no space is present between the teeth and there is no recession of interdental papilla. Dental floss can be used by rotating around the fingers or they also can be used with a floss holder.

Type of interdental space	Interdental cleaning device to be used
Narrow interdental space with intact interdental papillae	Dental floss or toothpick
Little interdental space with slight papilla recession	Dental floss, toothpick or small interdental brush
Wide interdental space with complete loss of interdental papilla	Interdental brush
Wide interdental space with diastema of teeth	Uni-tufted brush or gauze strip

Table 2.
Interdental space present and interdental aid to be used.

Toothpicks: toothpicks are used in the tight interdental areas and it can be used as normal cleaning instrument anywhere required. Toothpicks have been used to clean teeth since ages; they come in different designs and varieties.

Interproximal brushes: Miniature interproximal brushes are available and they can be used in the interdental areas with slight papillary recession. Interproximal brushes are designed like a miniature bottle cleaning brushes are used in to and fro direction in the interdental areas.

Uni-tufted brush: Uni-tufted brushes are used in wide interdental areas with open embrasure and adjacent teeth with no contact. They help in cleaning of the open contact and make them plaque free.

Water jet/piks: water jets are the instruments which spray water with pulsations and pressure. Water jets have shown to be effective in removing debris from the interdental areas in patients who avoid the use of dental floss. Mouthwashes can also be used instead of the water; this increases its action due to the anti-plaque nature of the mouthwash.

4.5 Tongue cleaners and mouthwashes

Tongue cleaners are used to clean the dorsal surface of the tongue, which harbors maximum number of microorganisms. Tongue cleaners are usually flat surfaced made up of wood or plastic to scrape the surface of the tongue.

An oral rinse help in promotion of good oral hygiene, reduce oral discomfort, provide moisture to oral tissues and reduce bad breath [1, 15]. Mouthwashes are essential to completely rid of microorganisms from all the parts of oral cavity. ADA advocates use of mouthwash for regular maintenance of oral hygiene. Many mouthwashes with different chemical formulations are available in the market. Chlorhexidine containing mouth washes are considered gold standard. Other chemicals used are Bisguanides, Hydrogen Peroxide, Sodium Hypochlorite, Salt and Herbal mouthwashes.

Rationale for the use of mouthwashes:

Antiseptics present in mouthwashes are effective against the bacteria found within dental plaque, when they are in a planktonic form; they show both bacteriostatic and bactericidal activity.

Mouthwashes have a number of advantages:

- They are available without prescription.
- They have a good safety record.
- No significant bacterial resistance has been reported.
- They require little skill and motivation on behalf of the patient.

Mouth rinses serve a variety of purposes

- Antiplaque/Anti gingivitis Rinses
    1. Therapeutic Antiseptics
        - Phenol products: Listerine, Chloraseptic
        - Chlorhexidine products: Peridex, Corsodyl
        - Sanguinaria products: Viadent
    2. Cosmetic antiplaque rinses: Plax, Close-Up Anti-Plaque
- Therapeutic Anti cavity Fluoride Rinses
  Act+, Fluorigard+, Listermint with Fluoride.
- Cosmetic Breath Freshening Mouth Rinses
  Cepacol, Lavoris, Scope, Signal, Clear Choice, Rembrandt Mouth Refreshing Rinse.
- Others
    a. Topical antibiotic rinses
    b. Enzyme rinses
    c. Artificial saliva rinses
    d. Rinses that control tartar

Types of mouthwashes.

1. First generation anti-plaque agents
    - Capable of reducing plaque scores by 20–50%.
2. Second generation anti-plaque agents
    - Overall plaque reduction by 70–90% and exhibit slow release properties.
3. Third generation anti-plaque agents
    - Exhibit better retentive properties over second generation agents.

Triclosan and Chlorhexidine mouthwashes have been widely used in recent times. Triclosan delays plaque maturation and inhibits formation of prostaglandin leukotrines which is a key controller of inflammation. Chlorhexidine acts against plaque and bacteria.

5. Oral hygiene maintenance in deciduous dentition

The primary dentition is fragile compared to the permanent dentition. The parent or the caregiver has to be delicate and gentle while brushing of teeth. It is advised to use a soft bristle brush in circular motion to clean the teeth. In the area of trauma and teeth with trauma, extra care should be given not to hurt and cause more pain and complications to the child.

In the area of injury during the healing phase, a cotton swab dipped in 0.12% chlorhexidine or antiseptic mouthwash can be used to clean the teeth and soft tissues. The cleaning of teeth and soft tissues should be carried out twice daily morning and night.

Use of mouthwashes in children is not advised as they may swallow the mouthwash instead of rinsing. In the area, where sutures are placed toothbrush usage should be avoided and gentle cleaning with a cotton swab is advised, so that the sutures do not get disturbed. After traumatic injuries of the primary dentition, most complications are associated to infection due to caries [30]. Post trauma after complete healing of the soft tissues radiographic assessment should be carried out to see any damage to the tooth buds of permanent teeth. Decidious teeth are not usually splinted to avoid disturbance to the permanent tooth buds. If splinting of deciduous teeth is carried out than the interdental areas below the splint fiber or wire should be kept clean by the use of interdental brushes in to and fro motion.

6. Oral hygiene maintenance in mixed dentition

The mixed dentition is the period when maximum dental trauma cases occur. Professional oral hygiene like scaling and root planning can be rendered to the patients in this age group.

Tooth brushing with soft bristled brush with caution in the traumatic areas is advised. Dental flossing to keep the interdental areas clean and prevent inter dental plaque accumulation has to be incorporated in the oral hygiene practice. It is important to check for the trauma to the tooth buds of permanent teeth and render treatment accordingly. If the patient is accustomed to using powered toothbrush, he or she needs to be careful while brushing around teeth with dental trauma. The use of mouthwashes to reduce plaque growth helps in easy oral hygiene maintenance. If the teeth are splinted for stabilization during healing phase, use of interdental brushes such as proxa brush is advised to keep the interdental regions clean.

7. Oral hygiene in dental trauma of permanent dentition

In the permanent dentition oral hygiene around the traumatized teeth becomes vital and post trauma care is essential for long term prognosis. The teeth with traumatic injuries may have cracks, fractures, luxation or may be replanted and this alters the natural shape and structure of the teeth. Many different oral hygiene methods have to be followed to maintain hygiene around these teeth. It is better to have supragingival prosthesis of the fractured tooth as subgingival placement of the crown margin is plaque accumulating and leads to periodontitis if not well maintained.

8. Oral hygiene maintenance in special situations

Oral hygiene maintenance methods have to be modified to meet the special clinical situations.

8.1 Splinted teeth

The splint should be placed on the buccal surfaces of the maxillary teeth to enable lingual access for endodontic procedures and to avoid occlusal interference [31–34].

Splinting up to four months is advised in root fractures at the cervical third [13]. The use of semi rigid splint and flexible splints is more indicated than the rigid one as per The International Association of Dental Traumatology (IADT), and splinting done for long periods can cause root resorption or ankylosis of teeth [35, 36].

Care must be taken in teeth which are splinted during the healing phase. Interdental cleaning under and over the wire or fiber splint can be carried out with an interproximal brush.

8.2 Teeth with ligature wiring splint

Brushing must be done carefully and mouthwash should be advised to be rinsed regularly to stop the plaque growth. Interdental brush or proxa brushes are best suited for use under the wire of splints and interdental areas.

The interdental area between the teeth harbor's plaque and it has to be cleaned with interdental aids using dental floss, interdental brushes or unitufted brushes.

Dental floss a thread like material is used to clean interdental area with tight interdental contact. The dental floss is inserted or passed between the two teeth and moved in to and fro motion to clean the interdental area below the gum papilla. Dental floss is passed between every interdental area between teeth and activated to get rid of plaque. **Figure 1** shows the use of dental floss between upper right lateral incisor and canine.

Interdental brushes have shown to be the best in interdental cleaning. The use of interdental bushes can only be accomplished, if slight spacing is present between adjacent teeth either due to spacing or minimal gingival recession. **Figure 2** shows the use of interdental brush in between two central incisors.

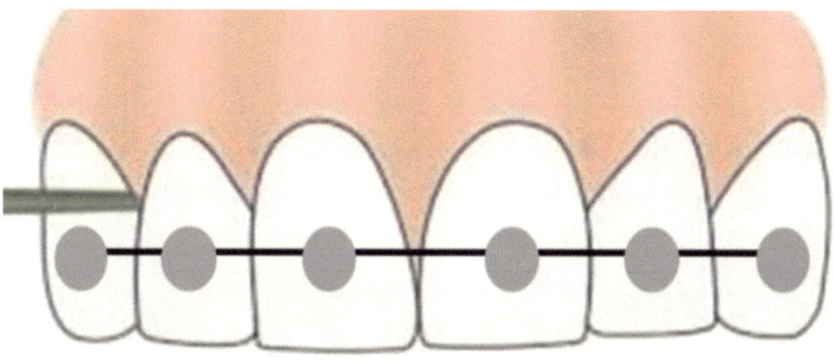

Figure 1.
The use of dental floss between upper right lateral incisor and canine.

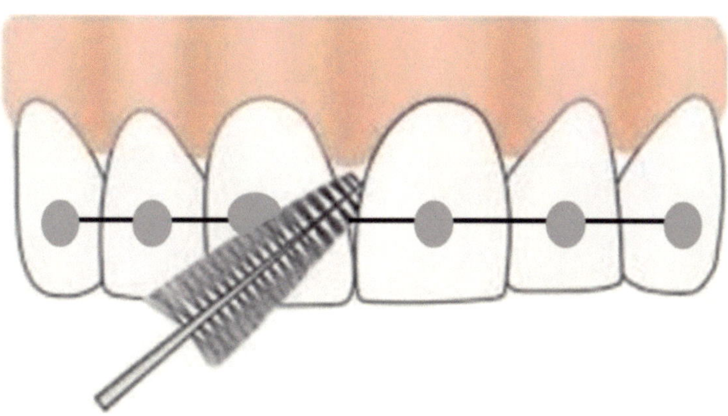

Figure 2.
The use of interdental brush between two central incisors.

Unitufted or single tufted brushes are advocated in patients with spacing between teeth or severe gingival recession. Unitufted brushes are easy to use and effective in cases with big interdental space. **Figure 3** shows the use of unitufted brush between the two central incisors. **Figure 4** shows the use of unitufted brush on the lingual side under beneath the ligature or fiber splint.

8.3 Sub gingival fracture

Teeth with sub gingival fracture line should be observed closely and maintained plaque free otherwise, gingivitis and periodontitis can develop and jeopardize the prognosis of the tooth.

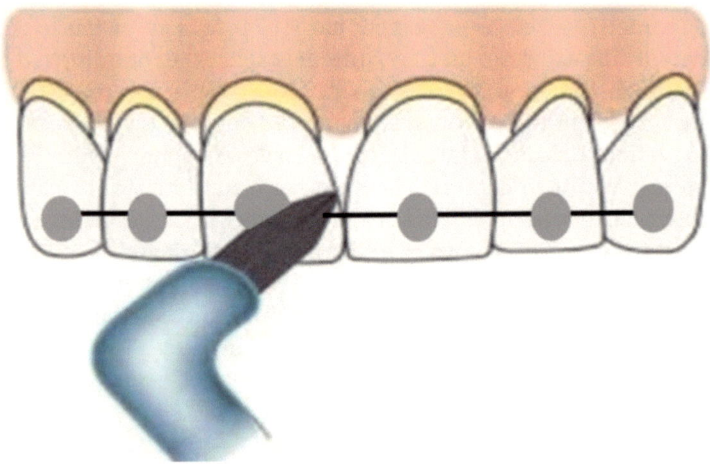

Figure 3.
The use of unitufted brush between two central incisors below the dental splint.

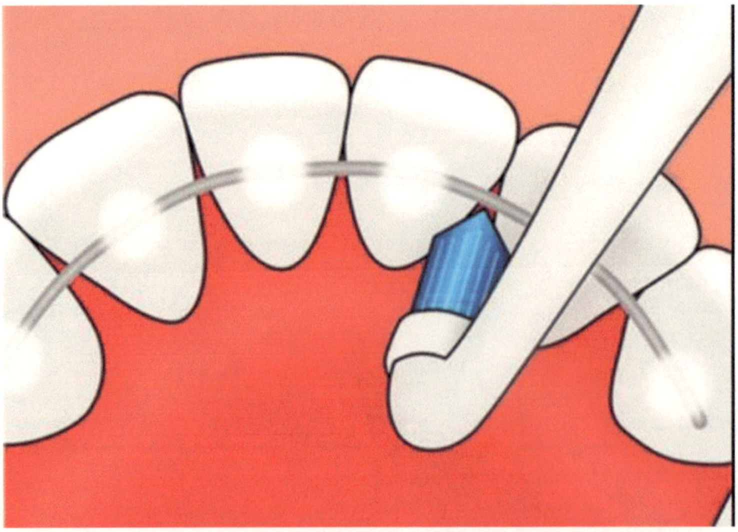

Figure 4.
The use of unitufted brush on the lingual surface of mandibular anterior teeth below the dental splint.

8.4 Teeth with prosthesis

Teeth with crowns and bridges should be monitored regularly for excess cement or leakage of the cement, which can be plaque accumulating. The margins of prosthesis should be placed supra gingivally whenever possible and have to be monitored regularly for periodontal health.

8.5 Composite restoration

Brushing on the teeth with composite build-up, inlay or onlay restoration should be carried out with caution. These teeth should not be brushed vigorously to avoid abrasion of the composite material and exposure of fracture line.

8.6 Removable denture

Removable dentures and any device or bite guard used by the patient should be removed and cleaned after every meal to avoid bacteria, fungi, plaque and tartar growth. The oral mucosa covered by the prosthesis, including the palate, must be cleaned at least once a day with a soft toothbrush. Mechanical cleaning of prosthesis under running water with help of denture brush should be done both on outer and inner surfaces [3].

8.7 Permanent tooth avulsion ('Knock Out of tooth')

- Hold the tooth by its crown (white part). Do not touch the root (Yellow part).
- Wash the teeth for ten seconds under cold tap water. Do not scrub.
- Replant the tooth in the original socket in jaw.
- Bite on handkerchief (to hold in position).
- Refer to the dental office for fixation and antibiotics.
- If the tooth cannot be replanted, place the tooth in cold milk and refer to the dental office immediately (within 20 min) [3].

8.8 Long term maintenance of TDI's

- The teeth that undergo TDI's have to be maintained for a long time as there may be occurrence of complications such as pulp necrosis, root resorption and root ankylosis.
- Regular follow-up and prompt treatment will improve the overall prognosis and improve the quality of life in the affected individual.
- Follow up of TDI's up to 5 years has been advocated by International Association of Dental Traumatology [37].

9. Conclusion

The research of published data suggests that there is a lack of proper knowledge on emergency dental first-aid among the parents, care givers, school authority and general public. In most of the countries worldwide, no attempt has been made by the government or other dental organizations to educate people on the management of dental trauma. TDI's are an important general and public health issue and public awareness of its importance should be bolstered to enable equitable access for injury care. Greater emphasis on prevention and the significance of emergency care for dental injuries will reduce the financial burden of the individual and improve the quality of life [6].

Research conducted to assess the treatment and management of TDI's have shown that the treatments provided at emergency care units are often inadequate and patients remain unsatisfied with care provided. The International Association of Dental Traumatology (IADT) has given a comprehensive guidelines management of TDI's, which can be accessed via Internet (www.iadt-dentaltrauma.org) [38]. The IADT recently developed a core outcome set (COS) for traumatic dental injuries (TDI) in children and adults, these guidelines should be followed and, even in extreme situations, replantation of teeth should always be considered [39]. Interactive website has been introduced for clinicians (Dental Trauma Guide, www.dentaltraumaguide.org) which can be used by dentist and health care workers either via computer or smart phone during a trauma situation [40]. Mobile phone based free App was introduced by IADT (IADT ToothSOS Mobile App) to help user to take care of a dental trauma at the scene of an accident.

Dental injuries cause both periodontal and pulpal complications. The delay in dental consultation for TDI's increases the amount of complications that develop later during the maintenance. Time lapse between the TDI's and the date of dental consultation is a decisive element in the therapeutic choice and influences the prognosis [5]. The parents and individuals should be educated to consult a dentist immediately after trauma and take prompt treatment for the TDI's to reduce the complications that develop at the later date.

There is need for refinement of dental curriculum for the management of TDI's in terms of design, content, teaching methodology and long term maintenance for better prognosis of the patients with dental trauma [41].

The prevalence of TDI's in Europe and many other continents is one in five school going children and if untreated they affect the quality of life of children. The environment of the school and action taken towards management of TDI's is very crucial. Schools with supportive social and physical environment have fewer occurrences of TDI's. Schools should adopt health and safety policies, improvements in the physical environment and closer supervision of children while playing will reduce the occurrence of TDI's [42]. School teachers and physical instructors should be educated about emergency management of TDI's and consult child specialist and dentist at the earliest to lessen post traumatic complications. Studies have pointed out that health promotion policies, safe environment at the schools, correction of predisposing risk factors of TDI's and use of protective intraoral and extra oral devices while physical activity will lessen the financial burden caused by TDI's [43]. Conducting health educational programs to improve the level of general knowledge about prevention and managing TDI's at the schools is necessary [44].

Parents, Education authorities, and children involved with sports and recreation activities should be educated about the risk factors involved and management of TDI's. Screening programs to identify children with high anatomic (incisal over jet and inadequate lip coverage) and behavioral risk for occurrence of traumatic injury and necessary corrective measures (preventive orthodontic treatment and use

DOI: http://dx.doi.org/10.5772/intechopen.96043

of Mouth guards) will help reduce the occurrence of injury among children [45]. Mounting posters, leaflets at public places along with media campaigns using television, social networking sites and internet will educate people for managing avulsed permanent teeth [1]. The teachers and school management should be educated about TDIs and emergency care and referral to dentist as schools with good physical structures and promote health activities had lesser prevalence of TDIs [46, 47].

The dentist treating TDIs must involve other specialists including Oral Radiologist, Pediatrician, Paedodontist, Endodontist, Periodontist, Prosthodontist, Orthodontist and Oral maxillofacial Surgeon. Dentist must capture good quality photographs of the TDIs and lesions and can use them to discuss the treatment protocol with specialists. Studies have proved that photographic assessment method of dental trauma was valid and reliable as compared to the oral clinical examination [48].

Dentist must be aware of different types of TDIs and its immediate treatments [49]. Dentist should educate good oral hygiene maintenance techniques to the patients suffering from TDIs. During the healing and splinting of teeth, oral hygiene cleaning with interdental brushes will help the patients.

Complications even with the best of treatment guidelines followed occur occasionally and pulp necrosis is the most observed complication [12]. Dentist must refer the patient to other specialists whenever deemed necessary. Combined efforts of different specialists will improve the prognosis of the teeth and soft tissues.

Conflict of interest

"The authors declare no conflict of interest."

Notes/thanks/other declarations

We would like to thank Dr. Reema Shah and Dr. Harshada Zagade postgraduate students in Periodontology for editing and preparation of the figures.

Acronyms and abbreviations

TDI's	Traumatic Dental Injuries
OHRQoL	Oral Health-Related Quality of Life
PDL	Periodontal Ligament
IADT	International Association for Dental Traumatology
CNS	Central Nervous System
IOPA	Intraoral periapical radiographs
OPG	Orthopantomogram
CBCT	Cone beam computed tomography
TT	Tetanus Toxoid
ADA	American Dental Association
NSPT	Non-Surgical Periodontal Therapy

Author details

Girish Suragimath[1*] and Ashwinirani SR[2]

1 Department of Periodontology, School of Dental Sciences, Krishna Institute of Medical Sciences Deemed to be University, Karad, Maharashtra State, India

2 Department of Oral Medicine and Radiology, School of Dental Sciences, Krishna Institute of Medical Sciences Deemed to be University, Karad, Maharashtra State, India

*Address all correspondence to: drgirishsuragimath@gmail.com

References

[1] Pujita C, Nuvvula S, Shilpa G, Nirmala S, Yamini V. Informative promotional outcome on school teachers' knowledge about emergency management of dental trauma. J Conserv Dent. 2013 Jan;16(1):21-7. doi: 10.4103/0972-0707.105293. PMID: 23349571; PMCID: PMC3548340.

[2] Andreasen JO, Lauridsen E, Gerds AT, Ahrensburg SS. Dental Trauma Guide: A source of evidence-based treatment guidelines for dental trauma. Dent Traumatol. 2012;28:142-147.

[3] DiAngelis AJ, Andreasen JO, Ebeleseder KA, Kenny DJ, Trope M, Sigurdsson A, Andersson L, Bourguignon C, Flores MT, Hicks ML, Lenzi AR, Malmgren B, Moule AJ, Pohl Y, Tsukiboshi M. Guidelines for the Management of Traumatic Dental Injuries: 1. Fractures and Luxations of Permanent Teeth. Pediatr Dent. 2016 Oct;38(6):358-368. PMID: 27931478.

[4] Ghosh, R., Gopalkrishnan, K. and Adirajaiah, S. Association of dental injuries with maxillofacial fractures: a 10-year retrospective study. Oral Surg. 2017:10: 210-215. doi:10.1111/ors.12253

[5] Kallel I, Douki N, Amaidi S, Ben AF. The incidence of complications of dental trauma and associated factors: a retrospective study. Int J Dent. 2020;2020:2968174.

[6] Milani AJ, Alves NF, Espirito-Santo TM, Ribeiro LG, Ammari MM, Antunes LS et al. Impact of Traumatic Dental Injuries on Oral Health-Related Quality of Life of Preschool Children and Their Families Attending a Dental Trauma Care Program. Port J Public Health. 2019;37(1):19-25. doi: 10.1159/000501525

[7] Glendor U. Epidemiology of traumatic dental injuries – a 12 year review of the literature. Dent Traumatol 2008;24: 603-611.

[8] Das M, Reddy L V, Singh S. Prevalence of traumatic dental injuries among 5-16 years-old children and knowledge of teachers in the management of dental injuries. J Indian Assoc Public Health Dent 2019;17:328-332.

[9] Al-Ansari A,Nazir M. Prevalence of dental trauma and Receipt of Its Treatment among Male School Children in the Eastern Province of Saudi Arabia. Scientific World Journal. 2020;2020:1-6. doi:10.1155/2020/7321873.

[10] Andreasen JO, Ravn JJ. Epidemiology of traumatic dental injuries to primary and permanent teeth in a Danish population sample. Int J Oral Surg. 1972;1(5):235-239. doi: 10.1016/s0300-9785(72)80042-5. PMID: 4146883.

[11] Chadwick BL, White DA, Morris AJ, Evans D, Pitts NB. Non-carious tooth conditions in children in the UK, 2003. Br Dent J. 2006 Apr 8;200(7):379-384. doi: 10.1038/sj.bdj.4813424. PMID: 16607325.

[12] Govindarajan M, Reddy VN, Ramalingam K, et al. Prevalence of traumatic dental injuries to the anterior teeth among three to thirteen-year-old school children of Tamilnadu. Contemp Clin Dent 2012;3(2):164-167. DOI: 10.4103/0976-237X.96819.

[13] Levin, L, Day, PF, Hicks, L, et al. International Association of Dental Traumatology guidelines for the management of traumatic dental injuries: General introduction. Dent Traumatol. 2020; 36: 309-313. https://doi.org/10.1111/edt.12574

[14] Keels MA, Section on Oral Health, American Academy of Pediatrics. Management of dental trauma in a primary care setting. Pediatrics. 2014 Feb;133(2):e466–e476. DOI: 10.1542/peds.2013-3792.

[15] Emerich K, Gazda E. Review of recommendations for the management of dental trauma presented in first-aid textbooks and manuals. Dent Traumatol. 2010 Jun;26(3):212-216. doi: 10.1111/j.1600-9657.2010.00900.x. PMID: 20572837.

[16] Fouad AF, Abbott PV, Tsilingaridis G, Cohenca N, Lauridsen E, Bourguignon C, et al International Association of Dental Traumatology guidelines for the management of traumatic dental injuries: 2. Avulsion of permanent teeth. Dent Traumatol. 2020 Aug;36(4):331-342. doi: 10.1111/edt.12573. Epub 2020 Jun 13. PMID: 32460393.

[17] Azodo CC, Erhabor P. Management of tooth mobility in the periodontology clinic: An overview and experience from a tertiary healthcare setting. Afr J Med Health Sci 2016;15:50-57.

[18] Dental Trauma Guide. IADT treatment guidelines, Avulsion- First aid for avulsions 2019. Available from: https://dentaltraumaguide.org/free-dental-guides/permanent-teeth/avulsion/. [Accessed 05 October 2020].

[19] Day PF, Kindelan SA, Spencer JR, Kindelan JD, Duggal MS. Dental trauma: part 2. Managing poor prognosis anterior teeth--treatment options for the subsequent space in a growing patient. J Orthod. 2008 Sep;35(3):143-155. doi: 10.1179/146531207225022590. PMID: 18809778.

[20] Diangelis AJ, Andreasen JO, Ebeleseder KA, Kenny DJ, Trope M, Sigurdsson A, Andersson L, Bourguignon C, Flores MT, Hicks ML, Lenzi AR, Malmgren B, Moule AJ, Pohl Y, Tsukiboshi M; International Association of Dental Traumatology. International Association of Dental Traumatology guidelines for the management of traumatic dental injuries: 1. Fractures and luxations of permanent teeth. Dent Traumatol. 2012 Feb;28(1):2-12. doi: 10.1111/j.1600-9657.2011.01103.x. Erratum in: Dent Traumatol. 2012 Dec;28(6):499. PMID: 22230724.

[21] Andersson L, Andreasen JO, Day P, Heithersay G, Trope M, Diangelis AJ, et al. International Association of Dental Traumatology. International Association of Dental Traumatology guidelines for the management of traumatic dental injuries: 2. Avulsion of permanent teeth. Dent Traumatol. 2012 Apr;28(2):88-96. doi: 10.1111/j.1600-9657.2012.01125.x. PMID: 22409417.

[22] Andreasen JO, Andreasen FM, Bakland LK, Flores MT, Andersson L. *Traumatic dental injuries, a manual*, 3rd edn. Chichester, West Sussex: Wiley-Blackwell; 2011. p. 48-53.

[23] Soares TR, Luiz RR, Risso PA, Maia LC. Healing complications of traumatized permanent teeth in pediatric patients: a longitudinal study. Int J Paediatr Dent. 2014 Sep;24(5):380-386. https://doi.org/10.1111/ipd.12082

[24] Hirschfeld I. Tooth-brush trauma recession: A clinical study. J Dent Res. 1931;11:61-63.

[25] Fotinos S. Panagakos and Cesar A. Migliorati (February 19th 2014). Concepts of Oral Hygiene Maintenance that Would Apply for the Different Groups of Patients, Diagnosis and Management of Oral Lesions and Conditions: A Resource Handbook for the Clinician, Cesar A. Migliorati and Fotinos S. Panagakos, IntechOpen, DOI: 10.5772/57597. Available from: https://www.intechopen.com/books/diagnosis-and-management-of-oral-lesions-and-conditions-a-resource-handbook-for-the-clinician/concepts-of-oral-hygiene-maintenance-that-would-apply-for-the-different-groups-of-patients.

[26] Scannapieco FA, Gershovich E. The prevention of periodontal disease-An overview. Periodontol 2000. 2020 Oct;84(1):9-13. doi: 10.1111/prd.12330. PMID: 32844421.

[27] Heasman PA, McCraken GI. Powered toothbrushes: a review of clinical trials. J Clin Periodontol 1999;26:407-420.

[28] Singh G, Mehta DS, Chopra S, Khatri M. Comparison of sonic and ionic toothbrush in reduction in plaque and gingivitis. J Indian Soc Periodontol. 2011 Jul-Sep; 15(3): 210-214. doi: 10.4103/0972-124X.85662

[29] Slot DE, Dörfer CE, Van der Weijden GA. The efficacy of interdental brushes on plaque and parameter of periodontal inflammation: a systematic review. Int J Dent Hyg. 2008; 6:253-264.

[30] Flores MT. Traumatic injuries in the primary dentition. Dent Traumatol. 2002 Dec;18(6):287-298. doi: 10.1034/j.1600-9657.2002.00153.x. PMID: 12656861.

[31] Von Arx T, Filippi A, Lussi A. Comparison of a new dental trauma splint device (TTS) with three commonly used splinting techniques. Dent Traumatol 2001; 17: 266-274.

[32] Kathariya R, Devanoorkar A, Golani R, Shetty N, Vallakatla V, Bhat MY, *et al.* To splint or not to splint: The current status of periodontal splinting. J Int Acad Periodontol 2016;18:45-56.

[33] Jamal S, Motiwala MA, Ghafoor R. Conventional and contemporary approaches of splinting traumatized teeth: A review article. J Pak Med Assoc. 2020 Feb;70(Suppl 1)(2):S53-S59. PMID: 31981337.

[34] Geeta T, Preethi S. Managment of complex crown root fracture using fibre post – A case report. Endodontology 2014;26(3):211-216.

[35] Nicolau B, Marcenes W, Sheiham A. The relationship between traumatic dental injuries and adolescents' development along the life course. Community Dent Oral Epidemiol 2003;31:306-313

[36] Goswami M, Eranhikkal A. Management of Traumatic Dental Injuries Using Different Types of Splints: A Case Series. Int J Clin Pediatr Dent 2020;13(2):199-202.

[37] Sharif MO, Tejani-Sharif A, Kenny K, Day PF. A systematic review of outcome measures used in clinical trials of treatment interventions following traumatic dental injuries. Dent Traumatol. 2015; 31: 422-428.

[38] Lopes LB, Botelho J, Machado V. Severe Case of Delayed Replantation of Avulsed Permanent Central Incisor: A Case Report with Four-Year Follow-Up. Medicina (Kaunas). 2020 Sep 25;56(10):503. doi: 10.3390/medicina56100503. PMID: 32992684; PMCID: PMC7599862.

[39] Kenny KP, Day PF, Sharif MO, Parashos P, Lauridsen E, Feldens CA, et al. What are the important outcomes in traumatic dental injuries? An international approach to the development of a core outcome set. Dent Traumatol. 2018;34:4-11.

[40] Andersson L. Epidemiology of traumatic dental injuries. J Endod. 2013;39(3 Suppl):S2–S5.

[41] Mahmood IA, Morshidi DNA, Hamzah SH, Baharuddin IH, Ahmad MS. Malaysian Dental Students' Knowledge of Managing Dental Trauma in Children. Eur J Dent Educ. 2020 Nov 20. doi: 10.1111/eje.12632. Epub ahead of print. PMID: 33217767.

[42] Malikaew P, Watt RG, Sheiham A. Prevalence and factors associated with traumatic dental injuries (TDI) to anterior teeth of 11-13 year old Thai children. Community Dent Health 2006;23:222-227.

[43] Patel M C, Sujan S G. The prevalence of traumatic dental injuries to permanent anterior teeth and its relation with predisposing risk factors among 8-13 years school children of Vadodara city: An epidemiological study. J Indian Soc Pedod Prev Dent 2012;30:151-157

[44] Rouhani A, Movahhed T, Ghoddusi J, Mohiti Y, anihashemi E, Akbari M. Anterior Traumatic Dental Injuries in East Iranian School Children: Prevalence and Risk Factors. Iran Endod J. 2015;10(1):35-38.

[45] Suhad H. Al-Jundi Dental emergencies presenting to a dental teaching hospital due to complications from traumatic dental injuries. Dent Traumatol.2002;18:181-185.

[46] McIntyre J.D. Lee J.Y. Trope M. et al. Effectiveness of dental trauma education for elementary school staff. Dent Traumatol. 2008; 24: 146-150.

[47] Quezada-Conde, MDC, Alvarez-Velasco, PDL, Lopez, EF, et al. Influence of school environment on occurrence of traumatic dental injuries in 12 years old children. Dent Traumatol. 2020; 36: 510-517. https://doi.org/10.1111/edt.12559

[48] Pinto, G.d.S., Goettems, M.L., Brancher, L.C., da Silva, F.B., Boeira, G.F., Correa, M.B., dos Santos, I.d.S., Torriani, D.D. and Demarco, F.F. Validation of the digital photographic assessment to diagnose traumatic dental injuries. Dent Traumatol. 2016;32: 37-42. doi:10.1111/edt.12204

[49] Namdev R, Jindal A, Bhargava S, Bakshi L, Verma R, Beniwal D. Awareness of emergency management of dental trauma. Contemp Clin Dent. 2014;5:507

Chapter 9

The Role of the Dental Therapists and Oral Hygienists in the Immediate Response to Traumatic Dental Injuries

Tshakane R.M.D. Ralephenya, Sizakele Ngwenya and Kelebogile A. Mothupi

Abstract

Dental Therapists and Oral Hygienists receive training in dental trauma in their curriculum. When they are in their workspace however, many are not confident enough to provide treatment for patients presenting with dental trauma in the oral health setting. As members of the dental team they play an important role in the management of patients who present with traumatic dental injuries. It is therefore important that guidelines are developed for them to understand the role they need to play when providing oral health treatment. The chapter will focus on the etiology of dental trauma to assist the oral health clinicians to prepare for a diagnosis. The classification of traumatic dental injuries will be explained. This will lead to the description of the classified injuries and their management. Clear guidelines and management for the patients will thereafter be provided. The prevention of traumatic dental injuries will also be discussed so that the treatment provided to the patients is improved.

Keywords: dental trauma, traumatic dental injuries, soft tissue injuries, dento-alveolar injuries, oro-facial injuries

1. Introduction

Dental Therapists and Oral Hygienists are members of the dental team and dental professions who receive training in Traumatic Dental Injuries (TDI). However, many are not confident enough to provide treatment for patients presenting with TDI in the oral health setting. They are the first in line of response to provide treatment before referring to dentists and dental specialists. Anecdotal evidence indicates that the inability to treat TDI could be due to the fact that at times dental health care team members are not able to determine the source of TDI [1–3]. Based on this it is important to develop guidelines that will assist dental professionals to manage patients who present with TDI. [1, 2] It has been indicated that there is a need for treatment guidelines when oral health professionals provide treatment for TDI such as avulsed teeth [2]. Providing treatment guidelines will aid in ensuring that oral health care is delivered efficiently and in the best care possible [2, 3].

The consequences of not determining the source of TDI could at times lead to a failure in referring patients for further management. Knowledge of the appropriate treatments and management of patient presenting with TDI can reduce stress and anxiety for both patients and the dental professionals [3]. Therefore, it is important to promote awareness and recent information among the dental professionals as well as groups at risk regarding prevention and emergency treatment modalities. Correct application of these techniques immediately after the traumatic injury should improve both short- and long-term outcomes [1].

2. Rationale

Qualified Dental Therapists and Oral Hygienists have to develop lifelong learning to ensure optimal care for each patient. Part of the lifelong learning entails the ability to manage patients who present with TDIs. It is therefore important that there are guidelines established to improve their oral health practice [2, 3].

Objectives for professional practice include the ability to identify and care for the needs of patients with health problems that affect their oral hygiene [4]. Dental trauma has an impact on the oral hygiene of the patient thus it is critical for Dental Therapists and Oral Hygienists to be able to manage patients who present with those conditions [4–6]. This will enable them to maintain competency in their daily practice, apply scientific advances from new research, and provide patient care that is evidence based.

Based on the brief rationale it is therefore important to develop the objectives indicated in the next section for this book chapter.

2.1 Objectives

The objectives of this article are to:

- Classify traumatic dental injuries that can be observed in an oral health setting
- Provide clinical management strategies for patients presenting with dental trauma injuries
- Indicate the clinical guidelines to be followed by Dental Therapists and Oral Hygienists when managing dental trauma injuries

2.2 Methods

A computer data base research method was implemented to collate information for this chapter. Information was gathered through applied literature research articles from Google Scholar, Science Direct, Web of Science, Scopus, EBSOhost and PubMed.

3. Prevalence of traumatic dental injuries

Trauma has been reported as a major disease burden in lower- and middle-income countries such as South Africa [5, 6]. TDI often occur in association with and contribute significantly to other bodily injuries. With more than one billion people having experienced TDI, these injuries are increasingly becoming of great dental public health concern because of the associated negative impact on economic productivity and the quality of life of affected children and their families [5]. Children sustain 30% and 22% injuries to the primary and the permanent dentition, respectively [5]. It has been estimated that 50% of TDIs occur prior to children leaving school [5].

There is scarcity of data on the prevalence of TDIs in South Africa and Africa at large. A report indicated that there is a TDI prevalence of 16% in primary school children while another report indicated TDI prevalence of 6.4% in children aged 11–13 years old in South Africa [6, 7]. The prevalence of dental trauma varies from 6.1 to 62.1% in pre-school children and from 5.3 to 21% in schoolchildren [6, 7]. A recent review study which sought to estimate the global frequency and incident rates for TDI reported a prevalence of 15.2% and 22.7% in permanent and primary dentition, respectively [6]. Furthermore, the study reported a prevalence of 18.1% in 12-year-old children and an incidence rate of 2.82 per 100 person-years [7].

The variation in the prevalence of TDIs may be attributed to various factors including the study design, geographical location, different diagnostic criteria as determined by the trauma classification used, behavioral and cultural diversity [8].

Soft tissue injuries such as luxations and subluxations are more frequently seen in primary dentition while fractures of the crown involving enamel and dentine are seen more commonly in permanent dentition [8]. The most commonly injured teeth in primary mainly from falls in children and sport activities in adolescents.

The strongest association has been demonstrated between TDIs and gender as well as TDIs and age. Males experience TDIs more frequently than males with the ratio ranging from 1.3:1 to 2.5:1 [9, 10]. The ratio has however been decreasing over the years as more females participate in sport activities. TDIs are mainly sustained in young adults, preschool and school going children. Twenty five percent of school going children experience TDIs as a result of physical and behavioral factors [9–11].

4. Etiologic factors for traumatic dental injuries

There are many studies that have been conducted that provide the epidemiology of maxillofacial trauma throughout the world [12–15]. This is important as they provide etiological factors which vary, depending on the age of the patient in question, as well as cultural and socio-economic factors [12, 16].

Among the most common causes of the TDIs are: traffic accident involving motor vehicle, motorcycle, or bicycle; day-to-day activities and sports; as well as a fall from a height [17, 18]. Knowing the etiology of the maxillofacial trauma provides an understanding of people's behavior in a region and the need for adoption of preventive policies [12, 13, 16].

Traumatic dental and facial injuries are frequent in sports and often cause esthetic, functional, psychological, and economic problems [3–20]. Dental injuries are the most frequent orofacial injury related to participation in sports activities [19, 20].

The main causes of traumatic dental injuries are falls and collisions with people or objects, which are very common in contact sports [19, 20]. Participation in sports, especially contact sports, greatly increases the risk of traumatic dental injury.

5. Classification systems for dental trauma

Dental Therapists and Oral Hygienists need to be aware of how TDI are classified so that they can provide treatment for patients presenting with the conditions. Many classifications of TDI have been presented over the years [21].

The currently accepted system is based on the Application of International Classification of Diseases to dentistry and stomatology by the WHO (1995), and was modified by Andreasen and Andreasen (2011) [22–24].

The conditions to be observed in the two classifications include the following: crown infraction; uncomplicated and complicated crown fracture; uncomplicated and complicated crown-root fracture; root fracture; concussion; luxation; avulsion; and lacerations.

The modified Andreasen classification is more comprehensive and contains and explains more conditions to be observed when studying dental trauma. **Table 1** indicates the differences in the two classification systems and will prepare us to review and formulate a structure to guide dental professionals.

Based on the classification described in **Table 1** detailed descriptions of the injuries is provided. The injuries are categorized into soft tissue injuries (**Table 2**); Dento-alveolar Injuries (**Table 3**); and Oro-Facial Bony Injuries

Andreasen and Andreasen (2011)	World Health Organization (1995)
Crown infraction, incomplete fracture of the enamel	Fracture of enamel of tooth
Uncomplicated crown fracture: a fracture confined to the enamel or dentine but not exposing the pulp	Fracture of crown without pulpal involvement
Complicated crown fracture: a fracture confined to the enamel and dentine and exposing the pulp	Fracture of crown with pulpal involvement
Uncomplicated crown-root fracture: a fracture involving enamel, dentine cementum, not exposing the pulp	Fracture of root of tooth
Complicated crown-root fracture: A fracture involving enamel, dentine, cementum and exposing the pulp	Fracture of crown and root of tooth
Root fracture: a fracture involving dentine, cementum, and the pulp	Fracture of tooth, unspecified
Concussion: injury without abnormal loosening or displacement but with marked reaction to percussion	Luxation of tooth
Subluxation (loosening): injury with abnormal loosening but without displacement of the tooth	Intrusion or extrusion of tooth
Intrusive luxation (central dislocation)	Avulsion of tooth
Extrusive luxation (peripheral dislocation, partial avulsion)	Other injuries including laceration of oral soft tissues
Lateral luxation	
Exarticulation (complete luxation)	
Comminution of alveolar socket	
Fractures of facial or lingual alveolar socket wall	
Fractures of alveolar process with and without involvement of the socket	
Fractures of the mandible or maxilla with and without involvement of the tooth socket	
Laceration of gingiva or oral mucosa	
Contusion of gingiva or oral mucosa	
Abrasion of gingiva or oral mucosa	

Table 1.
Andreasen and Andreasen (2011) and WHO classification (1995) of TDI.

Soft tissue injuries	Description	Management
Abrasion	Wound caused by superficial damage to the skin	Area to be cleansed through irrigating with saline solutions to remove irritants
Contusions	Hematoma of the tissue without a break in the surface	Often resolve on their own but ice or pressure dressing could decrease swelling
Lacerations	Any tear in the soft tissue (skin or mucosa)	Treatment varies but the area could be cleansed with copious saline irrigation to remove foreign debri
Soft tissue avulsions	An injury in which a structure is forcibly detached from its normal Point of insertion	Hemostatic control with direct pressure and alleviation of pain, followed by copious saline irrigation to help determine the severity of the injury

Table 2.
Summary describing common soft tissue injuries and their management (Patel et al.*, 2014).*

Dento-alveolar Injuries	Description	Management
Crown fracture	Injury on the coronal portion of the teeth affecting the enamel or dentin and/or the pulp	Depending on area, enamel does not need acute treatment, dentine involvement needs referral for a restoration by dental therapist or dentist
Crown-root fracture	Crown-root fractures involving the crown and root of the tooth, with or without involvement of the pulp	Restorations by dental therapist or dentist if the pulp is not involved and does not and extend far apically into the root. Root Canal Therapy or tooth extraction if there is pulpal involvement. Extraction delayed to allow healing of bony fracture.
Root fracture	Root fractures involving the root or roots of teeth. Radiographs could aid in diagnosis.	Root Canal Therapy, post and core, and crowns for fractures close to the crown; depending on the severity immobilization, extraction or apical fragment to be left in socket.
Tooth concussion	Teeth sensitive to touch or percussion and patient does not experience tooth mobility or displacement	Acute treatment not needed and relieve provided through occlusal contact relief of the sensitive tooth via enameloplasty on the opposing tooth
Tooth subluxation	Mobility on the tooth or looseness without tooth displacement	Extent of tooth mobility to determine treatment needed. Mild mobility can be treated as tooth concussion with occlusal contact relief and significantly mobile teeth may be splinted and immobilized by dental therapist or dentist.
Tooth displacement	Teeth could be displaced in any direction, but the most common displacement are in a buccal-lingual direction and mesiodistal direction. There is a possibility for intrusion or extrusion.	Depending on the extent of the displacement. Repositioning of the teeth could be provided along with splinting and immobilization for a minimum of 2 weeks depending on severity. Further management could include medication and referral to Maxillo-Facial and Oral Surgeons.
Intrusion	Maxillary teeth often involved and if severe the teeth appear missing. The tooth is displaced into the socket.	Treatment could be controversial and management taken on a case by case basis.

Dento-alveolar Injuries	Description	Management
Extrusion	The tooth is displaced out of the socket.	The displaced tooth could be pushed back into the appropriate position within their sockets, and could require splinting and immobilization. Depending on the severity Root Canal Therapy could be recommended.
Tooth Avulsion	Complete displacement of the tooth out from its alveolar socket.	Management varied and depends on extra-alveolar time, pulpal health and periodontal health.
Alveolar bone fracture	Injury to the alveolar process in the presence or absence of teeth.	Referral to Maxillo-Facial and Oral Surgeon for proper repositioning and stabilization. Splinting, copious irrigation and soft tissue suturing could be included in the treatment plan.

Table 3.
Summary describing common dento-alveolar injuries and their management (Patel et al., 2014).

Oro-facial bony injuries	Description	Management
Orbital Fracture	Involves fracture of the medial and lateral orbital walls, orbital roof and floor, and orbital rim. Clinical findings may include maxillary (midface) paresthesia, peri orbital edema, subconjunctival hemorrhage, diplopia, and impaired extraocular movements	Orbital fracture repair is usually indicated with enopthalmus greater than 2 mm, diplopia, floor defect greater than 1 cm, and ophthalmoplegia.
Nasal Fracture	Determined by physical examinations and clinical findings may include nasal edema, ecchymosis, epistaxis, septal deviation, mobility, crepitus, and nasal deformity.	Optimal within 1–2 days but waiting 7 to 10 days is recommended to allow for resolution of soft-tissue swelling.
Maxillary Fracture	Divided into LeFort I, II, and III, depending on the extent of the midfacial fractures.	Maxillary LeFort fractures often treated with open reduction and internal fixation. Maxillomandibular fixation (MMF) may be required for fracture reduction.
Mandibular Fracture	Occur in multiple locations based on injury type, force and direction of trauma.	Open or closed reduction.

Table 4.
Summary describing common oro-facial bony injuries and their management (Patel et al., 2014).

(**Table 4**). The tables will also include the management to be provided for the TDIs as guidelines for dental professionals.

6. Discussion

The information compiled above shows that it is very crucial for Dental Therapists and Oral Hygienist to have a clear ability to formulate a diagnosis and oral hygiene care plan based on the assessment of the oral cavity [22–24]. Literature available tends to focus on TDI being diagnosed and managed by dentists and dental specialists [2, 3]. This is not always feasible as the first in line for the provision of oral health services are Dental Therapists and Oral Hygienists. The future of oral health services shows a need to empower all oral health professionals in the provision of TDI so that patients get optimal oral health services. With the number of auxiliary oral health professionals increasing, it is very important that their role in providing critical and emergency oral health services as emphasized.

Dental Therapist and Oral Hygienists provide treatment in a Primary Health Care setting and could therefore be the first in line to provide treatment when patients present in developing countries [6, 7, 9]. Hence it is crucial that they be provided with clear guidelines and information to diagnose and manage TDI. This will be done through the ability to classify the various TDI indicated in **Table 1**. The scope of practice for Dental Therapists and Oral Hygienists indicates that there should be a focus on dental trauma when clinical services are provided (**Tables 2–4**).

Table 5 provides a brief schematic template that indicates that during practice the Dental Therapists and Oral Hygienists should be able to identify whether patients present with soft tissue, dento-alveolar or oro-facial bony injuries when they provide dental treatment for adults and pediatric patients [25, 26]. This is important as they will be able to monitor the patient's progress towards achieving desired oral health outcomes.

When the patients present in the clinical environment there should be adequate clinical reasoning skills to know how to manage the TDI. The information provided in the middle column of **Tables 2–4** provides detailed descriptions of the TDI so that the Dental Therapists and Oral Hygienists can have clear guidelines of what to expect in practice. The middle circle of **Table 5** provides a relevant scheme to be

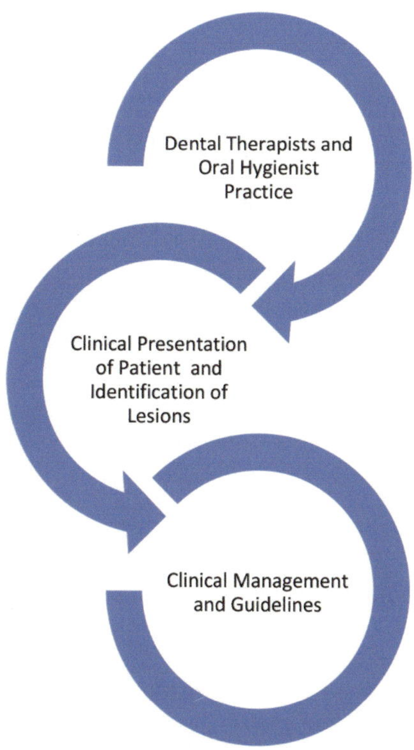
Dental Therapists and Oral Hygienist Practice
Clinical Presentation of Patient and Identification of Lesions
Clinical Management and Guidelines

Table 5.
Applying the clinical findings in dental therapist and Oral hygiene practice.

followed that they should use to have a clear description of the possible lesions. This is essential for the provision of evidence of adequate consultation when needed and leads the clinicians to have adequate and clear written responses should the information be requested by other members of the dental team or health team [25–28]. This is a key factor to be considered as they also need to refer the lesions to the appropriate dental team members based on the scope of practice [27, 29, 30].

Clinical service and oral hygiene patient care is improved if the TDI are managed efficiently and effectively [31, 32].

The crucial step to be followed during all the phases is to ensure that there is appropriate documentation of self-care education, status of patient compliance, failed or canceled appointments, postoperative instructions provided, modification made in care plan and supportive facts, referrals and continued care schedule when the TDI are managed [4, 33].

The appropriate management will assist all clinicians to ensure that the individual patients' potential state of oral health and maintenance is achieved [33]. This leads to optimum oral health service that is crucial for the patients.

7. Conclusions

Ultimately, knowing how to effectively diagnose and start treating dental emergencies early will lead to better clinical outcomes and greater patient satisfaction. Availability of easily accessible dental emergency manual/guidelines provide an overview of effective management strategies for dental emergencies which is essential for Dental Therapists and Oral Hygienist [34].

It is very important to select appropriate clinical responses when patients present with dental trauma as discussed [35, 36]. It is also crucial to note as discussed, that relevant approaches to diagnostic testing and evaluation when treating dental emergencies will build confidence and enable Dental Therapists and Oral Hygienists to effectively manage dental trauma.

A recommendation for developing protocols for the different categories of patients such as pediatric patients is suggested for further development. There is further room for a broader schematic template that shows how the inter and multi-disciplinary team can play a role in providing oral health services for patients presenting with TDI.

Conflict of interest

The authors declare no conflict of interest.

Author details

Tshakane R.M.D. Ralephenya*, Sizakele Ngwenya and Kelebogile A. Mothupi
School of Oral Health Sciences, University of the Witwatersrand, Johannesburg, South Africa

*Address all correspondence to: tshakane.ralephenya@wits.ac.za

References

[1] Batista, A.M., Marques, L.S., Batista, A.E., Falci, S.G.M., Ramos-Jorge, M.L., 2012. Urban-rural differences in oral and maxillofacial trauma. *Brazilian Oral Research* 26, 132–138. https://doi.org/10.1590/S1806-83242012000200008

[2] Cohenca, N., Forrest, J.L., Rotstein, I. 2006. Knowledge of oral health professionals of treatment of avulsed teeth. *Dental Traumatology*; 22: 296–301)

[3] Levin, L., Day, P.F., Hicks, L., O'Connell, A., Fouad, A.F., Bourguignon, C., Abbott, P.V., 2020. International Association of Dental Traumatology guidelines for the management of traumatic dental injuries: General introduction. *Dental Traumatology* 36, 309–313. https://doi.org/10.1111/edt.12574

[4] Darby, M.L. and Walsh, M.M. (2015) *Dental hygiene theory and practice.* (4th Edition) Missouri: Saunders

[5] Hardcastle, T.C., Oosthuizen, G., Clarke, D. Lutge, E. (2016) Trauma, a preventable burden of disease in South Africa: review of the evidence, with a focus on KwaZulu-Natal. *South African Health Review*, 1, 179-189

[6] Hargreaves, J.A., Matejka, J.M., Cleaton-Jones, P.E., Williams, S. (1995) Anterior tooth trauma in eleven-year-old South African children. *ASDC journal of dentistry for children*, 62(5), 353.

[7] Naidoo, S., Sheiham A., Tsakos, G. (2009) Traumatic dental injuries of permanent incisors in 11- to 13-year-old South African schoolchildren *Dental Traumatology,* 25: 224–228; doi: 10.1111/j.1600-9657.2008.00749.x

[8] Anderson, L. (2013) Epidemiology of traumatic dental injuries. *Journal of Endodontics,* 39(3 Suppl): S2-5. DOI: 10.1016/j.joen.2012.11.021.

[9] Lam, R., Abbott P., Lloyd, C., Lloyd, C., Kruger E., Tennant, M. (2008) Dental trauma in an Australian rural centre. *Dental Traumatology*, 24(6), 663-670.

[10] Mahmoodi, B., Rahimi-Nedjat, R., Weusmann, J., Azaripour A., Walter, C., Willershausen,B. (2015) Traumatic dental injuries in a university hospital: a four-year retrospective study. *BMC Oral Health,* 15(1), 139.

[11] Milani, A.J., Alves N.F., do Espiroto-Santo T.M., Ribeiro L.G., Ammari M.M., Antunes L.S., Antunes L.A.A. (2019) Impact of Traumatic Dental Injuries on Oral Health-Related Quality of Life of Preschool Children and Their Families Attending a Dental Trauma Care Program. *Port J Public Health,*37:19–25. DOI: 10.1159/000501525

[12] Al-Ansari, A., Nazir, M., 2020. Prevalence of Dental Trauma and Receipt of Its Treatment among Male School Children in the Eastern Province of Saudi Arabia. *The Scientific World Journal* 2020, 1–6. https://doi.org/10.1155/2020/7321873

[13] Ali S.N.A., Algarawi SA, Alrubaian AM, Asma I. Alasqah AI. (2020) Knowledge of General Dental Practitioners and Specialists about Emergency Management of Traumatic Dental Injuries in Qassim, Saudi Arabia. *International Journal of Pediatrics*, 2020, Article ID 6059346, 7 pages https://doi.org/10.1155/2020/6059346

[14] Al Sari, S., Kowash, M., Hussein, I., Al-Halabi, M., 2019. An Educational Initiative for Dubai School Nurses and Physical Education Teachers on the Management of Traumatic Dental Injuries. *The Journal of School Nursing* 35, 359–366. https://doi.org/10.1177/1059840518780306

[15] Eigbobo, J.O., Orikpete, E.V. Traumatic dental injuries among a

selected population of adolescents in Southern Nigeria. *Journal of Dentistry and Oral Hygiene* 12(1): 11-15, January-June 2020 DOI: 10.5897/JDOH2020.0247

[16] Petti, S., Ulf Glendor, U, Lars Andersson L. (2018) World traumatic dental injury prevalence and incidence, a meta-analysis-One billion living people have had traumatic dental injuries. *Dental Traumatology* Apr;34(2): 71-86. doi: 10.1111/edt.12389.

[17] Aras, A., n.d. Evaluating the Levels of Knowledge and Attitudes of Emergency Medical Technicians and Paramedics toward Traumatic Dental Injuries

[18] Basha, S., Mohamed, R.N., Al-Thomali, Y., Ashour, A.A., Zahrani, F.S. A., Almutair, N.E., 2021. Traumatic dental injuries in special health care needs children and association with obesity. *Annals of Saudi Medicine* 41, 51–58. https://doi.org/10.5144/0256-4947.2021.51

[19] Çalışkan, S., Delikan, E., Kızılaslan, S., Özbek, Ö., 2021. Knowledge of Dental Avulsion Among Emergency Physicians: A Survey Study. *The Journal of Pediatric Research* 8, 62–68. https://doi.org/10.4274/jpr.galenos.2020.98705

[20] Prabhu, A., Rao, A.P., Govindarajan, M., Reddy V., Krishnakumar, R., Kalaiperumal, S. (2013) Attributes of dental trauma in a school population with active sports involvement. *Asian Journal of Sports Medicine,* 4(3), 190.

[21] Bastone E.B., Freer T.J., Mc Namara J.R., 2000 Epidemiology of dental trauma: A review of literature. *Australian Dental Journal* 45:2-9

[22] Patel, P.B., Stanton, D.C., Granquist, E.J., 2014. Common Dental and Orofacial Trauma. *Medical Clinics of North America*; 98: 1261-1279 https://doi.org/10.1016/j.mcna.2014.08.003

[23] Douglass, A.B., Douglass, J.M., 2003. Common Dental Emergencies 67, 7.

[24] Dure-Molla, M., Fournier, B.P., Manzanares, M.C., Acevedo, A.C., Hennekam, R.C., Friedlander, L., Boy-Lefèvre, M., Kerner, S., Toupenay, S., Garrec, P., Vi-Fane, B., Felizardo, R., Berteretche, M., Jordan, L., Ferré, F., Clauss, F., Jung, S., Chalendar, M., Troester, S., Kawczynski, M., Chaloyard, J., International Group of Dental Nomenclature, Manière, M.C., Berdal, A., Bloch-Zupan, A., 2019a. Elements of morphology: Standard terminology for the teeth and classifying genetic dental disorders. *American Journal of Medical Genetics Part* A 179, 1913–1981. https://doi.org/10.1002/ajmg.a.61316

[25] El-Kalla, I., Shalan, H., Bakr, R., 2017. Impact of dental trauma on quality of life among 11–14 years school children. *Contemporary Clinical Dentistry* 8, 538. https://doi.org/10.4103/ccd.ccd_428_17

[26] Kurt, A., Güdük, Ö.F., Erbek, Ş.M., Baygın, Ö. Tüzüner, T., 2019. Retrospective evaluation of patients admitted to Karadeniz Technical University Pediatric Dentistry clinic due to trauma. *European Oral Research* 53. https://doi.org/10.26650/eor.20195236

[27] Malcolm, N., Boyd, L., Giblin-Scanlon, L., Vineyard, J., 2020. Occupational stressors of dental hygienists in the United States. *Work* 65, 517–524. https://doi.org/10.3233/WOR-203106

[28] Prevalence of Tooth Injuries Among Children 2 To 13 Years of Age Reporting to Dental Hospital- An Institutional Based Retrospective Study, 2021. *Journal of Contemporary Issues in Business and Government 26*. https://doi.org/10.47750/cibg.2020.26.02.020

[29] Shockley, L.W., Legome, E., 2011. *Trauma: A Comprehensive Emergency*

Medicine Approach, Cambridge Medicine. Cambridge University Press, Cambridge.

[30] Vlok, J.L., Worthington, E.M., Hindson, J.A., Davidson, L.E., Thomson, W.M., Drummond, B.K., 2011. Young people's perceptions of photographs of dental trauma: Young people's thoughts on dental trauma. *Dental Traumatology* 27, 109–112. https://doi.org/10.1111/j.1600-9657.2010.00969.x

[31] Welbury, R., n.d. *IADT Guidelines 2020* An Update 21.

[32] Yee, R., Chay, P.L., Tham, L.P., 2020. Safety and effectiveness of intramuscular ketamine sedation in the management of children with oro-dental trauma in a paediatric emergency department. *Dental Traumatology* 36, 19–24. https://doi.org/10.1111/edt.12497

[33] Cagetitti, M.G., Marcoli, P.A., Berengo, M., Cascone, P. Cordone, L, Defabianis, P. De Giglio, O., Esposito, N., Federici, A., Laino, A., Majorana, A., Nardone, M., Pinchi, V. Pizzi, S., Polimeni, A., Grazia, M., Privetera, M. G., Talarico, V. Zampogna, S. 2019 Italian guidelines for the prevention and management of dental trauma in children. *Italian Journal of Pediatrics* 45: 157, 1-14. https://doi.org/10.1186/s13052-019-0734-7

[34] Arikan, V., Sari, S. Sonmez, H. 2010 The prevalence and treatment outcomes of primary tooth injuries. *European Journal of Dentistry* 4(4), 447-453

[35] Atabek, D., Alacam, A., Aydintug, I., Konakoglu, G. 2014 A retrospective study of traumatic dental injuries. *Dental Traumatology* 30(2), 154-161

[36] Glendor, U. 2008 Epidemiology of traumatic dental injuries – a year review of the literature. *Dental Traumatology* 24: 603e11

Chapter 10

Signs of Child Abuse and Neglect: A Practical Guide for Dental Professionals

Aneesa Moolla, Tshakane Ralephenya, Sizakele Ngwenya and Sankeshan Padayachee

Abstract

Children are the future of society. Society should, in turn protect their dignity and wellbeing by ensuring that they are treated with respect and care. Dental practitioners are often the first health professionals to come into contact with victims of child abuse and neglect, not only to render treatment to abuse victims but also to serve as their first line of defense. As part of a larger human community, dental practitioners are responsible for identifying evidence of intentional harm befalling children and reporting it to law enforcers. Physically abused children predominantly present with injuries to the maxillofacial and oral regions. It is therefore important for dental practitioners to be aware of the intra-oral and extra-oral signs that may be indicative of child abuse and neglect in order to champion the fight against child abuse.

Keywords: physical abuse, sexual abuse, emotional abuse, dental trauma, dental neglect

1. Introduction

Evidence from the United States of America (US) indicates that there was an estimated number of 656,000 (rounded) victims of child abuse and neglect in recent years [1]. These statistics indicate that the victim rate for child abuse and neglect is 8.9 victims per 1000 children in the US population [1]. Information from the World Health Organization (WHO) (2020) shows that globally, nearly 3 in 4 children - or 300 million children - aged 2–4 years regularly suffer physical punishment and/or psychological violence at the hands of parents and caregivers [2, 3]. It is therefore important to be aware that victims of child abuse and dental neglect could present in the dental office. 65% of physical abuse to children involves injuries to the head, face, neck, or mouth and dental professionals could be the first health professionals to render treatment to abuse victims as well as being their first line of defense [4]. Hence, there should be an awareness of pediatric patients who are withdrawn or present with a hostile demeanor accompanied by tell-tale bruises, bite-marks, scars, swollen lips and severely decayed teeth [4–6]. These could be red flags that could alert the dental professional that the pediatric patient has experienced child neglect and gross physical, verbal or sexual abuse [5].

Dental professionals – including general dentists, dental specialists, dental hygienists, dental therapists and dental assistants – are all afforded a unique lens

IntechOpen

into the lives of children who pass through their dental offices [4, 5]. It is thus both an obligation and mandatory for dental professionals to ensure that they are knowledgeable on both outward extra-oral and oral clinical clues, which may preclude dental injuries and trauma as a result of child abuse and neglect [7, 8].

This guide thus offers a practical outlook on signs of neglect and trauma that intends to signal cases of abuse and neglect to assist dental professionals identify and recognize those signs.

It is advised that all dental patient examinations should follow a holistic assessment and analysis [9–11]. The dental professional's jurisdiction for such signs may go beyond dental and oral signs, particularly when seeking to identify victims of abuse. This would imply the need for increased vigilance related to visible physical injuries with suspicious appearance, location and origin, inconsistent verbal testimonies as well as the outward behavior and demeanor of the potentially neglected or abused child [9–11]. It is also important to consider the details that would be required to form a comprehensive report in order to support or warrant alerting the relevant authorities for further investigations [9–11].

2. Understanding abuse

It is crucial for dental professionals to have a clear understanding of abuse and the important terminology linked to neglect. The WHO (2020) defines child abuse as "maltreatment and neglect that occurs to children under 18 years of age". The definition includes "all types of physical and/or emotional ill-treatment, sexual abuse, neglect, negligence and commercial or other exploitation, which results in actual or potential harm to the child's health, survival, development or dignity in the context of a relationship of responsibility, trust or power" [2].

To provide a broad perspective of the key terms that define child abuse and neglect (**Table 1** is included).

Abuse and neglect can be defined and categorized as follows:

- **Physical abuse** takes place when there are incidents that cause physical harm to a child [9]. This is not limited to, but also includes incidents where the symptoms of disease are concocted, or children's illnesses are deliberately induced [12–16]. It further refers to non-accidental injuries which are deliberately inflicted and result in physical injury or death [17]. Physical abuse or use of excessive force can manifest as bruises, scars, fractures, burns or bite marks [12].

- **Emotional abuse or ill-treatment** is at times referred to as psychological maltreatments and occurs when a child is harmed emotionally by their parent or guardian [10–12]. It is observed when there is persistent emotional harm to a child and includes failure to meet a child's need for affection, attention or stimulation [12]. Constant verbal abuse, rejection, threats of violence or attempts to frighten the child also constitute emotional abuse [13, 14], as do social isolation and humiliation [15].

- **Sexual abuse** involves "sexually molesting or assaulting a child; allowing a child to be sexually abused or assaulted; encouraging, inducing or forcing a child to be used for the sexual gratification of another person; participating or assisting in the commercial sexual exploitation of a child" [6].

- **Neglect** is the failure to meet a child's physical and or psychological needs [15]. This is the most common form of maltreatment and involves continuous failure

Category of abuse	Definition	Manifestation or symptom of abuse
Physical abuse	Physical harm to a child including fabricating the symptoms of or deliberately inducing illnesses.	Bruises, scars, fractures, burns or bite marks.
Emotional abuse or ill-treatment	Psychological abuse due to failure of a parent or caregiver to provide a developmentally appropriate and supportive environment for a child.	Poor hygiene. Sudden change in self-confidence. Headaches or stomach-aches with no medical cause.
Sexual abuse	Involving a child in sexual activity that s/he does not fully comprehend, is unable to give informed consent to, or for which the child is not developmentally prepared.	Lacerations of the tongue, buccal mucosa or palate. Lingual and labial frenal tears. Teeth that are fractured, displaces, avulsed or non-vital Radiographic evidence of fractures in different degrees of healing.
Neglect	Failure by a parent, guardian or family member to provide for the development and well-being of a child.	Malnourishment Failure to gain weight Desperately affectionate behavior
Dental neglect	Failure by a parent or guardian to seek provision of oral health treatment for a child.	Rampant caries; untreated dental and gingival disease;

Table 1.
Categories of abuse, definitions and manifestations or symptoms of abuse.

Type of abuse or neglect	Behavioral indicators
Physical abuse	Aggression and withdrawal Fear of caregiver/guardian/parent Cautious of adult contact Uneasy when others cry Reports abuse by parent / caregiver/guardian Frightened to return home
Emotional abuse or ill-treatment	Habits including sucking or rocking Antisocial and destructive Sleep disorders Phobias, obsessions, compulsions Behavior extremes Developmental lags and suicide attempts
Sexual abuse	Will not change in front of peers Fantasy or immature behavior Mature sexual awareness Reports sexual abuse
Physical neglect	Begging or stealing food/drinks Arrives early to school and stays late Constantly tired Alcohol/drug abuse States there is no caregiver
Adapted from Ref. [5].	

Table 2.
Types of abuse and behavioral indicators.

to protect a child from exposure to any danger, cold, starvation or substance abuse [13]. It can also include failure to carry out important aspects of childcare which could impact on a child's emotional, psychological or physical development [13–15]. Poor supervision of a child could also bean indication of neglect [16].

- **Dental neglect** is defined as the "wilful failure of parent or guardian to seek and follow through with treatment necessary to ensure a level of oral health essential for adequate function and freedom from pain and infection" [15].

As noted, abuse and neglect take on many different forms and this may be obvious or not obvious at all to anyone. However, by becoming more knowledgeable about all these warning signs indicated in **Table 2** above, dental professionals may inadvertently save the childhood or even the life of an abused child who has nobody to turn to for help and lacks the capacity to understand where to seek help in the very first place.

3. Guidelines to signs and symptoms of child abuse and neglect

From the time that a child enters a dental office, there are warning signs that could signal potential malice against their well-being. These warning signs may include the following factors which will likely overlap across the different types of abuse:

3.1 Physical appearance, behavior and demeanor of a child

The dental clinical environment provides a unique platform with the benefit of close engagement with patients [2, 5, 12]. One of the key aspects to successful dental treatment is the formation of trust between the dental professional and the patient [12, 13]. Dental professionals should be experienced in this regard and need to be well-equipped to identify clues and make deductions from obvious and non-obvious signs of potential abuse [12, 13].

From this vantage point, dental professionals should approach pediatric patients by observing both subtle and gross signs during their consultation and clinical examination, whereby the practitioner should be observing and analyzing the pediatric patient's outward appearance and demeanor, their behaviors and mannerisms and their response to the environment [13, 15].

It should be noted that there are several considerations that make suspicion of abuse challenging. The first is that children often have within their nature the tendency to be shy with strangers, have difficulties with expression, a difference in response to new environments - particularly to a dental environment, which society has portrayed as a place for fear [12, 13]. These are thus usually intrinsic to the behavior of children. Also, children tend to often engage in boisterous play, and are thus prone to more injuries than adults [13, 15]. Another key factor is that there are different forms of abuse, such as neglect, physical and sexual abuse [12–16]. These may have different manifestations and highlight the difficulty with separating suspicion of abuse from the mundane [13, 15].

Below is a description of the observations of outward and non-clinical signs of child maltreatment that dental professionals need to be aware of.

3.1.1 Poor hygiene and attire

Whilst many children are notorious for challenging parents regarding their choice of clothes and bath routines, and with consideration for the socio-economic restrictions, there is a level of hygiene and tidiness that most parents can achieve with their children [11]. If this level is not attained, it can raise concerns about neglect [11, 16].

Dental professionals should commence any consultation by first evaluating a child's overall hygiene, their physical appearance and their dressing and attire [5, 15]. They should assess whether the child appears unkempt and if the child's clothing is appropriate for the current weather conditions [12]. Clothing that appears to be inappropriate could be used to cover bites, scars and wounds [12]. It is important to also note however, that this factor could be related to poor socio-economic and cultural status and thus as discussed, all individual factors should never be considered in isolation but as part of a far bigger conglomerate of issues [12, 15].

3.1.2 Signs of malnourishment

Children could be left to starve if neglected or being punished [16]. This has long term consequences if it is a common occurrence. It has been reported that at times individuals who were malnourished as infants tend to display higher levels of physical neglect during their late childhood [13, 16]. This has been observed in relationships that remained statistically significant even after accounting for childhood standard of living [13, 16]. It may not be as evident to non-health professionals but dental professionals should consider common signs of malnutrition to be discerned through and discussed with the parent or caregiver and the child [5, 13, 16]. The signs include: lack of interest in food, poor appetite, getting ill often with a slow recovery rate, poor concentration, feeling cold all the time, moodiness, not growing or putting on weight at the expected rate for their age and they tire very easily [5, 13, 16].

3.1.3 Developmental delays

According to the Committee on Child Maltreatment Research, Policy, and Practice for the Next Decade: Phase II (2014), "children who have experienced abuse and neglect are at an increased risk for a number of problematic developmental, health, and mental health outcomes, including learning problems" [17]. The examples of the problems that the children experience include "inadequate attention and deficits in executive functions, problems relating to peers (example, peer rejection), internalising symptoms (example, depression, anxiety), externalising symptoms (example, oppositional defiant disorder, conduct disorder, aggression), and post-traumatic stress disorder (PTSD)" [17]. As adults, these children continue to show increased risk for psychiatric disorders, substance use, serious medical illnesses, and lower economic productivity [17]. Dental professionals should therefore, be able to observe the delays in overall development that are not accounted for by parents or caregivers [17]. This includes both these social and behavioral signs that are noted here and that may be noticeable over a period of subsequent visits [17].

3.1.4 Injuries at different stages of healing

Dental professionals need to observe if a pediatric patient presents with any bruises, burns or wounds on the face or body that are at different stages of healing.

The most common presentation on physical abuse that can be observed in children are bruises [11]. Children who have been abused physically tend to experience bruises or injuries on the buttocks, extremities and ears [18, 19], and injuries of soft tissue which do not cover bone [18]. Observations on the face show that the cheeks are indicated to be the most frequently traumatized part in physical abuse [18]. The physically abused child will present with bruises in the shape of a fingertip especially in the neck region which are usually indicative of a "gripping" action [13]. If a child is physically abused with objects such as belts there will be distinctive marks on the skin [12] which can raise suspicions of deliberate injury. A handprint may present as parallel linear spaced marks [11]. Multiple bruises of different colors are indicative of various stages of healing and could be as a result of protracted abuse [12, 20].

Figure 1 has an illustration of a slap to the cheek. In the drawing one can observe the imprint of one slap to the cheek. The slap forces the blood from the impact site of the fingers and deforms tissues between the fingers [2]. A histamine reaction occurs along the margins [2]. This bruise can last from a few minutes to a few hours or even a day depending on the force of the blow and the resiliency of the child's system [2, 6].

Dental professionals who suspect physical abuse should examine the pediatric patient's head and neck for asymmetry, swelling and bruising; inspect the scalp for signs of hair pulling; check the ears for tears, abnormalities and scars during the extra oral assessment [2, 12]. The dental professional should examine the face for bruises and abrasions that have different colors, which could be an indication of the different stages of healing. The extra oral examination should include observations of any distinctive pattern marks on skin left by objects such as belts, cords, hangers or cigarettes [2, 12]. The dental professional should also observe if there are any bite marks, which could present on the pediatric patient as a result of uncontrollable anger by the adult or another child [12]. Bite marks in areas that cannot be the result of self-inflicted wounds are not usually accidental. The extra oral examination should include assessment of the middle third of the face for bilateral bruising around the eyes, petechiae (small red or purple spots containing blood) in the sclera of the eye, ptosis of the eyelids, or a deviated gaze, a bruised nose, deviated septum or blood clot in the nose [12].

Figure 2 shows bruises on the skin due to bite marks. In the picture one can observe the distinctive shape of the teeth on the skin with areas of perforation caused by the intensity of the bite being clearly visible.

Physical abuse could also lead to burns as a result of electrical, thermal or chemical substances being used as forms of punishment [11, 20]. In some instances, children could experience accidental burns and it is thus important to determine the age and overall development of the child when analyzing the basis of the injury [11]. Cigarette burns are very unique in appearance [20] and can present as an oval or round lesion 5 mm to 10 mm in diameter [21]. Conversely, other abnormalities such as those triggered by impetigo or varicella could have a comparable form and hence those possibilities should be omitted [11]. A cigarette that has been stubbed out on the body can leave an injury or scar with an uneven outline [21] as demonstrated in the **Figure 3**.

These will most often be explained away as being frequent accidental injuries or accidents. However, it is important to note that certain parts of the body are more

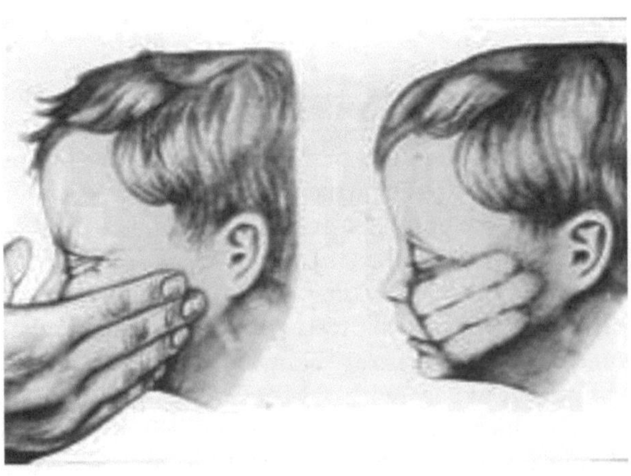

Figure 1.
Slap to the cheek.

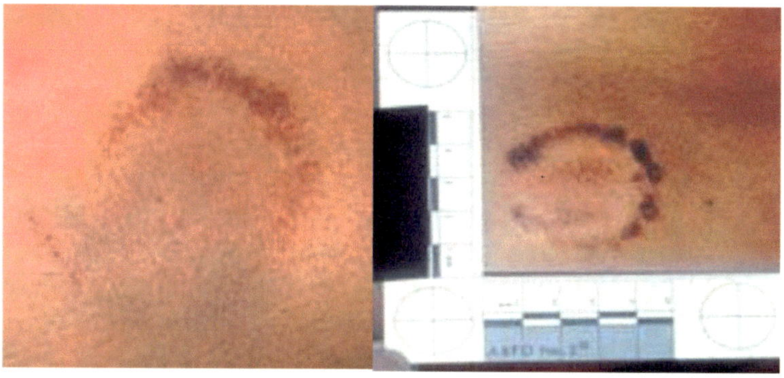

Figure 2.
Bite marks.

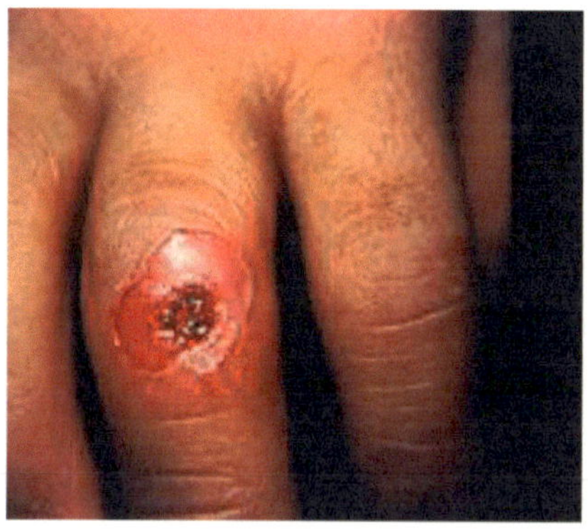

Figure 3.
Cigarette burn.

prone to sustain accidental injuries [21, 22]. These include the knees, elbows, shins, and forehead [22]. It should be noted that protected parts of the body such as the back, thighs, genital area, buttocks, backs of legs, and face, are more common as the sites of non-accidental injury which may constitute physical abuse [22].

3.2 At every dental visit, observe child patient for changes in behavior

It is very important to note that abused children are often scared to reach out for help and do not trust most people [12]. Their extended families and people who are in regular contact with them play a crucial role in identifying if there is abuse as they are the first point of reference to observe any behavioral changes [13, 23].

Individuals with whom the child comes into contact with regularly play an essential role in identifying probable abuse cases as they may be the first to become conscious of any noticeable fluctuations in behavior [23]. Any cautioning signs of potential abuse which are noted should be immediately and meticulously documented [13, 23].

There should be an awareness of how the pediatric patient respond to others. Abused children may act aggressively by showing inappropriate anger and loss of control, or they may be sullen, stoic or withdrawn [2, 5]. Psychological indicators include avoidance, fear, anxiety, low self-esteem, and depression as indicated in **Table 2**. These psychological indicators are usually clearly visible and the victim is highly withdrawn [23]. Behavioral indicators of abuse may also include: child not making eye contact, is wary of parents, demonstrates fear of touch or an intense fear of being examined, dramatic mood changes, withdrawal or aggressiveness, has a history of suicide attempts and running away [5, 13].

3.3 Testimonies

Testimonies to be observed include inconsistent explanations of how the trauma occurred. Careful attention needs to be paid to any strange behavior being displayed by caregivers and in these cases, this comes through with unconvincing accounts about how the child had been injured and sometimes no reasons being offered when asked about the visible injuries [24]. There can even be various justifications offered and upon closer inspection of the records, it may often be found that there is confirmation or a trail of proof of previous similar injuries. In addition, there would also often be substantial periods of delay or a long interval between the injury episode and the date at which the injured child is booked and brought in for assistance and treatment.

Descriptions of behavior that a suspected abuser may display includes the following [24]:

- Is dispassionate to the point of indifference about the state of the child, and will often be dismissive about the events leading up to the injury [11].
- Has a dominating spouse or partner, often male, who never wants the mother to be left unaccompanied with the examining clinician; and who directly responds to any queries directed at the mother of the injured child [11].
- Provides an overstated, self-justifying response to questioning [13], and often comes across as having an antagonistic or forceful attitude [13].
- Is an authoritative, uncompromising and dominating parent [24].
- Provides an ambiguous indistinct explanation whilst offering up sparse information relating to the specifics of the cause of the child's injury or injuries [24].
- Offers varying accounts of how the child got injured [24].
- Waits for a long interval after the injury episode before seeking dental or medical treatment for the child [25].
- Provides an account of events that fluctuates with time [25].
- For a mother bringing in a child with suspicious injuries, there may be the existence of a boyfriend who has moved in with the mother and child [26].

3.3.1 Assessment of associated risk factors

Clinicians should always ensure that a thorough history is taken for all children who are consulted. This must include all social, medical and psychological factors of the attending child patient. Clinicians must always take cognizance of the following points in order to assess a child holistically as these dynamics noted below are often the key risk factors which predispose a child to potential abuse or neglect:

- Households with a history of domestic abuse – this will not always be self-reported, however there will be anecdotal evidence that could be used parallel to the new information coming to light.

- Known or suspected parental substance misuse – the mouth will provide crucial markers to indicate substance abuse – which include staining and even localized soft tissue keratinization.

- Poor parental mental health – this may be self-reported but can also be gauged from testimonies given by these parents related to current circumstances.

- Parents with learning difficulties – this is also difficult to determine but the clinician should exhaust all sources and resources related to the case at hand in order to draw up as holistic a profile as possible.

- Children with disabilities – this will be visible or discernible by clinicians since they are usually monitoring the children during the routine dental visits.

- Families with history of child abuse – again this will not always be self-reported, however there will be anecdotal evidence that could be used parallel to the new information coming to light.

- Other risk factors include large burdens of stress that parents carry, lack of employment, low socio-economic status, living spaces that are congested with too many people and limited support structures.

3.4 Oro-facial trauma that may be indicative of abuse or neglect

Various reports indicate that injuries related to child abuse predominantly occur in the head and neck region, particularly the face [18, 27–29] as it is easily accessible and a psychologically important target area for abuse [18]. As school-age children commonly sustain accidental dental injuries [29], dental practitioners must have a heightened index of suspicion and practice vigilance in the examination of maxillofacial injuries in children to distinguish between abuse and non-abuse related injuries.

Physical abuse is more prevalent in younger males while sexual abuse is more common in younger females [18]. It is however important to also consider the possibility of outliers of these groups to ensure that no abused child is overlooked.

Dependent on the nature and the site of abuse, there may be a multitude of clinical manifestations of abuse that are encountered as described below. It is important to note that although these signs may alert the dental practitioner to the possibility of abuse, they should not be considered in isolation, but rather contextually [29].

3.4.1 Early childhood caries and neglect

Dental neglect is a subtype of physical neglect that is least likely to be considered during a dental consultation [30]. Dental neglect should be suspected in the presence of the following:

- Untreated early childhood caries that may be easily detected by a lay person [28];

- Untreated pain, infection, bleeding, or trauma affecting the orofacial region [28];

- A history of lack of continuity of care in the presence of identified dental morbidity [28].

Early childhood caries, although one of the main signs to neglect may be present as a of sequelae of environmental and social confounders such as drinking water, breast feeding habits, poor economic situations or unemployment of parents and lack of education [28, 31]. Furthermore, depending on the geographic region and socio-economic environment, early childhood caries may be commonly encountered in some parts of the world within the dental environment [31]. Untreated symptoms and a lack of continuity of care although considered to be negligent, may sometimes occur in the setting of caregivers who are unaware or unknowledgeable. This provides a challenge for the clinician who, whilst conducting a consultation and examination, must also deduce whether the failure of treatment is due to lack of knowledge, socio-economic difficulties such as access to health care and poverty, or is in fact due to a conscious failure to provide a child with adequate health care [14].

The presence of early childhood caries should therefore elicit a higher index of suspicion from the dental practitioner [28] followed up with a thorough investigation for external signs related to behavior, dressing and appearance; but also other intra-oral signs such as early childhood caries in the setting of untreated or chronic oro-facial pain, a high bleeding index and poor or no plaque control may alert neglect and where appropriate dental care has not been sought despite previous advice received [29]. Under these circumstances, the caries must be contextualized and suspicion for abuse interrogated.

3.4.2 Injury to the soft tissues of the mouth

The most common abusive injury to the mouth is to the lips resulting in laceration, bruising or swelling of the lips [32, 33]. Intraorally, bruising is the most common form of injury, with lacerations being the third most common [18].

3.4.2.1 Lacerations, bruises and contusions to the soft tissues of the mouth

Lacerations presenting in the oral cavity and related to physical and sexual abuse may present as tears, penetrating mucosal wounds, cuts through the mucosa and bite marks.

The location of the injury is often the clue and may assist a dental practitioner to distinguish suspicious cases of abuse from the mundane.

Lacerations of the mucosa in the vicinity of the commissure of the mouth could result from gagging with a rope or cloth [34], suggestive of injuries that are often related to forms of physical and sexual abuse. Lacerations to the tongue are also commonly reported [18]. Penetrating injuries to the vestibule, floor of the mouth and more common and less commonly the palate can occur with forcible insertion of objects such as feeding utensils or pacifiers in the mouths of young infants [35].

Laceration may also occur in the form of bite marks with recorded cases of adult bite marks on a child's tongue [36]. A bite mark pattern, generally appearing as a central area of hemorrhage found between markings of the upper and lower dental arches is suggestive of physical or sexual abuse. In the context of the head and neck region, these are rarely reported intraorally but commonly reported on the cheeks of abused children [37].

Lacerations to the upper labial frenum with a tear of the frenum from the inner aspect of the upper lip is an injury that is often quoted as an intraoral injury pathognomonic of abuse based on historical cases reported [13]. Whilst a torn frenum may result from forced feeding, gagging, violent rubbing or a direct blow, recent literature does not support a diagnosis of abuse from the presence of a torn labial frenum in isolation [29]. Contextualizing the situation to discern a suspected case of abuse from that of a non-abuse, such as in the case of a regular bump to the mouth or fall during the years that a child is learning to walk, is important. For instance, a frenal tear in a non-ambulatory neonate (< 1 year), or an older, more stable child (> 2 years) should raise one's suspicion as to the possibility of the injury being non-accidental [13] and to proceed with a full oral examination to screen for any further potential signs of abuse [32].

Intraoral contusions, ecchymoses and petechiae are commonly found in abuse cases. The location of the bruising, ecchymoses or petechiae may also allude to the presence and nature of abuse. An unexplained erythema, petechiae or ecchymoses at the junction of the hard and soft palate or elsewhere on the palatal mucosa potentially may be as a result of forced oral sex [14]. This bruising is usually non-ulcerated and may be a single lesion or be bilateral extending across the midline [38]. There have also been reports of ecchymoses on the alveolar mucosa in conjunction with avulsed teeth [33].

3.4.2.2 Burns

Burn injuries may be due to electrical, thermal and chemical sources and may represent any of the forms of abuse; being physical and sexual abuse as well as neglect [39]. Damage to the skin usually occurs in temperatures in excess of approximately 49°C and over a sufficient contact time, thereby resulting in mechanisms of cellular damage. It can be extrapolated, that due to the structure of oral mucosa, these burns may be easier to inflict on mucosal surfaces.

In general, injury sustained by burns can be scalds which are thermal contact burns from hot objects or fluids and flame burns. Burns may be inflicted by hot utensils or cigarettes as a sign of abuse and by hot food as a sign of neglect.

Electric burns from cables are also common injuries of infants but a dental practitioner should consider neglect if an electric burn is found in conjunction with any of the other signs mentioned in this chapter.

3.4.3 Injuries to the dentition

Injuries to the dentition related to physical abuse frequently present as fractured or avulsed teeth. This may be in setting of other soft tissue (lacerations, bruising) or hard tissue injuries (dento-alveolar fractures, skeletal fractures) or in isolation. Damage to the primary or permanent teeth can be due to blunt trauma [14, 33, 35]. Due to fractured or avulsed teeth commonly occurring with accidental injury in children, it is important to verify the explanation of the injury between the caregiver and the child, but also to look out for other signs such as other discolored teeth, inappropriately missing teeth and in the setting of any other sign of abuse [28].

3.4.4 Injuries to the facial bones

The dental practitioner is one who would be the first health professional to detect fractures, dislocations, avulsions or mobility related to teeth or within the jaws that are pathologic [28]. Furthermore, the mandible and maxilla can often show early, or previous fracture signs localized to the condyles, mandibular ascending ramus and mandibular symphysis which should alert to abuse [40]. It is important to screen for any previous fractures of teeth or the jaw bones and evidence of dental malocclusions as a result of a previous trauma.

3.4.5 Pathological lesions

The dental practitioner may be focused on diagnosing and managing the condition but may overlook the circumstance in which the condition occurs, and in turn overlook a lesion suggesting abuse.

Sexually transmitted infections in children are rare and their oral manifestation may suggest oro-genital contact and alert the practitioner to the suspicion of sexual abuse. Oral and peri-oral gonorrhea in children is pathognomonic of abuse [14] and may present as erythema, pharyngitis or itching but is often asymptomatic [40]. Gonococcal infection is more likely to be suspected and investigated in the setting of the more common manifestations of gonococcal infection such as those that are found in the urogenital or rectal region [40].

Whilst an HPV-induced infection of the oral cavity is transmitted through sexual contact, amongst children at pre-primary school, HPV spread may be due to close contact or sharing of utensils [41]. There are several oral lesions seen namely: Oral squamous cell papilloma, multifocal epithelial hyperplasia, verruca vulgaris and condyloma acuminatum are some of the oral lesions associated with HPV infection [41]. Condyloma acuminatum is spread via sexual contact and when it occurs in children, it alerts to possible sexual abuse [41]. Oral condylomas develop at the site of oro-genital sexual contact and are found commonly on the tongue, gingiva, soft palate and lips. Classically, the lesions present as broad based (sessile) exophytic masses with blunt projections [5, 41]. The other HPV-induced lesions listed above may not be as suggestive, however abuse should always be a consideration in their presence.

Manifestations of syphilis are less prevalent in abuse cases than other sexually transmitted infections such as gonorrhea and HPV-induced lesions, however, transmission of syphilis outside the neonatal period is almost always due to sexual abuse [41]. Syphilis in children manifests the same as it does in adults with presentations in three different phases [41]. The dental practitioner should thus be sensitive to lesions such as syphilitic chancres, mucous patches and condylomata lata that may indicate abuse [42].

3.5 Documentation and record keeping

Dental professionals should ensure that they document and make notes in patients' files on any deviations from the norm. Detailed information should be recorded in the dental file along with images and x-rays of the injuries [27, 43]. Information gathered in the dental record should include the time and date of the dental data i.e. radiographs and photographs [43]. In order to gauge size for records, a measurement scale ruler should be placed alongside an injury or bite mark when taking photographs [43]. In order to prevent distortion and give a more precise representation of the actual size of the injury, the camera lens should be held directly over the bite and perpendicular to the plane of the bite mark [20, 27]. The site, appearance, phase of healing and severity of the injury should be accurately and comprehensively recorded [13, 19, 20]. Each entry should be dated and signed. Diagrams for recording purposes are also useful [19]. It is important that handwriting on written documents is legible and that no abbreviations are used [19]. Wherever possible, information collated should be in the child, guardian or parent's own words [19].

Finally, it is imperative that consent should be acquired prior to collecting dental records and taking photographs. The pediatric patient has the right to exercise their voluntary participation and refuse photographs be taken and this refusal should be respected [19, 43]. The important factor to be noted is that such a refusal should be documented in the pediatric patient's file [19, 43].

In terms of appropriate referrals – this should be immediately done for the management of any injuries or lesions that are outside the scope of the consulting dental practitioner [21]. If child abuse is suspected, referrals should be made before discussing the issue of abuse with the parents. Making referrals after a discussion with parents or caregivers may negatively impact the treatment that the child receives as parents or caregivers may feel threatened [21]. Physicians and dental practitioners are obligated to detect cases of maltreatment or neglect, to meticulously and comprehensively document, to refer for appropriate treatment and to notify the relevant authorities as soon as possible [44].

4. Conclusion

Assessing a child for maltreatment should constitute an integral part of any clinical examination executed. Although many wounds are not caused by mistreatment, oral health professionals should always be alert during cases of traumatic injuries [5, 10, 44]. Due to the regularity of care offered, dental professionals are in an exclusive position to be able to monitor the caregiver-child relationship as well as fluctuations in the child's behavior [2]. Early warning signs include parents or caregivers bringing a child to the dental professional to have mobile or cracked teeth treated, but not seeking treatment from a medical doctor for other types of injuries [44].

It is also crucial to bear in mind that injuries can occur at any time to anybody for perfectly blameless reasons, and this is particularly the case for children of all ages who enjoy playing outdoors and engaging in sport activities. Certain sites on the body are also more prone to accidental injury. These include the knees, shins, elbows and forehead. However, sheltered body regions such as the thighs, genitals, buttocks, back, backs of legs, and face, are more common as the sites of non-accidental injuries [43].

It is for these very reasons that it is always best to ask a child or caregiver how the injuries were acquired, or how they are feeling, if there is a suspicion that abuse could be occurring. Dental professionals should therefore use their own initiatives and all the other information available to reach a conclusion about whether or not there is cause for concern.

Similarly, the presence of a single sign does not prove that child maltreatment or abuse is occurring in a household, but a closer look at all details may be necessary when these signs appear repeatedly or in combination with other signs described above. If a dental professional does indeed suspect that a child is being harmed, reporting these suspicions swiftly may safeguard the child and acquire assistance for the household. In these cases, dental professionals are urged to contact their local child welfare society and law enforcers for help in this regard and the process forward.

Author details

Aneesa Moolla[1,2*], Tshakane Ralephenya[1], Sizakele Ngwenya[3] and Sankeshan Padayachee[4]

1 Department of Oral Health, School of Oral Health Sciences, University of the Witwatersrand, South Africa

2 Faculty of Health Sciences, Department of Internal Medicine, School of Clinical Medicine, Health Economics and Epidemiology Research Office, University of the Witwatersrand, Johannesburg, South Africa

3 Department of Oral Pathology, School of Oral Health Sciences, Faculty of Health Sciences, University of Witwatersrand, South Africa

4 Department of Oral Medicine and Periodontology, School of Oral Health Sciences, University of the Witwatersrand, South Africa

*Address all correspondence to: amoolla@heroza.org

IntechOpen

References

[1] US Department of Health and Human Services, Administration for Children and Families, Administration on Children, Youth and Families, Children's Bureau. Child Maltreatment [Internet]. 2019. Available from: https://www.acf.hhs.gov/cb/research-data-technology/statistics-research/child-maltreatment [Accessed November 04, 2021]

[2] Shanel-Hogan KA, Roth JR, Balin M. A health issue that affects us all. Journal of the California Dental Association. 2004;**32**:297-298

[3] WHO. Child maltreatment factsheet statistics [Internet]. 2020. Available from: https://www.who.int/news-room/fact-sheets/detail/child-maltreatment [Accessed November 1, 2021]

[4] Hillis S, Mercy J, Amobi A, Kress H. Global prevalence of past-year violence against children: A systematic review and minimum estimates. Pediatrics. 2016;**137**(3):e20154079

[5] Wilkins EM. Clinical practice of the dental hygienist. 11th ed. Lippincott Williams and Williams: Philadelphia; 2017

[6] van As AB, Diederics R, Wallis LA, Naidoo S, Schaaf HS. Child abuse. In: van As S, Naidoo S, editors. Paediatric Trauma and Child Abuse. Oxford University Press Southern Africa (Pty) Ltd; 2006. pp. 45-63

[7] Cagetti M, Marcoli PA, Berengo M, et al. Italian guidelines for the prevention and management of dental trauma in children. Italian Journal of Pediatrics. 2019;**45**:157. DOI: 10.1186/s13052-019-0734-7

[8] Kellogg N, the Committee on Child Abuse and Neglect. Oral and dental aspects of child abuse and neglect. Pediatrics. 2005;**116**:6

[9] Children's Act 38 of 2005 [Internet]. Available from: http://www.justice.gov.za/legislation/acts/2005-038%20childrensact.pdf [Accessed December 12, 2020]

[10] Department of Social Development. The Children's Act explained. Booklet 3: The Courts and the Protection of Children [Internet]. Available from: http://www.dsd.gov.za/index2.php?option=com_docman&task=doc_view&gid=111&1temid=3 [Accessed December 10, 2020]

[11] Legano L, MT MH, Palusci VJ. Child abuse and neglect. Current Problems in Pediatric and Adolescent Health Care. 2009;**39**:31.e1-31.26

[12] Tsang A, Sweet D. Detecting child abuse and neglect-are dentists doing enough? Journal of the Canadian Dental Association. 1999;**65**:387-391

[13] Needleman HL. Orofacial trauma in child abuse: Types, prevalence, management, and the dental profession's involvement. Pediatric Dentistry. 1986;**8**(1):71-80

[14] Fisher-Owens SA, Lukefahr JL, Tate AR, American Academy of Pediatric Dentistry, Council on Clinical Affairs, Council on Scientific Affairs, Ad Hoc Work Group on Child Abuse and Neglect, American Academy of Pediatrics, Section on Oral Health Committee on Child Abuse and Neglect. Oral and dental aspects of child abuse and neglect. Pediatric Dentistry. 2017;**39**(4):278-283

[15] American Academy of Pediatric Dentistry. Definition of dental neglect [Internet]. 2010. Available from: http://www.aapd.org/media/Policies_Guidelines/D_DentalNeglect.pdf [Accessed December 10, 2020]

[16] Hock RS, Bryce CP, Waber DP, et al. Relationship between infant

malnutrition and childhood maltreatment in a Barbados lifespan cohort. Vulnerable Child Youth Studies. 2017;**12**(4):304-313. DOI: 10.1080/17450128.2017.1371817

[17] Committee on Child Maltreatment Research, Policy, and Practice for the Next Decade: Phase II; Board on Children, Youth, and Families; Committee on Law and Justice; Institute of Medicine; National Research Council. 4, Consequences of Child Abuse and Neglect. In: Petersen AC, Joseph J, Feit M, editors. New directions in child abuse and neglect research. Washington (DC): National Academies Press (US); 2014

[18] Naidoo S. A profile of the oro-facial injuries in child physical abuse at a children's hospital. Child Abuse & Neglect. 2000;**24**(4):521-534

[19] Maguire S, Mann MK, Sibert J, Kemp A. Are there patterns of bruising in childhood which are diagnostic or suggestive of abuse? A systematic review. Archives of Disease in Childhood. 2005;**90**:182-186

[20] American Academy of Pediatric Dentistry. Guideline on oral and dental aspects of child abuse and neglect. Clinical Guidelines. 2010-2011;**32**(6): 137-140

[21] Faller-Marquardt M, Pollack S, Schmidt U. Cigarette burns in forensic medicine. Forensic Science International. 2008;**176**:200-208

[22] Foster M. Noticing the signs of child abuse in dental patients. BDJ Team. 2018;**5**:18133. DOI: 10.1038/bdjteam.2018.133

[23] Sujatha G, Sivakumar G, Saraswathi TR. Role of the dentist in discrimination of abuse from accident. Journal of Forensic Dental Sciences. 2010;**2**(1):2-4

[24] Mohamed N, Naidoo S. A review of child abuse and the role of the dental team in South Africa. The Journal of the Dental Association of South Africa = Die Tydskrif van die Tandheelkundige Vereniging van Suid-Afrika. 2014;**69**:250-256

[25] Finger LM, van As S. Nursing care. In: van As S., Naidoo S. Paediatric Trauma and Child Abuse. Oxford University Press Southern Africa (Pty) Ltd, 2006; 40-44

[26] Schnitzer PG, Ewigman BG. Child deaths resulting from inflicted injuries: Household risk factors and perpetrator characteristics. Pediatrics. 2005;**116**:e687-e693

[27] Cairns AM, Mok JYQ, Welbury RR. Injuries to the head, face, mouth and neck in physically abused children in a community setting. International Journal of Paediatric Dentistry. 2005;**15**:310-318. DOI: 10.1111/j.1365-263X.2005.00661.x

[28] Baptista S, Laranjo E, Norton A, Andrade D, Areias C, Macedo A. Dental Neglect, one type of child abuse – Narrative review. Medical Express. 2017;**4**(3)

[29] Maguire S, Hunter B, Hunter L, et al. Diagnosing abuse: A systematic review of torn frenum and other intra-oral injuries [published correction appears in Arch Dis Child. 2008 May;93(5):453]. Archives of Disease in Childhood. 2007;**92**(12):1113-1117. DOI: 10.1136/adc.2006.113001

[30] Jessee SA. Risk factors as determinants of dental neglect in children. ASDC Journal of Dentistry for Children. 1998;**65**(1):17-20

[31] Postma TC, Ayo-Yusuf OA, van Wyk PJ. Socio-demographic correlates of early childhood caries prevalence and severity in a developing country - South Africa. International Dental Journal. 2008;**58**(2):91-97. DOI: 10.1111/j.1875-595x.2008.tb00182.x

[32] Welbury R. Torn labial frenum in isolation not pathognomonic of physical abuse. Evidence-Based Dentistry. 2007;**8**:71. DOI: 10.1038/sj.ebd.6400505

[33] Phillips VM, van Der Heyde Y. Oro-facial trauma in child abuse fatalities. South African Medical Journal. 2006;**96**(3):213-215

[34] Mathur S, Chopra R. Combating child abuse: The role of a dentist. Oral Health & Preventive Dentistry. 2013;**11**(3):243-250. DOI: 10.3290/j.ohpd.a29357

[35] British Dental Association (BDA). Physical abuse [Internet]. 2020. Available from: https://bda.org/childprotection/Recognising/Pages/Physical.aspx [Accessed December 12, 2020]

[36] Child Protection Evidence Systematic review on Oral Injuries. The Royal College of Paediatrics and Child Health (RCPCH) [Internet]. 2014. Available from: https://childprotection.rcpch.ac.uk/child-protection-evidence/oral-injuries-systematic-review/ [Accessed December 12, 2020]

[37] Jonson J, Wright F. Child Maltreatment: The Role of a Dental Professional [Internet]. Available from: https://www.dentalcare.com/en-us/professional-education/ce-courses/ce599/physical-abuse2020 [Accessed December 12, 2020]

[38] Arora R, Hartwig E, Kannikeswaran N. Oral lesion secondary to child abuse. Journal of Emergency Medicine. 2013;**45**(4):e139-e140. DOI: 10.1016/j.jemermed.2013.04.030

[39] Toon MH, Maybauer DM, Arceneaux LL, et al. Children with burn injuries--assessment of trauma, neglect, violence and abuse. Journal of Injury and Violence Research. 2011;**3**(2): 98-110. DOI: 10.5249/jivr.v3i2.91

[40] Little JW. Gonorrhea: Update. Oral Surgery, Oral Medicine, Oral Pathology, Oral Radiology, and Endodontology. 2006;**101**(2):137-143. DOI: 10.1016/j.tripleo.2005.05.077

[41] Prabhu SR, Wilson DF. Human papillomavirus and oral disease - emerging evidence: A review. Australian Dental Journal. 2013;**29**(1):2-10. DOI: 10.1111/adj.12020

[42] Rawstron SA, Bromberg K, Hammerschlag MR. STD in children: Syphilis and gonorrhoea. Genitourinary Medicine. 1993;**69**(1):66-75. DOI: 10.1136/sti.69.1.66

[43] Wakefield Safeguarding Children Partnership [Internet]. Available from: https://www.wakefieldscp.org.uk/getfile/wakefield-signs-indicators-primary-2+&cd=10&hl=en&ct=clnk&gl=za Accessed December 10, 2020

[44] Bower C. The role of non-medics in child abuse. In: van As S, Naidoo S, editors. Paediatric Trauma and Child Abuse. Oxford University Press Southern Africa (Pty) Ltd, 2006;69-78

Section 4

Statistics in Dentistry

Chapter 11

Probability and Sampling in Dentistry

Yasser Riaz Malik, Muhammad Saad Sheikh and Shakeela Yousaf

Abstract

Probability and sampling in dentistry are two fundamentals which have great importance in clinical research. Many research works in dentistry shows lack of proper understanding and use of these two factors. The definition of probability is incredibly significant in daily life. Statistical analysis is based on this particularly useful definition. In fact, the function of probability in modern science is that of substituting for certainty. Probabilities are numbers that represent the probability that a specific occurrence will occur. We learn about the odds of many daily cases, ranging from weather predictions (probability of rain or snow) to lotteries (probability of winning a major jackpot). In biostatistical applications, probability theory underlies the statistical inference. Statistical inference means drawing generalizations or inferences on unknown population parameters. After selecting a sample from the population of interest, we calculate the characteristics under analysis, summarize the characteristics in our sample, and then draw inferences about the population based on what we find in the sample. Population and sampling are two critical aspects of study design. The population is a group of individuals who share common relations. A sample is a population subset. The size of the sample is the number of individuals in the sample. The more representative the sample of the population, the surer the researcher can be about the validity of the data. In this module, we will explore sampling methods, basic principles of probability, and applications of probability theory. The definition of probability is introduced, and the function of probability distributions is discussed in the statistical theory, with reference to the normal distribution and its characteristics. Sampling and sampling variations are defined, along with the sampling error, the standard error of the mean and the confidence intervals for determining the likely magnitude of the population mean. Medical study typically includes patients with an illness or disorder. The generalization of clinical research results is focused on several factors linked to the internal and external validity of the research methods. The sampling process is the key methodological problem that affects the generalizability of clinical research results. In this educational article, we also clarify the various methods of sampling in clinical research.

Keywords: probability, sampling, dentistry, restorative, statistical analysis, clinical research, biostatistics, confidence interval, standard error, probability, non-probability, normal distribution, sampling errors, sampling types, probability distribution

1. Introduction

The theory of probability was developed in the 17th century. It has got its origin from game of poker after a dispute. It led two famous French mathematicians, Blaise Pascal and Pierre de Fermat to create a theory of probability. Antoine Gombaud, Chevalier de Méré, a French nobleman with an interest in gaming and gambling questions, called Pascal's attention to an apparent contradiction concerning a popular dice game. The game consisted of tossing a pair of dice 24 times; the issue was determining whether to bet even money on the occurrence of at least one "double six" during the 24 spins. A seemingly well-established gambling law led de Méré to conclude that betting on a double six in 24 spins would be profitable, but the reverse was implied by his own estimates. Based on questions posed by de Méré, Pascal began to correspond with his friend Pierre Fermat about these problems, in which the basic concepts of probability theory were drawn for the first time. While a few special gambling problems had been resolved by some Italian mathematicians in the 15th and 16th centuries, no general theory had been developed before this famous correspondence. The Dutch scientist Christian Huygens, Leibniz's teacher, heard of this correspondence and shortly afterward (1657) wrote the first book on probability, De Ratiociniis in Ludo Aleae, a treatise on gambling-related problems. Thanks to the innate appeal of gambling, probability theory soon became popular and the subject developed swiftly in the 18th century. The key contributors to this time were Jakob Bernoulli (1654–1705) and de Moivre (1667–1754).

In 1812, Pierre de Laplace (1749–1827) applied several new theories and mathematical methods to his book, Théorie Analytique des Probabilités. Prior to Laplace, the theory of probability was concerned primarily with the development of a statistical study of gambling. Laplace has applied probabilistic principles to a variety of theoretical and practical problems. The theory of errors, actuarial mathematics, and statistical mechanics are examples of some of the main applications of probability theory that have been developed. Gornband took an initiation and an interest in this area in 1954. After him, many statistical authors have tried to reshape the idea of the former. The quest for a generally accepted meaning lasted almost three centuries and was marked by a great deal of controversy. The problem was eventually addressed in the 20th century by approaching probability theory on an axiomatic basis, by a Russian mathematician A. Kolmogorov [1].

2. Objective

This module would discuss the techniques of sampling, the fundamental concepts of probability, and the applications of probability theory. The role played by probability in modern science is that of a substitute for certainty, therefore definition of the probability is added, and the function of the probability distribution is discussed in the statistical theory, with reference to the normal distribution and its characteristics. Normal distribution is of great value in evaluation and research in both psychology and education, because it helps us to predict that where cases will fall within a distribution probabilistically. Variations of sampling and sampling types will be explained, along with the error of sampling, the standard error of the mean and the confidence intervals for determining the likely magnitude of the population mean. Generally, sampling allows researchers to obtain enough data to answer the research question(s) without having to query the entire population - saving time and money. For this reason the major types of probability sampling methods and their characteristics would be addressed.

3. Probability

"Probability" has become one of the key methods for statistics in dentistry. Often statistical analysis is paralyzed without theory of probability [2].

The probability of an event is its chance of occurrence, measured on a scale from 0 (never occurs) to 1 (always occurring). There are two views we may take of probability. One is that it is the long-term frequency of an event, e.g., in a long series of coin tosses, heads should occur about half of the time, so we write P (Head) = 0.5. The second and broader, view is that probability is a subjective measure of our belief in the chances of an event occurring, e.g., "I believe that there is a 30% chance of a practical AIDS vaccine by the year 2025". Here, because the event can only occur once, there is no sensible long-term relative frequency view, but such subjective probabilities are useful when making decisions, e.g. planning future medical facilities. Of course, such subjective probabilities are most likely to be accurate when based on good long-term relative frequency information [3]. Predictions are taking the form of probabilities. We use probabilities to predict the likelihood of an earthquake, rain, or whether you are going to get an A in exams. Dentists use percentages to assess the risk of appliance that may trigger gum disease to use alternates. The investment schemes use the probability to determine the rate of return on the investment of the client. You could use the chance to decide whether to purchase a profitable commercial land. In your analysis of statistics, you will use the power of mathematics through probability calculations to evaluate and interpret your results [4].

4. Probability distributions

A probability distribution is a function that describes the probability of obtaining the possible values that a random variable may assume. In other words, the variable values differ depending on the distribution of the underlying probability. In Statistics, the probability distribution gives the possibility of each outcome of a random experiment or occurrences [5].

Suppose you take a random sample and measure the weight of the subjects. You will establish a distribution of weights when you calculate weights. This form of distribution is useful when you need to know the outcomes are most likely to occur, the spread of possible values, and the probability of various outcomes [6].

The probability distributions suggest the probability of an occurrence or result. Statistics use the following notation to define the probabilities:

$$P(X) = \text{the probability that the random variable will have a particular value of } X.$$

A probability model needs a measure of the probability, typically written to P. This probability measure must allocate a probability to each case A, a probability P(A).

We require the following properties:

1. P(X) is always a nonnegative real number, between 0 and 1 inclusive.

2. P (Ø) = 0, i.e., if X is the empty set Ø, then P(X) = 0.

3. P(S) = 1, i.e., if X is the entire sample space S, then P(X) = 1.

4. P is (countably) additive, meaning that if X1, X2,... is a finite or countable sequence of disjoint events, then P(X1 ∪ X2 ∪⋯) = P(X1) + P(X2) + ——.

The sum of all probabilities for all potential values must be equal to 1. In addition, the likelihood for a particular value or set of values must be between 0 and 1 [7].

The probability distributions define the dispersion of random variable values. Consequently, the type of variable determines the type of distribution of the likelihood [8]. For a single random variable, the statisticians split the distributions into the following two types:

- Discrete probability distribution
- Normal/Continuous distribution

4.1 Discrete probability distribution

A discreet distribution of probability is made up of discrete variables. Specifically, if a random variable is discreet, the probability distribution would be discreet. For a discrete probability distribution, each potential value of a discrete random variable can be correlated with a non-zero probability [9, 10]. Therefore, a discrete probability distribution is also provided in tabular form.

The following example shows that the probability (relative frequency) of someone randomly chosen from the operating theater staff being a non-smoker is 0.45 (**Table 1**).

Note that in the right column, the frequencies (counts) have been turned into relative frequencies (percentage). How you do this:

1. Count the total number of items. In this chart the total is 60.
2. Divide the count (the frequency) by the total number. For example, 27/ 60 = 0.45 or 17/ 60 = 0.28

4.2 Types of discrete distribution

According to the properties of data, there are other types of discrete probability distributions to display different kinds of data.

a. Binomial distribution to model binary data.

b. Poisson distribution to model count data.

4.2.1 Binomial distribution

The binomial distribution is a probability distribution that summarizes the probability that a value will take one of two impartial values under a given set of parameters or assumptions [11].

Smoking habit	Frequency	Relative frequency (%)
Non-Smoker	27	45
Ex-Smoker	17	28
Current smoker	16	27
Total	**60**	**100**

Table 1.
Smoking habit of maxillofacial surgery theater staff.

Consider a dichotomous variable, where the outcome for everyone is one of two types (A or B).

1. Sex at birth: M or F.

2. Disease status: diseased or not diseased.

3. Drug response: responded or did not respond.

4. Comparison of two treatments.

4.2.2 Poisson distribution

The Poisson distribution is another discrete distribution, i.e. it applies to a discrete variable. But unlike the binomial there is no strict upper limit to the possible values of the variable. The variable is the count of several independent events that occur randomly in a fixed interval or time or space [12, 13].

1. The number of radioactive emissions from a given source in a given time.

2. The number of particles in a given volume of fluid, samples from a well-mixed bulk quantity.

3. The number of cases of a particular disease that a doctor sees in a week.

4. The number of still births occurring in a hospital per month.

5. Normal distribution

Continuous probability functions are also known as probability density functions or *conjugate prior* [14]. We know that we have a continuous distribution if the variable can assume an infinite number of values between any two values. Continuous variables are often measurements on a scale, such as height, weight, and temperature. Unlike discrete probability distributions where each value has a non-zero likelihood, specific values in continuous distributions have a zero probability. For example, the likelihood of measuring a temperature that is exactly 28 degrees is zero [15, 16].

Just as there are different types of discrete distributions for different kinds of discrete data, there are different distributions for continuous data. Each probability distribution has parameters that determine the shape of the distribution. Most distributions have between 1 and 3 parameters [17]. Specifying these parameters sets out the structure of the distribution and all its probabilities entirely. These parameters reflect the fundamental characteristics of the distribution, such as the central tendency and the variability [18].

The most common is normal distribution which is often also referred to as the Gaussian distribution [19]. The normal distribution has two main features:

- It is symmetrical about its mean.

- It is bell shaped.

The normal distribution is the most important distribution in statistics. One reason is that many continuous variables, such as height, seems to have this distribution

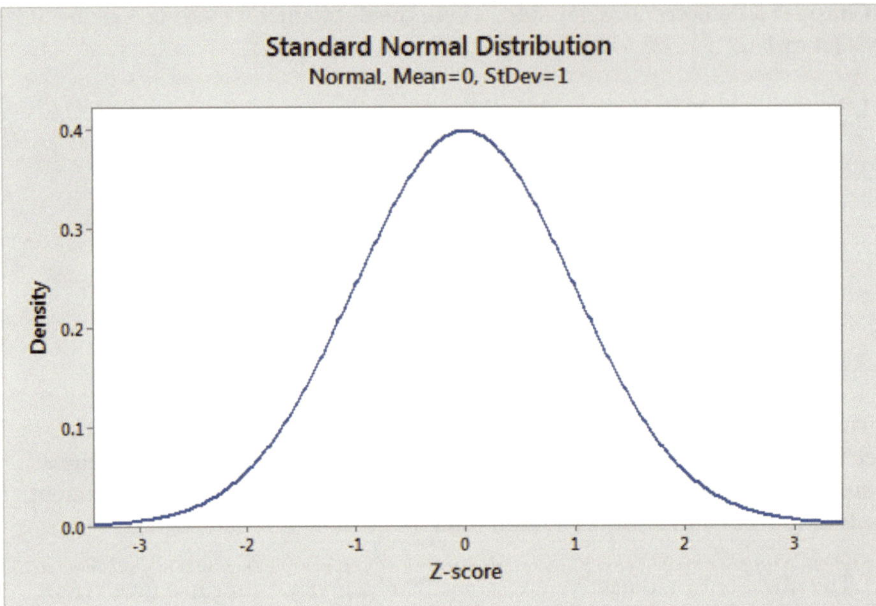

Figure 1.
The standard Normal distribution (source: https://statisticsbyjim.com/basics/normal-distribution).

[20]. But the main reason is because of what is known as the central limit theorem. This theorem states that if a random sample is taken from any distribution then the distribution of the sample mean x will be approximately Normal. The approximation becomes better as n gets larger [21]. The implication of this result is that inferences, from sample to population, can be based on the Normal distribution [22].

A Normal distribution may be summarized by its mean u and variance σ^2. It is often necessary to be able to find the areas under specified parts, particularly the tails, of Normal distribution curve.

This can be done by referring to published tables, which are given in most statistical texts. In order to use these tables, it is necessary to standardize the variable x. This can be done by calculating a standardized Normal deviate z by the formula (**Figure 1**) [23]:

$$Z = (X - \mu)/\sigma \text{ (Standardized Normal Deviate SND)} \tag{1}$$

(where Z is the value on the standard normal distribution, X is the value on the original distribution, μ is the mean of the original distribution, and σ is the standard deviation of the original distribution.)

The standard score is the number of standard deviations above or below the mean where a given observation falls. For example, a standard score of 1.5 means that the observation is 1.5 standard deviations above the average. On the other hand, the negative score is below the average. The mean is a Z-score of 0.

6. Sampling

A population in any collection of individuals in which we may be interested, e.g. all people in Saudi Arabia, all females in Hail Region, all diabetic children in Sydney Hail City under 12 years of age. Usually the population is too large for us to examine every individual, so we take a *sample* from the population. If the sample is **representative** of the population, we can then make *inferences* about the population from the sample.

For example, in a study of the incidence of schistosomiasis in a particular region, the population would be all adults living in the region and might consist of many thousands of individuals. The sample might be a few hundred people from the total population, and we wish to be able to generalize from the sample to the population [24]. The advantage of studying just a sample is a saving of labour and costs. The disadvantage of a sample is that precision is lost by not observing the complete population. The sample mean is unlikely to equal exactly the population mean; that is, the sample estimate will have some error [25].

It is useful to distinguish two kinds of error: sampling errors and non-sampling errors.

7. Sampling errors

Sampling errors are statistical errors, they arise because only a fraction of population has been observed. Different samples will give different results. Sampling errors become less important as the sample size increases [26].

$$\text{Sampling Error} = Z\,x\,\left(\sigma/\sqrt{n}\right) \tag{2}$$

(sampling Error is calculated by dividing the standard deviation of the population by the square root of the size of sample and then multiplying the resultant with the Z score value which is based on confidence interval).

Step by Step Calculation of Sampling Error:

Collected all the data set called the population. Calculate population mean and population standard deviation.

↓

Now, it is important to decide the size of the sample, and further, the size of the sample must be less than the population, and it should not be larger.

↓

Determine the confidence level and, as a result, the value of the Z score can be calculated from its table.

↓

Now multiply the Z score by the population standard deviation and divide the same by the square root of the sample size in order to arrive at an error margin or an error in the sample size.

8. Non-sampling errors

They arise if the sampling procedure is not representative of the total population. Such errors do not necessarily decrease as sample size increases. Examples of this type of error are the failure to include people with no permanent home because their existence is not recorded, or the refusal of some individuals to participate in the study. These errors constitute *bias* [27].

9. Types of sampling methods

Methods of sampling are as follows:

9.1 Probability sampling

Probability Sampling is a method in which each member of the population has the same chance of being part of the sample. Probability or random sampling is the most impartial but can be the most expensive sample in terms of time and energy for a given amount of sampling error [28].

9.2 Simple random sampling

A simple random sample means that each case in the population has the same probability of being included in the sample. This approach is the most straightforward of all probability sampling methods, because it includes only a single random sample and requires no specialized knowledge of the population. Since randomization is used, any research conducted on this sample should have a high internal and external validity.

Simple random sampling can be difficult to implement in practice. There are some prerequisites for using this method:

I. If chosen, you can contact or access each member of the population.

II. You have the time and resources to collect the data from the appropriate sample size.

III. Standard errors of estimators may be high and a complete framework (a list of all units in the whole population) is needed [29].

Simple random sampling works best if you have a lot of time and resources to carry out your study, or if you are studying a limited population that can be easily sampled (**Figure 2**).

9.3 Stratified sampling

Stratified sampling is where the population is divided into sub-groups and a random sample is collected from each sub-group.

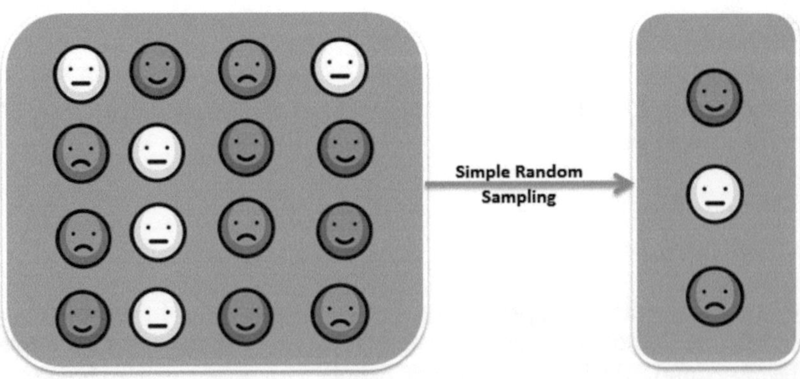

Figure 2.
Simple random sampling (source: https://www.datasciencemadesimple.com/simple-random-sampling-in-sas/).

(Stratified sampling formula)

$$\text{Stratified random sampling} = \text{Total Sample size/Entire population} \times \text{Population of subgroups.}$$

Mostly used when the population is heterogeneous and includes a variety of different classes, some of which are related to the subject of the analysis. The advantage of stratified sampling that it ensures a high degree of representativeness of all strata or strata in the population. Disadvantage is that it increases the work for planning and analysis for keeping the uncertainty within an acceptable level (**Figure 3**) [30].

9.4 Cluster sampling

Cluster sampling is where the entire population is divided into clusters or groups. Subsequently, a random sample of these clusters is taken, all of which are used in the final sample [31, 32].

It is simple and convenient, but the downside is that the members of the groups can be different from each other, decreasing the efficiency of the techniques (**Figure 4**).

9.5 Systematic sampling

Systematic sampling is the selection of a sample on an orderly basis. To build a sample, look at the target population and choose every fifth, tenth, or twentieth name, based on the size of the sample.

Systematic sampling can be used by statisticians if they want to save time or are disappointed with the results obtained from a simple random sampling process. If a fixed starting point has been established, the statisticians choose a constant interval to encourage the selection of the participant.

It ensures a high degree of representativeness, and no need to use a table of random numbers. Disadvantage is that it is Less random than simple random sampling (**Figure 5**) [33].

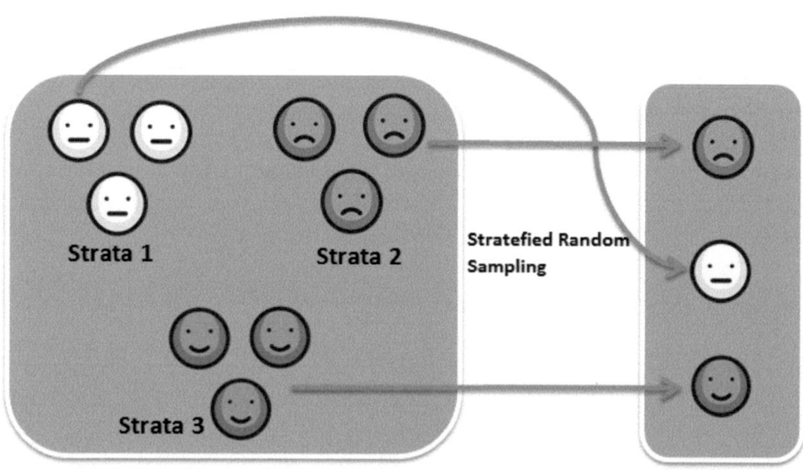

Figure 3.
Stratified sampling–(source: https://www.datasciencemadesimple.com/stratified-sampling-in-sas/).

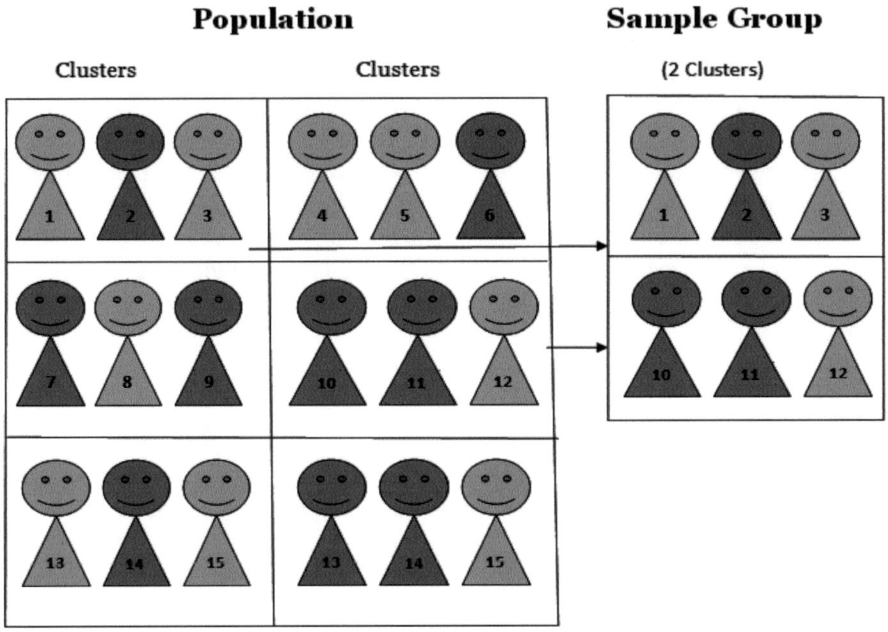

Figure 4.
Cluster sampling (source: https://research-methodology.net/sampling-in-primary-data-collection/cluster-sampling/).

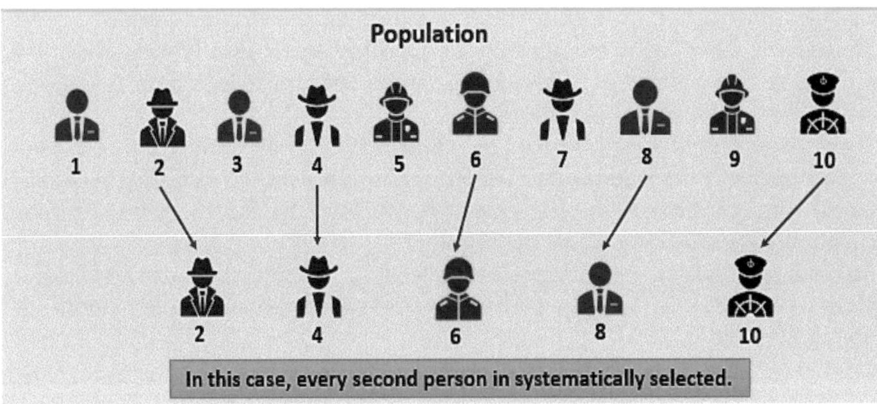

Figure 5.
Systematic sampling (source: https://www.wallstreetmojo.com/systematic-sampling/).

9.6 Non-probability sampling

Non-probability Sampling is a process in which each member of the population has no fair chance of being chosen. If the researcher chooses to choose participants selectively, non-probability sampling shall be considered [34].

9.7 Quota sampling

Quota sampling is a non-random sampling method in which participants are selected based on predetermined characteristics such that the total sample will have the same distribution of characteristics as the larger population. Selection of participants who meet certain characteristics, such as gender, age, fitness, etc. Scientists will also go back over the preferred sample population to guarantee that subgroups are represented to the same degree as those in the wider population.

There are several drawbacks to quota sampling since a subgroup's meanings are usually limited to a few characteristics. Other characteristics associated with the population could also become over-expressed (**Figure 6**) [35].

9.8 Purposive sampling

Pre-selected research hypotheses criteria are used to classify research subjects, such as a lung cancer study for individuals having repeated exposure to asbestos. That is where the researcher includes cases or participants in the study because they think they should be included. The purposive sampling approach may prove to be successful when only a limited number of people can serve as primary data sources due to the nature of the research design and objectives.

Purposive sampling is one of the most cost-effective and time-effective sampling methods available. The disadvantages of purposive sampling are vulnerability of errors of judgment by the researcher, poor level of reliability and high degree of bias and inability to generalize the results of study (**Figure 7**) [36].

9.9 Snowball sampling

Participants in the study are referred to the researcher by other individuals who match the characteristics needed for the study. This method is most applicable to

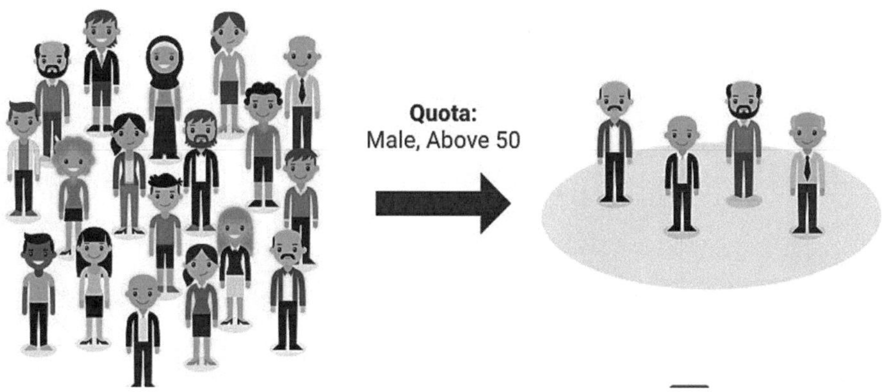

Figure 6.
Quota sampling (source: https://deepai.org/machine-learning-glossary-and-terms/quota-sample).

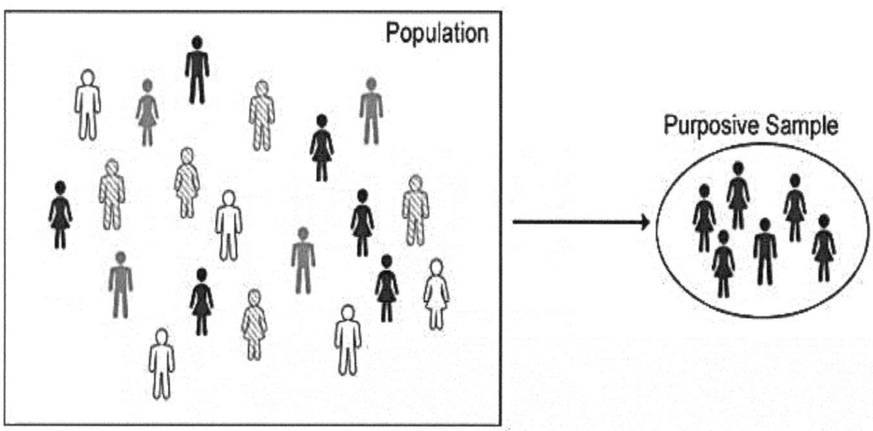

Figure 7.
Purposive sampling (source: https://research-methodology.net/sampling-in-primary-data-collection/purposive-sampling/).

small communities that are difficult to reach dur to cultural professional or other reasons.

Snowball sampling is also sometimes referred to as chain-referral sampling. Snowball sampling is low-cost and easy to implement. Snowball sampling is low-cost and easy to implement. It does not require a research team to hire recruiters for the study since the initial subjects act as the recruiters who bring in additional subjects. The disadvantage is that sampling bias can occur because, when initial subjects recruit additional subjects, it is possible that several subjects may share similar characteristics or characteristics that may not be representative of the broader population under research (**Figure 8**) [37].

9.10 Convenience sampling

Convenience sampling appears to be a favorite sampling technique among students, as it is cheap and simple compared to other sampling techniques. It is collection of participants since they are often readily and conveniently available.

Convenience sampling is not the preferred form of sampling for successful research as samples are taken from a particular segment of the population, so the degree of generalizability is questionable (**Figure 9**) [38].

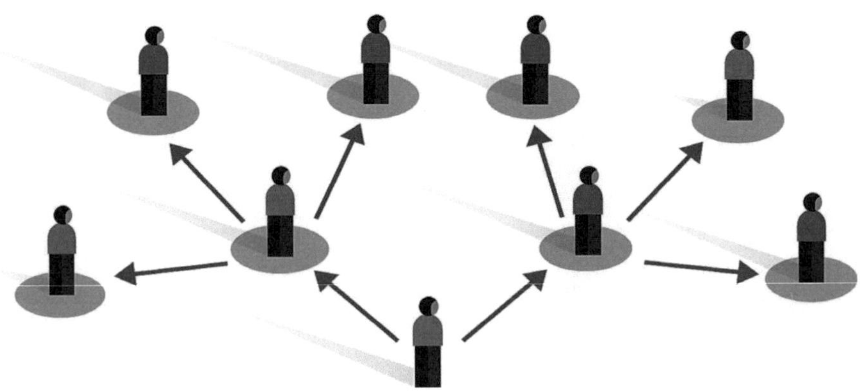

Figure 8.
Snowball sampling (source: https://cuttingedgepr.com/find-mobilize-unofficial-opinion-leaders/).

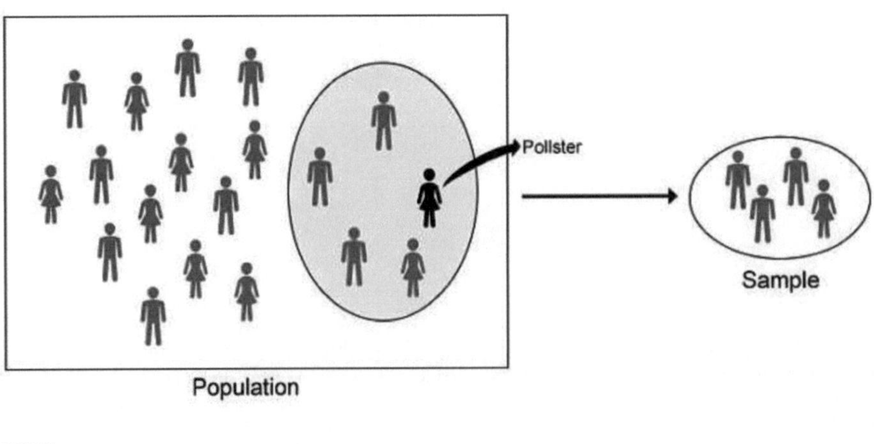

Figure 9.
Convenience sampling (source: https://www.mathstopia.net/sampling/convenience-sampling).

DOI: http://dx.doi.org/10.5772/intechopen.97705

10. Standard error of a sample mean

Suppose we have taken a sample of n measurements of some continuous variate, such as blood pressure or hemoglobin level. The sample mean $\boldsymbol{x}$ may be different from the population mean because it is based on a sample. Different samples of the same size $\boldsymbol{n}$ would give different values of the mean. These differences are due to sampling error. The sample mean therefore has its own distribution.

If the distribution of $\boldsymbol{x}$ in the population has mean $\boldsymbol{\mu}$ and standard deviation $\boldsymbol{\sigma}$ and a sample of size $\boldsymbol{n}$ is taken, then the *sampling distribution* of the sample mean $\boldsymbol{x}$ has the following properties:

1. The mean of the distribution of $\boldsymbol{x}$ is the same as that of the whole population, i.e.

$$\mathbf{E}(\bar{\boldsymbol{x}}) = \boldsymbol{\mu} \text{ (see Appendix for proof)}$$

or the sample mean is an unbiased estimate of the population mean.

2. The standard deviation of $\boldsymbol{x}$ is equal to $\boldsymbol{\sigma}/\sqrt{\mathbf{n}}$. The standard deviation of an estimate is referred to as the standard error (SE). The standard error of the mean is therefore [39]

$$\mathbf{SE}\ (\bar{\boldsymbol{x}}) = \boldsymbol{\sigma}/\ \mathbf{n}$$

3. By the central limit theorem, $\boldsymbol{x}$ is approximately Normally distributed, i.e. the distribution of $\boldsymbol{x}$ tends to be Normal even if the distribution in the population is markedly non-Normal. The distribution of means becomes closer to the Normal distribution as $\boldsymbol{n}$ increases.

The standard error of the mean is a measure of the sampling error [40]. For example, consider the measurement of lung function, forced expiratory volume, measured in liters. This is known to have a standard deviation of 0.5 in a population. If we select various sample sizes from this population, we have:

$$n = 1\ \mathrm{SE}(\bar{x}) - 0.5/1 = 0.50$$

$$n = 9\ \mathrm{SE}(\bar{x}) - 0.5/3 = 0.17$$

$$n = 25\ \mathrm{SE}(\bar{x}) = 0.5/5 = 0.10$$

$$n = 100\ \mathrm{SE}(\bar{x}) = 0.5/10 = 0.05$$

The larger the sample size, the smaller the sampling error. The standard error of the mean is used when we want to indicate how precise our estimate of the mean is. The standard deviation s, on the other hand, is used to show how widely spread our measurements of x are.

11. Confidence intervals

From property (3) above, and using tables of the Normal distribution, it can be stated that there is a 95% probability that x (the sample mean) will be no further than 1.96x SE(x), from $\boldsymbol{\mu}$, the (unknown) population mean. There is also a 99% chance that it will be within 2.58 SE(x) of u. The quantities 1.96 x SE(x) and 2.5 x SE(x) are referred to as the *maximum likely error*.

11.1 Known standard deviation

The foregoing statements describe a property of the sample mean in terms of the population mean. But the sample mean is known, and the population mean unknown, so we require a statement describing the population mean in terms of the known sample mean.

This is achieved by reversing the statement above, viz., if the sample mean is within 1.96 x SE(x) of the population mean, then the population mean is within 1.96 x SE(x) of the sample mean. That is, for 95% of samples it is true that μ lies in the interval.

$$\bar{x} - 1.96\text{xSE}(\bar{x}) \text{ to } \bar{x} + 1.96\text{xSE}(\bar{x})$$

This interval is called the 95% confidence interval for u and the ends of the interval are called the 95% *confidence limits*. The single value x is called a *point estimate* of the population mean μ, in contrast with the above interval *estimate*.

Example 1

The respiratory health of a sample of 25 men exposed to fumes in a dental laboratory was assessed by measuring the forced expiratory volume (FEV). The sample mean was 3.20 liters. From previous work it is known that the standard deviation of FEV is 0.5 liters.

$\bar{x}$ = 3.20

SE ($\bar{x}$) = 0.5/ $\sqrt{n}$ = 0.1

95% confidence interval for x is 3.20 ± 1.96 x 0.1 liters

=3.00 to 3.40 liters

Conclusion We are 95% confident that the interval 3.00 to 3.40 liters contains the unknown population mean μ.

99% confidence interval for x is 3.20 ± 2.5 x 0.1 liters

=2.94 to 3.46 litres

Conclusion We are 99% confident that the interval 3.00 to 3.46 liters contains the unknown population mean μ.

Note: The 99% confidence interval is wider because of the extra confidence that the interval contains the population mean μ.

11.2 Unknown standard deviation

In the above it was assumed that the standard deviation in the population was known. In many practical situations this will not be the case and the standard deviation has to be estimated from the sample data. It therefore seems natural to replace σ by its estimate s and argue exactly as above. However, there is a loss of precision because the standard deviation has its own sampling error. This extra imprecision is included by widening the confidence intervals by using larger constants than 1.96 (for 5%) or 2.58 (for 1%).

Example 2. In (example 1) the values of FEV were:

2.82	3.49	2.72	2.59	2.30
2.64	3.16	3.59	2.44	4.10
3.66	3.35	3.62	3.24	2.82
2.79	2.92	4.20	3.21	3.80
3.62	4.00	3.53	2.76	2.68

$\bar{x}$ = 3.20 *s* 0.54 (24*df*).

The sample mean is 3.20 liters and the sample standard deviation 0.54 liters. The standard error of the mean is 0.11 liters. The estimated standard deviation has 24 degrees of freedom and the 5% and 1% points of the *t* distribution with 24 df are 2.06 and 2.80 respectively.

Thus the 95% confidence interval is:

3.20 2.06x0.11 = 2.97 to 3.43 liters

and the 99% confidence interval is:

3.20 2.800.11 = 2.89 to 3.51 liter.

12. The significance of choosing an effective method of sampling

Sampling determines the outcome of analysis. However, with the variations that may be present between the population and the sample, there may be errors in the sample (**Figure 10**).

Sampling bias happens because certain members of the population are more likely to be included in a survey than others. It is often referred to as determination bias in medical fields. *Sampling frame error* occurs when a sample is having a certain type of possible respondent relative to the population of interest. *Systematic errors* mostly affect the precision of the calculation. It is of prime importance to use the most appropriate and useful form of sampling to attain accurate outcome of research.

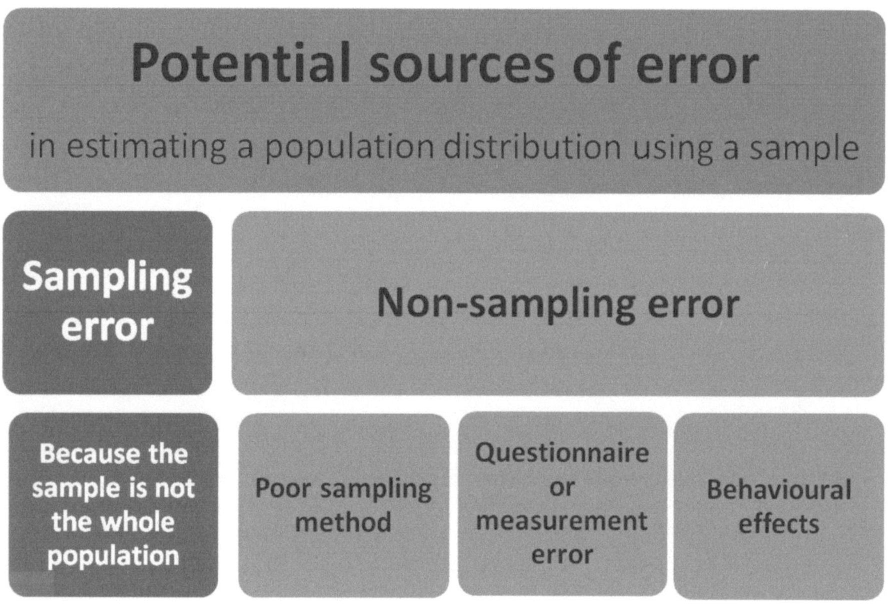

Figure 10.
Sources of error (source: https://creativemaths.net/blog/sampling-and-non-sampling-error/).

A. Appendix

A.1. Proof of the basic formulae of statistical inference

$$E(x) = E[(x1, + x2 + \ldots + xn)/n]$$
$$= [E(x1) + E(x2) + \ldots + E(xn)]/n$$
$$= \mu, \text{ since } E(xi) = \mu \text{ for all } i.$$

$$Variance(x\ ) = [var(x1) + var(x2)) + \ldots + var(xn)]/\ n^2$$
$$= [\ n\sigma^2]/\ n^2?$$
$$= \sigma^2/\ n$$
Therefore Standard error of x is: $SE(x\ ) = to\ \sigma\ /\ \sqrt{n}$

Author details

Yasser Riaz Malik[1,2]*, Muhammad Saad Sheikh[3] and Shakeela Yousaf[4]

1 Department of Preventive Dentistry, Dental Public Health, University of Hail, Hail, Saudi Arabia

2 Department of Community Dentistry, Sir Syed College of Medical Sciences for Girls, Karachi, Pakistan

3 Department of Oral Biology, Sindh Institute of Oral Health Sciences, Jinnah Sindh Medical University, Karachi, Pakistan

4 Sir Syed College of Medical Sciences, Karachi, Pakistan

*Address all correspondence to: docyrm@gmail.com

References

[1] Apostol, T. M. (1969). *Calculus, Volume II.* (2nd edition, John Wiley & Sons.

[2] Smeeton, N. (2005). *Dental Statistics Made Easy.* Radcliffe Publishing.

[3] Martin, B. (2000). *Introduction to medical statistics 3rd edition.* oxford university press.

[4] Dean, B. I. (2013, July 18). Introductory Statistics. OpenStax.

[5] Frost, J. (2000). *Introduction to Statistics: An Intuitive Guide for Analyzing Data and Unlocking Discoveries.* James D. Frost.

[6] Charles Miller Grinstead, J. L. (2012). *Charles Miller Grinstead, James Laurie Snell.* American Mathematical Soc., 2012.

[7] Rosenthal, M. J. (2004). Probability Models. In *Probability and Statistics* (pp. 4-6). Macmillan.

[8] Armitage P, B. G. (2001). *Statistical methods in medical research. 4th edition.* Oxford: Blackwell Scientific Publications.

[9] Bryman, A. &. (2003). *Business research methods.* Oxford: Oxford University Press .

[10] Altman, D. G. (1999). *Practical statistics for medical research.* London: Champan & Hall.

[11] Barbara Illowsky, S. D. (2017). *Introductory Statistics.* Samurai Media Limited.

[12] Palmisano, A. (2018). *The Encyclopedia of Archaeological Sciences , S. L. López Varela (Ed.) (pp.1–4).* Wiley.

[13] Günter Last, M. P. (2017). *Lectures on the Poisson Process.* Cambridge University Press.

[14] Koch, K.-R. (2007). *Introduction to Bayesian Statistics.* Springer Science & Business Media.

[15] Catherine Forbes, M. E. (2010). *Statistical Distributions.* John Wiley & Sons.

[16] Wesolowski, D. J. (2018). *The SAGE Encyclopedia of Educational Research, Measurement, and Evaluation.* Thousand Oaks: SAGE Publications, Inc.

[17] Bryc, W. (2012). *The Normal Distribution: Characterizations with Applications.* Springer Science & Business Media.

[18] Jagdish K. Patel, C. B. (1982). *Handbook of the Normal Distribution.* M. Dekker.

[19] J.S.Chitode, D. (n.d.). *Digital Communication.* 2009: Technical Publications.

[20] DasGupta, A. (2010). *Fundamentals of Probability: A First Course.* Springer Science & Business Media.

[21] Agarwal, B. L. (2006). *Basic Statistics.* New Age International.

[22] Silvey, S. (2017). *Statistical Inference.* Routledge.

[23] Michael C. Fleming, J. G. (2000). *Principles of Applied Statistics.* Cengage Learning EMEA.

[24] Dhivyadeepa, D. E. (n.d.). *Sampling Techniques in Educational Research.* Lulu. com.

[25] Arijit Chaudhuri, H. S. (2005). *Survey Sampling: Theory and Methods, Second Edition.* CRC Press.

[26] Sedgwick, P. (June 2012). BMJ, 344.

[27] Slutsky, D. J. (November 2013). Statistical Errors in Clinical Studies. Journal of wrist surgery, 285–287.

[28] ZIKMUND. (2002). *Business research methods.* Dryden: Thomas learning.

[29] GHAURI, P. & GRONHAUG, K. 2005. *Research Methods in Business Studies*, Harlow, FT/Prentice Hall

[30] ACKOFF, R. L. 1953. *The Design of Social Research*, Chicago, University of Chicago Press

[31] WILSON, J. 2010. *Essentials of business research: a guide to doing your research project*, SAGE Publication

[32] DAVIS, D. 2005. *Business Research for Decision Making*, Australia, Thomson South-Western

[33] Michael Köhl, S. S. (2006). *Sampling Methods, Remote Sensing and GIS Multiresource Forest Inventory.* Springer Science & Business Media.

[34] Uprichard, E. (2011). Sampling: bridging probability and non-probability designs. . International Journal of Social Research Methodology - INT J SOC RES METHODOL. , 16(1):1–11.

[35] Moser, C. A. (1952). Quota sampling. *Journal of the Royal Statistical Society.* Series A (General) *Vol. 115, No. 3*, pp. 411–423 (13 pages).

[36] MAXWELL, J. A. 1996. Qualitative Research Design: An Intractive Approach London, Applied Social Research Methods Series

[37] Irina-Maria Dragan, A. I.-M. (2013). Snowball Sampling Completion. Journal of Studies in Social Sciences , *Volume 5, Number 2*, 160–177.

[38] Henry, G. T. (1990). *Practical Sampling Volume 21 of Applied Social Research Methods.* SAGE Publications.

[39] Allen, M. P. (2007). *Understanding Regression Analysis.* Springer Science & Business Media.

[40] Caldwell, S. (2012). *Statistics Unplugged edition 4.* Cengage Learning.